'A timely book addressing the opportun
excitement of art therapy in the independe
new for the profession and still widely co
the principles of the NHS. James has bro
of essays that explore and reflect on the specific concerns ...
taken into account by current and intending practitioners. Identifying, understanding and being able to put theory into practice will ensure a safe and effective service in our rapidly changing social conditions. A must for current art therapy training programmes.'

— *Professor Diane Waller OBE, Emeritus Professor of Art Psychotherapy and Hon. President British Association of Art Therapists*

'*Art Therapy in Private Practice* is an eye-opening collation of the experiences and developing approaches of art therapists in private practice in the United Kingdom. Composed of chapters written by experienced art therapists on specific and important subjects such as liaison with GPs, working with children and their parents, culture and diversity, financial and time restrictions, support networks and research methodology, this book shows how private practice necessitates additional clinical thinking to develop and respond to the context, contract, meanings and symbols that emerge in private work. It is an important addition to the literature and will be helpful to art therapists in both the public and private sectors.'

— *Brian Kaplan, MBBCh*

'This is a timely book offering a wealth of good practical advice and information. Experienced art psychotherapists debate current issues in a lively and engaging way. A variety of theoretical stances, enhance engaging case material, illustrating topical concerns in the profession. Art therapists considering a mixed public and private practice or of moving into private practice, will find it of great benefit and use. Thoughtful and engaging with current issues pertaining to the profession, this book is a significant addition to the literature.'

— *Caroline Case, Art Psychotherapist and Child and Adolescent Psychotherapist in Private Practice*

ART THERAPY IN PRIVATE PRACTICE

THEORY, PRACTICE AND RESEARCH IN CHANGING CONTEXTS

Edited by **James D. West**

Forewords by **Joan Woddis and Chris Wood**

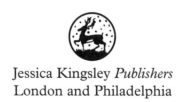

Jessica Kingsley *Publishers*
London and Philadelphia

First published in 2018
by Jessica Kingsley Publishers
73 Collier Street
London N1 9BE, UK
and
400 Market Street, Suite 400
Philadelphia, PA 19106, USA

www.jkp.com

Copyright © Jessica Kingsley Publishers 2018
Foreword copyright © Joan Woddis 2018
Foreword copyright © Chris Wood 2018

Front cover image source: Shutterstock®.

Library of Congress Cataloging in Publication Data
Names: West, James D., (Art psychotherapist)
Title: Art therapy in private practice : theory, practice and research in
    changing contexts / edited by James D. West.
Description: London ; Philadelphia : Jessica Kingsley Publishers, 2018. |
    Includes bibliographical references and index.
Identifiers: LCCN 2017023173 | ISBN 9781785920431 (alk. paper)
Subjects: LCSH: Art therapy.
Classification: LCC RC489.A7 A776 2018 | DDC 616.89/1656--
dc23 LC record available at https://lccn.loc.gov/2017023173

British Library Cataloguing in Publication Data
A CIP catalogue record for this book is available from the British Library

ISBN 978 1 78592 043 1
eISBN 978 1 78450 297 3

Printed and bound in Great Britain by Bell & Bain Ltd, Glasgow

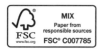

This book is dedicated to Don Rendell
(4 March 1926–20 October 2015)

For his lessons in music, theory, practice and Love,
and how it all fits together!

Contents

Part I: Contexts and Collaboration

Part II: Working with Children, Families and the Child in the Adult

Part III: Training and Transmission

Part IV: Governance and Supervision

Part V: Research

FOREWORD

—— JOAN WODDIS ——

At the heart of art therapy practice lies the act of externalising an individual's account of their existence, their emotions and their experience of others and to convert these inner thoughts and feelings into images which, crucially, can be shared. I do not believe it is too fanciful to connect this to the earliest evidence of our human ancestors who chronicled their lives on the walls of their caves and, stunningly, embodied their individuality in a single hand print. One can imagine the audience of these endeavours, many thousands of years ago, celebrating their creation and their sense of connection. We are all, in a sense, the inheritors of the work of these historic artists. The act of making events and experience tangible certainly precedes the sophisticated language of description. The development of art therapy has such events at its centre: the act of creation witnessed by another as it develops and takes shape. The process of bringing painful, even intolerable, feelings into a form exterior to oneself without the immediate necessity of explanation or rationalisation is in itself an engine of change. There are many striking examples from anthropology and art history available to us.

When we address the development of art therapy as a profession in the UK, for it is essential to contextualise the contents of this book, it will come as no surprise that its mainspring was the social change following the end of the Second World War, with the establishment of the National Health Service (NHS), the Beveridge Report on social care and the improvements contained in the Education Act of 1944. It is in this climate that the organised profession has its origins. By the early 1960s a number of artists were working with patients in the large psychiatric institutions of the day. They defined themselves as art therapists and in 1964 established the British Association of

Art Therapists (BAAT). The pressing need for discrete trainings for practitioners was acknowledged from the start, and by 1977 there were two postgraduate trainings in the discipline.

The next milestone was the establishment of an agreed career structure in the NHS, where the majority of art therapists practised. This was a source of great celebration in 1982 and was followed by an equivalent system in the custodial services some time later. The mood of the time was that art therapy, like all health care, should be free at the point of need. That clients should pay from their own pockets for their care was an anathema and was viewed by the majority of practitioners as a step backwards into inequality. The professional association's duty was always seen as being both to its members and their clients, in equal measure.

It was in this context that the profession committed itself to the task of securing state regulation for its members, as the prime function of regulation is public protection. In 1997 this was achieved and art, music and drama therapists became registrants of what was to become the Health and Care Professions Council.

Broadly speaking, this was the position of British art therapy at the beginning of the 21st century. There was recognition in health, custodial and much of social care, growth and improvement in the training courses, now at master's level, and much interest in the profession and its practice. The professional structures had expanded, there was a refereed learned journal, frequent publications, conferences, and special interest groups. The membership of the BAAT had increased enormously, for there are now ten training courses and consequently increased numbers of graduates seeking work every autumn and equally healthy numbers joining the courses to train.

However, as I write, there has been a profound change in the landscape in which art therapy flourishes. We can demonstrate that the majority of art therapists no longer work in the NHS as in the past, but many now work with children in schools, pupil referral units and charitably funded provision. Many practise independently in retirement and care homes. These practitioners often have no fixed contract and sometimes no discrete job description. They frequently experience high levels of vulnerability for their clients and themselves. Other art therapists report stringent cuts in social and community care for adult mental health service users. This is the background, the very arresting context of this book. Traditionally art therapy in the UK has had a radical culture, and for some the idea of private practice remains at odds with this. Whilst psychotherapy and often counselling have been routinely practised in the independent sector, private practice has been a new development for our profession, full of opportunities but not without hazard. For this reason BAAT, the professional guardian of our practice, advises all its members to have adequate employed experience before venturing into the field. It is argued that without it they lack a necessary component in their ability to function as a sole practitioner and BAAT will rarely consider registering an individual as a private practitioner without it.

It follows that without a tradition of private practice in the profession, clinical placements whilst on training will not provide an adequate learning experience in such a setting. They are most likely to include a period in a psychiatric ward or child mental health care which is vital in terms of the development of a clinician, but excludes any examination of art therapy in private practice, not solely in terms of practicalities. Consequently an art therapist will approach setting up a private practice having their sole experience of independent practice as that of their own personal therapy, a mandatory part of their training. This was, and continues to be, problematic. Support was needed, and a group of colleagues, already experienced in the independent and private sector, came together as a BAAT special interest group, pooling their experience, advice and hopes for the future. This book is one of the results of their collaboration.

The reader will find a wealth of information and solid practical advice on establishing a small private practice in art therapy here. The accounts are both discursive and reflective, and the theoretical base of the discipline is explored in some rich case material. The ongoing need for research into practice is thoroughly addressed and powerfully argued. The difficulties of practice in this area are not ignored or minimised, rather they are addressed and interrogated.

The development of the profession of art therapy in the UK can be seen as an evolutionary process, a response to changing societal conditions by adaptation, modification and change. The establishment of our practice in the private setting is the most recent move in a history spanning more than half a century. I hope that this book will persuade you that it is a timely, exciting and beneficial development.

FOREWORD

—— CHRIS WOOD ——

The ethos of public and third sector services in health care has been to help those who cannot pay. The term 'third sector' describes the range of organisations that are neither public nor private. It includes voluntary and community organisations, for example registered charities, associations, self-help groups, community groups, social enterprises and co-operatives. The ethos of private sector services has been to offer choice for those who are able to pay, and sometimes to offer a service when there is no prospect of it in the public sector. As with other forms of health and social care there are interwoven realms of art therapy practice in the public, third and private sectors.

In an increasingly complex world all three – public sector, third sector and private practice – are needed. For example, sometimes public services for children in need have no alternative other than to purchase private psychological care if they are to meet statutory requirements, whereas, during the Ebola outbreak, private health care in the US could not manage and needed to send patients with the virus into public hospitals, and internationally everyone's health depended on that being done (BBC News: US and Canada 2014). Organisations in the third sector develop different ways of responding to human need by raising money through agencies and charities in order that users of services do not pay for care or therapy at the point of its delivery, although many of the practitioners are still paid. Each realm of public, third and private sector provision is to some extent interdependent on the others. Knowledge and experience of practice are exchanged between the different sectors. The way in which this takes place is generally a response to the contemporary circumstances of a historical period. So in this period, since the banking crisis of 2008 which led to the world economic crash, many services and professions have seen resources cut. Nevertheless, rather than accept the loss of services, adaptations of practice and provision in different sectors have ensured that there is still a response to human need and human development.

Many things in this political and economic climate suggest that it is wise to avoid polarising the distinctions between public and private. A number of clear-thinking epidemiologists considering the physical, psychological, social and economic causes of ill health (Marmot 2015; Wilkinson and Pickett 2009) demonstrate that the health of national populations is interconnected across economic divides. It is expected that the health of those with least resources suffers in unequal societies; what is not anticipated is that the health of those with high resources also suffers in unequal societies. It seems fair in this light to indicate that public and private therapeutic practice are similarly interconnected.

This book, edited by James D. West, describes parts of a developing social history of art therapy. Contemporary professional practice exists within a spectrum of different contexts and approaches to therapy. It is evident in West's book that some art therapists in private practice adopt the conventions of private psychoanalytic practice, while others adopt different models such as the collaborative studio approach described in Chapter 3. Just as within public and third sector practice, there are different perspectives within private art therapy. Interestingly there is an overlapping use of technical terms, and this means that often the language of the hospital (patient, client, clinical) is used, despite practice being outside the hospital. This could sometimes be as a result of a historical lagging-behind in the use of language, or it could sometimes be too passive a conception of the service user. This makes for an interesting ongoing conversation. Art therapists working in different sectors are facing and working with challenges, and the people writing for this book are offering their contributions to the conversation-so-far about the private sector. The title of a talk, *From the couch to the council estate: Art therapy as meeting place* (Wood 2016), is my early attempt to describe what I understand of the changing spectrum of practice.

There are shared principles across different realms of practice. There are shared ideas about what contributes to quality in therapeutic work. Quality in many of the chapters here is seen as being dependent upon good training and research; clarity about boundaries; collaboration with service users; and supervision. Good standards of practice and good safeguards are also seen as important. The tenets of the Health and Care Professions Council (HCPC) now set the statutory boundaries for quality practice in a number of professions working with mental health: arts therapies, occupational therapy, psychology and social work. All of these professions are governed by statutory guidance in all three sectors: public, third and private.

Psychotherapy professions are also regulated by professional bodies, but regulation, although strict, tends not to be overtly statutory. Some art therapists have dual registration within both psychotherapy and art therapy systems ('art therapy' and 'art psychotherapy' are both protected titles in law).

Currently newly qualified art therapists are advised by the British Association of Art Therapists (BAAT), the professional association, to wait some years before entering private practice. This is intended as a safeguard for newly qualified therapists and for their service users. Technically the HCPC does not make a distinction between practitioners with different lengths of experience, but in the case of any dispute HCPC tends to seek guidance from professional associations.

All training organisations for art therapists are influenced by the BAAT guidance which advises the newly qualified to gain experience for some years before entering private practice. It is not possible to account for all the courses: all consider employment issues, but it seems few offer much direct training about private practice. The HCPC-validated training programme with which I am associated offers employment workshops within and post-training. A mixed economy is advocated; that is, to seek a combination of work: some work which pays the bills, and some work aimed at gradually developing a portfolio of art therapy practice. This art therapy experience tends initially to be in sessional work under the protective umbrella of organisations or agencies, and it is not private practice in the sense of an art therapist being a sole trader. It may well be that it is possible to establish private practice in ways that do not depend on therapists being sole traders. Experience will educate art therapists and be shared in ways that are sustainable. This book is part of that process.

Another part of the process is the growing body of experience within the art therapy profession as a result of trainees having to have their own private therapy whilst training. Student art therapists, all postgraduates, are often forthright in their opinions of the therapists they see whilst training. Shared guidance from students and course staff on seeking therapy is for trainees to ask early about the therapist's attitude to a range of issues (sexuality, ethnicity, class and culture, attitudes to student therapy, and to payments). The therapist's response to such questions, no matter what their approach, will inform the student's choice of therapist, as will cost. An art therapy trainee's experience of personal therapy lasts over periods of at least two years and for some it is three years. Trainers may hear snippets of student experience with their therapists (in a range of relevant modalities). Most accounts suggest that trainee therapy is of benefit and that it directly shapes the therapist that the trainee goes on to become. Some accounts suggest that therapists make mistakes (that they are human) and that some seriously transgress the boundaries in ways that require reference to governing bodies. Of course governance must be fair and yet also alive to the possibility of malicious complaints. All of this experience will increasingly inform and shape art therapy in private practice, but also in other areas of practice.

In relation to the discussion about research in this book, my approach is a little different. I tend to take a pragmatic approach which values highly both research rooted in the arts and humanities, and also empirical research which is systematic. The discussion of research by James D. West tends to be the former and that by Anthea Hendry presented here is the latter. Although employing both approaches to research can seem like riding two circus horses, with one foot on each, art therapy is an extraordinary discipline worthy of the challenge. It is nevertheless interesting that in the chapter on self-care for the private practitioner by West (Chapter 12), there is clear understanding that systematic research can provide guidelines that protect both therapist and their service user from 'burn-out'.

The book throughout has a questioning tone which is fitting as part of the development of approaches to practice: it advocates for private practitioners, but in the end it does not peddle illusions about what is involved.

As powerfully presented in the foreword by Joan Woddis, the art therapy discipline uses ancient knowledge that has been handed down through the ages. The art making is a gift in the way it provides mental space and shapes the therapy. The part of art therapy based in art making and imagination – and, where possible, studios – means that the therapeutic relationship is shaped in very particular ways in whichever realm of practice (public, third or private sector). Art therapy continues to learn from this.

References

BBC News: US and Canada (2014) 'Ebola crisis: Could the virus spread in the US?' 28 October 2014.

Marmot, M. (2015) *The Health Gap: The Challenge of an Unequal World.* London: Bloomsbury.

Wilkinson, R. and Pickett, J. (2009) *The Spirit Level: Why Equality is Better for Everyone.* London: Penguin.

Wood, C. (2016) *From the couch to the council estate: Art therapy as meeting place.* Talk given at Goldsmiths Conference, 'Finding Spaces, Making Places: Exploring Social and Cultural Space in Contemporary Art Therapy Practice', 14 April, University of London.

Acknowledgements

Thanks are due to my partner Pauline Johnson, my son Søren, my daughter Eve and my step-daughter Nadine Thomas, who have supported me through this project and forgiven me my absences. They have provided steady, constant love and humour when I occasionally lost the capacity for both and so they are the real heroes of this endeavour! In the longer story my sister Amanda and my brother Nick, both inspirational figures of my childhood, and, of course, my mother and father, with love and gratitude, for bringing me into this world in an era aspiring towards freedom and difference.

Supervisees, Colleagues, Friends

I would like to thank the arts therapists I have supervised and those who have advised me during the evolution of this manuscript prior to its publication, and particularly in the evolution of the modality chart developed in Chapter 12.

Art psychotherapists Marrianne Behm, Marika Cohen, James Cowie, Samantha Hunt and Ren Pesci.

Dance movement psychotherapists Claire Burrell, Sarah Boreham, Marina Rova and Dagmara Rosiecka.

Joan Woddis, art therapist, group analyst and supervisor, who with her casual genius has guided me for so many years showing me how to convert the muddiness of experience into practice gold through the guise of what seem deceptively like friendly chats. She has had the, sometimes unenviable, task of supervising me.

Thank you to the authors in this book who through the authors' meetings and the email list have given useful feedback throughout the project and given the book its direction and a real sense of it being a collective and collaborative work.

My colleague and friend Catherine Stevens whose faith in me has always bridged the gaps when I have failed in that faith in myself.

My friend David Spicer who has offered me so much useful and timely advice about the process of creative writing.

Marcela Vielman whose management of the Creative Therapies Project at the Copleston Centre offered me many opportunities for creative development, to the Reverend Edward Collier whose ongoing support for the project has enabled its continued community development as the Copleston Creative Therapies Project, and to Accuscript who now fund art therapy within the project.

Dr Chris Wood for the encouragements that led to a reflective workshop on private practice in Sheffield which subsequently led to the national development of the Private Practice Special Interest Group (PPSIG), and for her support for the development of ideas about how the skills of private practice can be integrated into the training of art therapists. Thanks are also due to the calm reflections and actions of Anthea Hendry, Debbie Michaels and Themis Kyriakidou for their ongoing support for development of practice in the North; and also Nigel Durkan who facilitated our meeting in Manchester.

Dr Val Huet, CEO of the British Association of Art Therapists (BAAT), who has often offered advice and direction, and who pointed us to the Dual Experiences Group as a forum for anonymous peer review allowing us to fulfil a self-imposed requirement to have all the chapters anonymously reviewed by mental health service users who are also peers. Thanks to the art therapist Julie Watson who coordinated the peer review for us and the psychotherapist Charles Brown who also helped us in this process.

Thanks to Tim Wright, Chair of BAAT, who sought the permission of BAAT Council for us to publish *The Core Skills and Practice Standards in Private Work*, which can be found in the appendices, and also to BAAT Council who have supported me with the complex issues that have arisen in relation to art therapy private practice in my role of PPSIG coordinator. Thanks to the 167 art therapists who are members of the PPSIG for the work done to develop the Core Skills document, and whose voluntary attendance and contributions to physical meetings, and online, have provided many notional grains of sand that have slowly formed into pearls in this book.

Thanks to Hephzibah Kaplan and Gary Nash from London Art Therapy Centre who over many years have offered a context for private practice and a reflective forum for many of the authors in this book at different times. Nothing can occur without a context. The centre continues to provide a creative context for private art therapy practice development. Gary's early work with me on preparing this project was vital to its final arrival, and his founding the PPSIG with Amanda Wright must also be acknowledged as a key development for the profession.

Dr Sandra Westland, Dr Tom Barber and Tina Tilmouth of the Contemporary College of Therapeutic Studies, whose critical reflections have both challenged and supported my personal and professional development and so also this project.

The editors at Jessica Kingsley Publishers who entrusted this project to us, and particularly the assistant editor Jane Evans who has guided both myself and the authors over the last two years.

Last, but certainly not least, I would also like to thank all the clients whose dilemmas are the grist of a therapist's practice and without whom practitioners would have no profession to consider. It is in their service that we exist as therapists. So for this a heartfelt 'Thank you!'

James D. West
Blackheath, London
31 March 2017

Throughout the book, all identifying features, locations and the names of clients have been anonymised, unless specific consent has been granted to do otherwise.

INTRODUCTION

—— JAMES D. WEST ——

The idea of this book arose through a growing recognition that the world view and lived experience of art therapy private practitioners is significantly different from that of art therapists within the state provision. It aims to identify and create a fair and balanced representation of the world of art therapy private practitioners and their clients, at a time when economic necessity is forcing many art therapists to consider, or reconsider, this practice option. Understanding the motivation of both the therapist and the client in seeking a private arrangement will be reflected upon throughout the chapters.

The Development of a Book as a Research Process

The structure of this book went through a number of phases of development that illustrate an emerging research project, aiming to represent and elucidate the field of art therapy private practice in the UK for the reader. It has been formed through numerous structurings and adjustments in many cycles of writing, rewriting, reading and dialogue, held between the authors, in conjunction with the anonymised peer review process, and with the wider profession. The initial structure of the book, as it first appeared in the original proposal, has changed significantly during the course of the writing, demonstrating what has been learned in the process of the exploration. Kim Etherington (2002) has eloquently outlined how an edited book can be considered as a valid process of inquiry and research.

Four authors' meetings were held in the course of the book's creation, to encourage cross-fertilisation and to avoid repetition and redundancy in the book. Where identifiable gaps were noticed in the manuscript the authors have aimed to address them individually or collectively. Below are some of the main themes identified during these meetings.

As a central defining issue of private practice, all the authors were asked to consider the fee and to illustrate and identify its significance as a central interaction of art therapy private practice.

We developed the Art Therapy in Private Practice Mind Map (see colour plate 1) as a responsive tool to consider the work as a whole with the aim of helping the authors and myself, as editor, to hold in mind the unfolding structure of its developing brief. The branches of the mind map were chosen in these discussions and they were also checked against the Health and Care Professions Council (HCPC) Standards of Proficiency (HCPC 2013), and both the British Association of Art Therapists (BAAT 2014) and HCPC (2016) Code of Ethics, and the BAAT (2017) *Core Skills and Practice Standards in Private Work* document (Appendix 1). The mind map continued to be developed within the authors' meetings and in relation to the forming chapters. It should now provide a useful visual guide to prospective art therapy private practitioners, outlining the main areas pertinent to their private practice.

All authors were asked to consider the epistemological question 'How do you know what you know?' to encourage a foregrounding of their research methodology and to promote the notion of practice as research. When concerns arose in the group around whether 'stories' could be part of this evidence, we agreed to be guided by the balance provided by Aristotle's three appeals of rhetoric: namely *logos* (reasoning), *ethos* (ethics) and *pathos* (passion). His conceptualisation of the art of persuasion encapsulates the communicative aims of the speaker, the reality of the context and the needs of the audience. It has withstood the test of time while addressing the importance of ethics and of the making of a reasoned case. The aim of this layered process of reflection and heuristic research has been to actively involve as many art therapy private practitioners as possible in a book that explores the topic of art therapy private practice through a range of lenses (professional, political, ethical, social and cultural, economic, psychological and aesthetic). The opportunity was widely advertised in the art therapy forums of research, the trainings and in the BAAT Private Practice Special Interest Group (PPSIG) to have a representative sample of practitioners within the authors' group and increase the likelihood of a fair representation of art therapy private practice occurring currently in the UK.

Peer Review

As a peer reviewer for the *International Journal of Art Therapy* (formally *Inscape*), I understand some of the benefits of peer review and so organised an anonymised peer review process for the authors. This was done by BAAT's Dual Experience Group, a group of art therapists who have lived experiences of mental health difficulties. The aim was to provide anonymous feedback, encourage greater reflection in the authors in the process of writing, and promote a consideration of the importance of the service user's and carer's voices in therapy, and to counter nepotism, which has historically been shown to be a hazard in professional psychotherapy associations. Two anonymous peer reviews for each chapter would have been preferable, but the time frame meant that this was not a practical possibility and so each chapter was read by one reviewer. In addition to this, it was formally arranged that each chapter received at least three additional readings by art therapist peers who would also offer feedback.

Contextual Epistemology

The contexts of practice and epistemology (theories of knowledge) have become central concerns of this book. In the history of psychoanalysis, a closely allied profession to art therapy, there have been many clashes and schisms: between Freud, a neurologist, and Jung, a psychiatrist, most notably. In these disputes, and in many other professional scenarios, tensions are often identified to persons – and yet, when we examine each case more deeply, it is noticeable that disputes are more often conflicts of discourse that evolve within different work settings and from varying client needs, rather than being simply personal or professional conflicts per se. This poses the question as to whether it is the setting that creates a way of knowing (the epistemology) and sets professionals against each other when knowledge territories become contested and financial resources become scarce. Gregory Bateson (2000) in his classic study of Alcoholics Anonymous as a transformative social space shows the importance of the social context to the everyday practices of individuals and considers how a self-help recovery group can facilitate a change of world view in its individual participants and thereby support recovery. An 'epistemological shift' occurs that brings about positive and creative change in the lives of its individual members. I would argue then that rather than promoting private practice ideologically, which would be difficult in a profession composed of socially aware artists, we could explore art therapy private practice as a particular socially transformative therapeutic context, with an observant eye to the epistemologies that are likely to be native to it and which may differ from those of art therapists in other contexts. This requires us to explore this practice contextually for its corresponding strengths and weaknesses. It has been one of the aims of this book to begin the process of exploration of this crucial and expanding field of practice and to consider its key role in the training and the supervision of the profession.

An Auto-Ethnography: My Journey towards Becoming a Private Art Therapy Practitioner

When I qualified through what was the first intake of the two-year full-time postgraduate diploma in Art Psychotherapy at Goldsmiths, University of London, in 1994, I was 30 years old. I had previously completed a BA in Art History and Studio Practice two years earlier. On qualification, the cohort of that year were faced with finding work at the tail end of a recession which was still playing out in the wider economy, removing art therapy departments wholesale from the National Health Service (NHS) and Social Services, where many of us would have sought work. Psychologically, following the training, I felt depleted and could not face the prospect of endless interviews with large groups of peers also seeking employment. As I continued to facilitate two groups for elders that followed from my training placement, I decided, and also felt pushed by my circumstances, to plough my own furrow and seek to build a self-employed practice. I decided to monitor this situation on a six-monthly basis and set myself the outcome that if my practice grew every six months I would continue on this path, and if it didn't, I would then submit myself to the more traditional route of employment and what was considered at the time as 'finding a proper job'. At the time, self-employed independent work was seen as a 'stop gap' or something to do 'on the side'. But for me, for all sorts of personal reasons, and partly as an expression of my nonconformism, I have no difficulty moving in a contrary direction to the larger group. I also felt strongly that being a professional means holding a set of values in whichever context you find yourself practising, and so my aim became more solidly to develop an independent professional practice if I could. However, the absence of a culture of private practice and adequate professional guidance meant that taking this route would occasionally be a very lonely road. One of the personal aims of this book is to offer guidance and encourage further sharing of the culture of art therapy private practice – making it a gift both to my retrospective, younger self and to offer something in sympathy to the now far greater number of art therapists facing this largely undelimited field. In the dark recessionary days of the early 1990s, a book like this, detailing the legal, professional and practical landscape, with tips from seasoned practitioners from the field, would have been a great help to me – and so I hope it will be 'that book' for those now facing the territory for the first time.

I continued to make slow but steady progress and 23 years later I am still following the self-employed route. It brings in a reasonable income, and while I have 'worked' in Social Services, charities and the NHS with clients of all ages, I have always done this as a 'consultant', 'sessional worker' or 'private practitioner', not as an employee. This choice was made partly as a consequence of my character and personal history, but as time has passed and as so many art therapists are now finding, it is increasingly less of a choice and more of a necessity due to our material, economic, historical and social circumstances. It now seems that, for the foreseeable future, most art therapists will have to choose at least a mix of self-employed and employed work, and this needs to be recognised and addressed. Speaking more positively, in addition to these necessary professional adjustments, it is important not to forget that there are also advantages for certain clients and therapists in choosing private practice. It is my hope that by the end of the book, the virtues of a mixed practice will be more clearly appreciated. This step will also bring art therapy into parity with other psychotherapeutic trainings that often orientate trainees primarily to private practice; this adaptation seems long overdue in art therapy training.

Soon after qualification I returned to working in a drug treatment rehabilitation centre where I had volunteered prior to training as an art worker, but this time as a qualified art psychotherapist offering group work. I also began offering services to young people and people with learning disabilities. It was in this varied work I learned the importance of balancing my energies with the dynamics of different clients and client groups by carefully timetabling interventions, which led me to develop a growing interest in the self-care of the therapist expressed in Chapter 12. I was subsequently asked to offer a yearly lecture on setting up independent and sessional work at Goldsmiths.

Being self-employed, I could juggle my time and gained an MA in Applied Psychoanalytic Theory. In my personal life this flexibility helped when I got divorced and subsequently became a single parent, and again I found through my self-employed status I was able to adapt to very new personal circumstances. Though perceived as insecure, self-employment is surprisingly malleable to life's slings and arrows. Looking back to this interface between the personal and the professional, I can now see that my father's experience of 'losing his money' inculcated in me the need to 'never have all my eggs in one basket', a world view which fits well with business notions of diversification in insecure times which seems an implicit aim in building a private practice. Similarly, as a consequence of negative experiences of boarding school, while I have a great interest in organisational dynamics and work well as a consultant to organisations and in staff support, I am not an 'organisational man'. I prefer to be on the outside. This ambiguous location is often the choice of artists who seek to be relevant to a community, yet try simultaneously to have an independent voice.

A mix of sessional institutional work, charity work, private supervision and private practice provides a sort of security, because it is unlikely that you will ever lose all your work at once with the devastating consequences I had witnessed personally early in life. There nonetheless remains one way that you can lose all your work in self-employment, and that is by not looking after your own health. Self-employment requires the practitioner to pay particular attention and show a kindness to oneself in reflections upon your own mind/body process and the relationships that sustain your wellbeing.

The last important development for me has been in the community, where I recently offered my service to a charity supported by the National Lottery for a number of years. After the funding was pulled I found myself seeking funding, eventually becoming a private practitioner even in community work for clients referred from the Health Service. I had previously seen myself in this context as an independent self-employed sessional provider. Where community services have in the last few years often completely vanished, this seems a necessary response to rapid and dramatic social change.

I hope that this brief auto-ethnography shows how the personal, professional and the social historical trends are closely interwoven. It remains for us to choose how we bring ourselves, with all our particular strengths and weaknesses, talents and character, into an engagement with the social realities of our times. Before the summary of the chapters, I will briefly paint a picture of some of the bigger wheels of historical and institutional social change to which we are responding as a profession and which present a dramatic background to the chapters of the book.

The Bigger Picture: Developments in the Profession and Change in the Organisational Structures around Art Therapy Private Practice

The book shows diverse perspectives on the wider social, economic and organisational frames in which art therapy private practice is currently situated. The timeline on the next double-page spread shows, in linear and condensed form, some of the major historical events that enable us to draw out trends.

What is shown by this timeline is a gradual acceptance of the place of private practice and independent work within the profession, alongside the larger political and historical movements that have encouraged these adaptations. It also reveals a gradual movement towards an autonomous professional stance held within both the state and community provisions, whether funded by the state or provided independently, or as a private practice. However, art therapists in all these contexts are offering a service by licence of the state regulation of our profession.

Art therapists remain the only *state*-regulated psychotherapists in the UK. It sometimes appears an irony that it is through its status as a profession 'supplementary to medicine' that art therapy has gained licence to practise beyond the state provision, at a time when other psychotherapeutic associations have sometimes fought hard against such regulation. State regulation has undoubtedly granted us a gift of relative autonomy, self-determination and professional independence as we now find ourselves well placed to meet the challenges of the current economic climate and those of our clients, both in and outside the statutory sector. We might not yet have fully recognised what this means and the possibilities it affords us now as a small independent profession. It is worth considering where the profession would be without state regulation in the current climate of austerity.

In *Becoming a Profession*, Waller (2013) offers an evolutionary metaphor of the art therapy profession growing from childhood to adolescence. It seems timely now to ask whether the recent developments since the 1990s represent further progress towards independence and maturity, in the journey from 'our home' in the state provisions of the NHS, Education and Social Services, and now finding our feet in the wider world. Through this metaphor, we could recall that leaving home brings potential risks as well as new freedoms. There is a need to find an independent identity and a way of speaking that better represents our lived experience. This process of self-discovery is always balanced with a necessary struggle for an independent identity, no longer bound by the aims of the previous generation, and the consequent risks of both loss of meaning and direction. The positive outcome of this process depends upon our being able to find, and/or invent, discourses that better fit the needs of the present. Eventually, we reach a secure but interdependent place amongst peers, from which we can eventually recognise both the value in the struggles of our antecedents and our real independence of them. Finally, there is a growing acceptance of a willingness to try 'to be' without the security of a dogma and a growing willingness, or even a desire, to partake in the sweet reveries of homecoming, a recognition of our roots, relishing again its favourite dishes but with the secure knowledge that we can leave before the demands for conformity begin, drawing us back into old routines. Through this dialectic tension between the search for the new and the respect for the past, we are formed and evolve as individuals and organisationally.

The setting up of an independent art therapy private practice demands of the profession that therapists develop a real sense of mature professional autonomy nurtured within a network of reliable others. This theme returns throughout these chapters, as we attempt to build professional routines within this relatively new field.

If we continue to extend the metaphor of the individual human lifespan to the art therapy profession, there is the other side of growth, which is decline. As individuals we each face old age and death; however, for a profession, while it may be prone to 'regressions' and 'maladaptive behaviour', demise is not a necessary condition, unless we make ourselves unavailable or irrelevant to the needs of our times. It is said and attributed to Hippocrates that art is long but life is short (*ars longa, vita brevis*) and so we can say art similarly seeks longevity. If we as artists, individually and organisationally, show our talents for creative adaptation, we rediscover an adaptable professional stance that is central to the therapy we offer to our clients, namely the capacity to play. The processes of the arts are inherently adaptable, and this *inter-play* provides clients with the possibility of change and reintegration, in the guise of the transforming metaphors and the metamorphoses evident in the physical and material processes of art making. We cannot elude our mortality – but we can employ the healing processes of the arts, an inheritance that continues now as it has done back to our untraceable human beginnings. It is in this spirit of playfulness and adaptation that this book presents art therapy in private practice, revealing our professional capacity to use and invent fitting metaphors in the face of challenge and change. I believe there is currently an urgent need to consider what metaphors of research and practice best suit our rapidly changing professional circumstances, and as we face a multitude of aesthetic and ethical dilemmas, sometimes being asked to submit the art and therapeutic process to discourses that may limit it in advance and stifle the free play necessary for both the art and the creative therapeutic process to flourish.

Seen in this light, art therapy in private practice can be seen as a vital sign for the profession by which we overcome the fearfulness of independence, while simultaneously facing the reality and challenges of our professional circumstances. In this book we hope to represent this current scene, the hopes and fears it represents to the profession as a whole, and some of our tentative forays into the future of theory and practice in this context.

Here is a summary of the chapters set out within the thematic areas that emerged in the process of the writing, to give readers a sense of the book as a whole.

TIMELINE OF SIGNIFICANT EVENTS

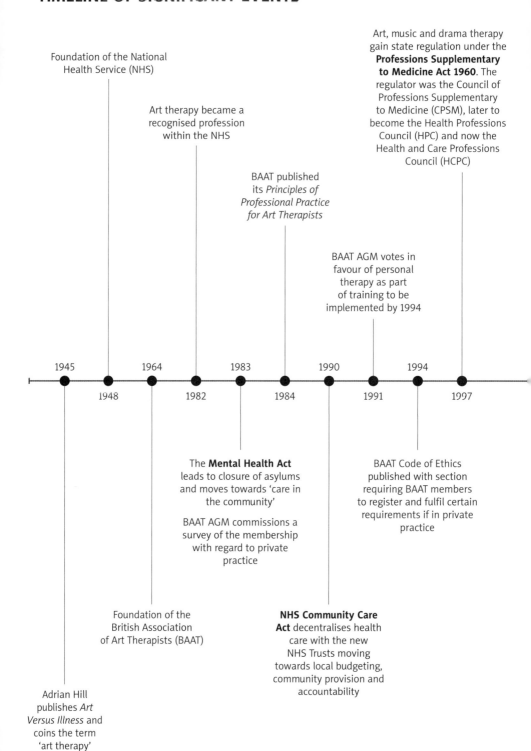

Foundation of the National
Health Service (NHS)

Art therapy became a
recognised profession
within the NHS

Art, music and drama therapy
gain state regulation under the
**Professions Supplementary
to Medicine Act 1960**. The
regulator was the Council of
Professions Supplementary
to Medicine (CPSM), later to
become the Health Professions
Council (HPC) and now the
Health and Care Professions
Council (HCPC)

BAAT published
its *Principles of
Professional Practice
for Art Therapists*

BAAT AGM votes in
favour of personal
therapy as part
of training to be
implemented by 1994

1945 1964 1983 1990 1994

1948 1982 1984 1991 1997

The **Mental Health Act**
leads to closure of asylums
and moves towards 'care in
the community'

BAAT AGM commissions a
survey of the membership
with regard to private
practice

BAAT Code of Ethics
published with section
requiring BAAT members
to register and fulfil certain
requirements if in private
practice

Foundation of the
British Association
of Art Therapists (BAAT)

**NHS Community Care
Act** decentralises health
care with the new
NHS Trusts moving
towards local budgeting,
community provision and
accountability

Adrian Hill
publishes *Art
Versus Illness* and
coins the term
'art therapy'

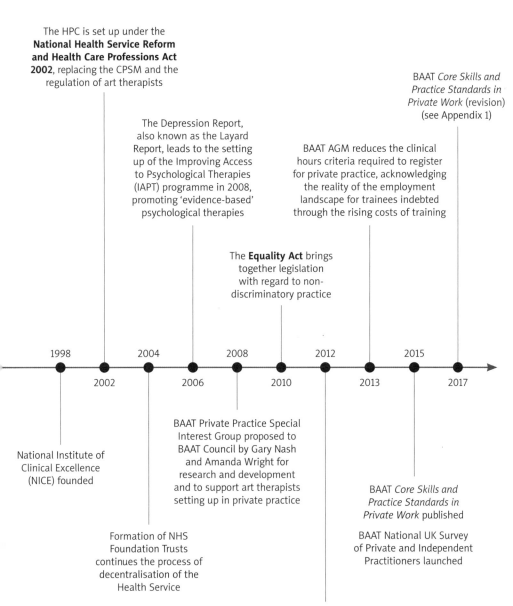

The HPC is set up under the **National Health Service Reform and Health Care Professions Act 2002**, replacing the CPSM and the regulation of art therapists

BAAT *Core Skills and Practice Standards in Private Work* (revision) (see Appendix 1)

The Depression Report, also known as the Layard Report, leads to the setting up of the Improving Access to Psychological Therapies (IAPT) programme in 2008, promoting 'evidence-based' psychological therapies

BAAT AGM reduces the clinical hours criteria required to register for private practice, acknowledging the reality of the employment landscape for trainees indebted through the rising costs of training

The **Equality Act** brings together legislation with regard to non-discriminatory practice

1998 2002 2004 2006 2008 2010 2012 2013 2015 2017

National Institute of Clinical Excellence (NICE) founded

BAAT Private Practice Special Interest Group proposed to BAAT Council by Gary Nash and Amanda Wright for research and development and to support art therapists setting up in private practice

BAAT *Core Skills and Practice Standards in Private Work* published

BAAT National UK Survey of Private and Independent Practitioners launched

Formation of NHS Foundation Trusts continues the process of decentralisation of the Health Service

Following the **Health and Social Care Act 2012**, NICE is renamed the National Institute for Health and Care Excellence on 1 April 2013, reflecting its new responsibilities for social care. It changes from a special health authority to an executive non-departmental public body (ENDPB) like the Care Quality Commission (CQC)

The NHS Commissioning Board and Clinical Commissioning Groups (Responsibilities and Standing Rules) Regulations 2012 prescribe 'payment by results' in the procurement of services

The HPC takes over the General Social Care Council and becomes the HCPC and subsequently broadens its remit into the community

Summary of Chapters

I have already mentioned how themes and chapter headings changed in the course of writing the book and new themes emerged. The themes eventually fell into four distinct areas that differed from the ones we had originally envisaged in the proposal. These themes subsequently became the five sections of the book, which are: Contexts and Collaboration; Working with Children, Families and the Child in the Adult; Training and Transmission; Governance and Supervision; and Research. Midway through the process the authors chose which area their work fell within and then continued to write and rewrite towards that emerging brief.

In **Part I: Contexts and Collaboration**, there is an exploration of private practice in four different practice contexts (the home setting, the community, the hospital and a therapy centre) which together give a sense of the diversity of art therapy private practice.

Julia Ryde provides a phenomenological exploration of working from a consulting room in a domestic setting through a single case study. The disappearance of a painting provides an opportunity to explore the nature of the therapeutic relationship, memory, loss and interpretation through a collaborative understanding of therapy. She encourages a close aesthetic attention to the art process and its objects and uses this to explore the therapeutic relationship and, crucially, what we mean by 'privacy' in private practice.

Frances Walton considers the art therapy profession and its relationship to the state provision, looking at it both historically, by representing the major changes that have occurred in the last decades, and autobiographically, in considering her own move into private practice. She explores the insights and opportunities offered within these discrete provisions, but finally recommends that we try to hold onto the best of both these 'worlds', understanding that the needs of clients will always require both, depending often on the intensity of those needs and the constantly changing political and social realities. She identifies the inter-systemic interplay of policy, context and economic and organisational factors and their impact on the therapeutic relationship. The adaptability of the art process is shown to provide a medium and containment for this many-levelled process of change and exploration.

Andrea Heath and Catherine Stevens give an account of their long involvement with a self-organised arts community. Their aim is to show the therapeutic value of an independent private provision, which can provide both a platform for a constructive critique of what is currently on offer and a vision of an alternative transformative art therapy provision, built through sharing skills and resources. Frances Walton also suggests that an independent provision can support independence and self-esteem and encourage the growth of relative autonomy, interdependence and creativity for both clients and therapists.

Hephzibah Kaplan considers the dynamics of faith, culture and diversity in the context of a London private practice and reflects, through a literature review, and with an eye to practice and process, how a close examination of the course of a therapy can provide opportunities to consider the identities and differences that appear in an art therapy intervention. She shows how this inevitably intercultural exchange can help the client and also provide the therapist with opportunities for professional development. While raising questions about the 'one size fits all' approach to therapeutic provision, she encourages us to consider the 'culture' of therapy and suggests we all make the journey together towards 'advanced cultural competence', raising the level of our individual and collective consciousness.

In **Part II: Working with Children, Families and the Child in the Adult**, Nili Sigal and Stephen Radley consider working with children (inner and actual) in art therapy private practice.

Nili Sigal first describes her private clinical work with children and their families, where she pays particular attention to the negotiations around boundaries with the family unit and the systems that surround the child, examining the complex dynamics that can follow in private practice. She then presents a case study and considers the wider impact of this type of clinical work by incorporating the perspectives and experiences of the parents, who are often the paying customers, but, importantly, *are not the clients*. Useful questions in relation to legislation and accountability are also raised, making this an informative piece for any therapist considering working with children in private practice.

Stephen Radley then provides an insight into the psychoanalytic training experience of infant observation, which has a long tradition in psychoanalytic training in the UK. Exploring psychoanalytic notions of 'the aesthetic', he examines the therapeutic relationship, transference, aesthetic pleasure and conflict which can arise within the private art therapy engagement, encouraging us to notice the 'aesthetic reciprocity' that can build within the therapy, and thereby acknowledging our common experience of being parented into existence. He does not seek to apply the value of infant observation prescriptively to the art therapy profession, but points to its notional value in the ongoing evolution of the understandings that underpin art therapy practice.

Both these chapters highlight the significance of object relations and attachment theory in the ongoing training of art therapists, theories that continue to provide some of the foundational ideas in our understanding of our practice, and also a framework of ideas to understand our clients' representations, behaviour and needs within therapy. In addition, Nili draws on systemic theory in her writing about the realities of art therapy private practice with children and its potential impact on the family unit.

In **Part III: Training and Transmission**, Themis Kyriakidou's and Dave Rogers' chapters consider the development of art therapy training programmes towards private practice that is being forced by economic circumstances, and the part played in the training of art therapists by private art therapists in the provision of training therapy.

Themis Kyriakidou begins with a historical narrative of the development of a collaborative learning experience that is supported by the Art Therapy Northern Programme in Sheffield, run in partnership with local universities in Leeds and Sheffield, and the local region 11 BAAT membership group. It provides employment workshops for programme students and for therapists who have already qualified. These workshops have developed to include a supplementary training preparing therapists for private practice. This shows how the professional association and its regional groups, in conjunction with the trainings, can build learning experiences, which could contribute to filling any existing gaps for art therapists approaching private and independent work. Themis explores how this gap has appeared historically and the way the Northern Programme has sought to bridge it. This chapter, in describing the curriculum of the training, provides a 'how to' element within this book that includes advice about negotiating contracts and fees, tax, risk assessment, marketing, registrations and pointers to other useful sources of professional support. Themis also offers theoretical reflections on the process of practical learning that is very necessary in the development of private practice. This book as a whole is also a response to this identified professional need.

Dave Rogers then considers the place of the private provision of personal art therapy for training art therapists. He shows the importance of considering this complex interaction theoretically, as an intense network of relationships and investments. He emphasises the importance of contracting and the setting of clear boundaries within training therapy, using four case study vignettes to illustrate the process. As a senior practitioner he usefully shows the value of understanding the place of error in the process of learning, how to 'hold' these complexly situated clients, and the importance of supervision in supporting this process. He draws a specific aesthetic attention to the particular dynamics of the art process in containing, supporting, illustrating and facilitating this process.

Together, these two chapters cover the two formative processes of art therapy training and show us how art therapy private practice must necessarily be considered as central to the future evolution of the profession during these testing times.

In **Part IV: Governance and Supervision**, Kate Rothwell, Colleen Steiner Westling, David Edwards and I (James D. West) address the issues of governance of art therapy private practice in terms of practice management, risk assessment, supervision and self-care, respectively, with pointers to the relevant professional codes of practice and the literature.

Kate Rothwell considers the governance and management of a small private practice through two case studies. She emphasises both the quality and the potentially longer timescale available in private practice and compares and contrasts this with services available in the state sector. She stresses the skills of ongoing assessment that are necessarily involved in safe practice and considers the structures and governance that surround art therapy private practice, especially in relation to relevant legal and professional codes and guidance. The importance of supervision in these reflections is identified once again.

Colleen Steiner Westling considers risk assessment in art therapy private practice, first through an exploration of the neurology and physiology of fear and stress reactions, and then looks toward the wider systems, the societal, regulatory norms and literature, which includes relevant BAAT, HCPC and Information Commissioner's Office's guidance and requirements. The value of supervision in the process of risk assessment is emphasised. Colleen's final position is to encourage us to take an open and informed, but nonprescriptive, stance towards risk assessment but shows how this sometimes runs contrary to our instinctual, individual and group reactions.

The centrality of supervision in the provision of safe and ethical clinical practice is also taken up by David Edwards, who considers art therapy supervisors as private practitioners themselves and then in their role as supervisors of private art therapists. He thoroughly examines the concepts of clinical and managerial supervision as they relate to ways the private practitioner can 'learn, develop and provide a safe service'. He explores a broad range of literature and professional documents that pertain to this professional requirement for art therapy practice. In this way, he provides a detailed picture of the private provision of supervision and the supervision of private art therapy practice.

In Chapter 12, I critically explore the notion of self-care in art therapy private practice in relation to our obligation to maintain 'fitness to practise'. Looking initially at the evidence of the prevalence of vicarious and secondary traumatisation in therapists through their work, and then identifying the means by which the private art therapy practitioner can monitor their own, and their client's, wellbeing as part of 'ongoing joint assessment', this chapter raises questions about how therapists can evaluate and reflect on the therapeutic process collaboratively with clients. To this end, I offer a number of practice-based tools to assist in this process of reflection and practice-based research.

This section is illustrated throughout with case studies and clinical vignettes from practice that reassert the importance of practice-based research, a theme that is taken up in the research section that follows.

In the final section, **Part V: Research**, the 2015 survey of BAAT private and independent members is analysed by Anthea Hendry, who then uses the survey to draw attention to the information we have about art therapists who identify themselves as private practitioners. There are currently 2093 state-regulated art therapists.[1] Of these, 1609 are members of BAAT and 383 are registered with BAAT for private practice. The numbers suggest that a BAAT survey is very representative of the profession as a whole, both in the high numbers that participated in the survey and due to the fact that BAAT currently represents the vast majority of art therapists in the UK. Anthea goes on to usefully explore and clarify the terms 'self-employment', 'independent practice', 'freelance' and 'private practice', presenting an overview of our demographic and some of its identifiable features as a professional group. She also makes

---

1   Based on a freedom of information request recorded on the HCPC website in 2016.

relevant links to data and information provided by other academic and professional surveys, to draw further inferences from the survey.

In Chapter 13, I raised further questions about current research and show how art therapists in private practice can and should be actively engaged in practice research as well as being part of 'bigger' professional research projects. Private practice draws attention to the need to reestablish practice-based research, which may evolve more naturally and with greater congruence from within the field of its therapeutic practice. It may be of greater value in drawing attention to specific clients' needs and in supporting appropriate and relevant professional development. It is vital for our practice to encourage greater practitioner engagement in research to revitalise the research debate from which many practitioners have become alienated. I argue that this disengagement can present risks to clients and to the health of therapists but, most significantly, that it potentially loses the most informative data of practice for the client, the practitioner and the profession.

Conclusion

I hope you will enjoy reading all the dedicated and considered work that has gone into this book. It was created to represent a view of art therapy private practice in the UK during this crucial time of change. While you can fruitfully read discrete chapters as they relate to your own practice, the book was conceived to try to represent as complete a view as possible of art therapy private practice at this time and so it also warrants being read as a whole. I hope it will be of continuing value in the stages of first building and then the ongoing development of your own art therapy private practice.

References

BAAT (2014) *Code of Ethics and Principles of Professional Practice for Art Therapists.* London: BAAT.

BAAT (2017) *Core Skills and Practice Standards in Private Work.* London: BAAT. Accessed on 29 June 2017 at www.baat.org/Assets/Docs/Protected/BAAT%20Private%20Practice%20Standards%20of%20Practice.pdf.

Bateson, G. (2000) 'The Cybernetics of "Self": A Theory of Alcoholism.' In *Steps to an Ecology of Mind.* Chicago, IL: University of Chicago.

Etherington, K. (2002) *Working Together: Editing a Book as Narrative Research Methodology.* Bristol: University of Bristol.

HCPC (2013) *Standards of Proficiency: Arts Therapists.* London: HCPC. Accessed on 22 May 2017 at www.hpc-uk.org/assets/documents/100004FBStandards_of_Proficiency_Arts_Therapists.pdf.

HCPC (2016) *Standards of Conduct, Performance and Ethics.* London: HCPC.

Waller, D. (2013) *Becoming a Profession.* New York: Routledge.

Part I

CONTEXTS AND COLLABORATION

1

HOW PRIVATE IS PRIVATE PRACTICE?

—— JULIA RYDE ——

Introduction

'How Private is Private Practice?' is a play on the word 'private', which I explore in terms of inner and outer realities. How much are we as therapists able to achieve privacy for those we work with, and for ourselves, and what does it mean in terms of a practice which is private, with the connotations of private sector work, money and accountability?

There are both external and internal pressures that affect the therapist and the patient, and their relationship, in all therapeutic practice. In thinking about writing this chapter for a book about art therapy in private practice, I found I wanted to explore the intricate combinations of these pressures, how they interact, and the tensions that they bring which become an essential part of the clinical work. I will travel from concrete realities to the extremes of unconscious activity. In doing so I want to convey how the therapeutic relationship and the art work become part of the aesthetic of practising outside of an institution.

To bring this alive clinically, one particular painting will be the focus for this. It is a painting out of the many paintings that were executed as part of a therapy. It was painted at a time in the therapy when a dog came into my life. As is often the case with images, they can hold a range of emotions. The painting, however, was lost, neither the patient nor I could find it, but it went on having a life in the mind of us both, which meant it became similar to a dream image.

Before I write about the painting, I will set the scene, covering aspects of my practice, and what I offer.

The Setting

I have a consulting room which contains two chairs, a couch, a plan chest with unused white and coloured paper in it, a table and chair, a basket by the table with art materials in it, and a small chest with drawers for pencils, pastels and so on. These are the concrete objects in the room.

The setting, which can also be referred to as the frame, includes the fact that I see someone on a regular basis, at set times each week, and I will give good warning for any changes to what is initially agreed to, and to holiday breaks. At the beginning of each month I give an invoice for the money owed for sessions.

Over the years since I began a private practice in 1996, there have been changes. I have now gone paperless and send my invoices by email, and the bills are paid by bank transfer or sometimes cash but rarely by cheque any more. It is a very different kind of exchange which has its own advantages and disadvantages, uses and abuses.

I have changed consulting rooms once. During the time in my current room I have always had the chairs and couch in the same positions. The furniture has come and gone and been replaced, the walls have changed colour and the room has gradually morphed into how it is now.

Outside of the Consulting Room

There is a hallway and then the front door and then the outside world.

Anyone wanting to use the lavatory will have to venture past an inner door in the hallway and go upstairs to the first floor. I mention this because, again, these are the concrete realities but they take on inner realities once the work starts.

For some there is a curiosity about going deeper into the house, for others a nervousness and feeling of dread that they will bump into someone. And how might that person see them? As someone in need of help and therefore shameful or as a possible rival who might engender hostility?

One particular patient comes to mind who was sensitive to any intrusion into the space around the consulting room from where she tied her bike up outside to when she got into the consulting room, about a ten-metre radius. Bumping into other people coming in or out of the house or hearing anyone going past in the hallway was a disaster for her. She would be furious with me, accusing me of not protecting the space.

Perhaps a similar but totally opposite reaction to the 'field' around the consulting room was in the case of a patient constantly wanting to get me out of the boundaried space and do the session outside.

In both cases this could be about wanting to deny that I had other patients and other people in my life.

Going further afield, there is the question of bumping into patients outside of sessions: in a shop, in the park. Do they see you, or have you seen them? If we have seen each other, I always wait to see if they want to acknowledge me before I respond. Then how it is brought back into the sessions is important to think about. Again, is there a wish for some reason to keep it separate from the therapy work, or perhaps an excited sense of having 'got' something more of you?

Working in an institution there are regulations: fire regulations, health and safety ones, security. Over the years, I have had experience of working in a psychiatric hospital and a day hospital run as a therapeutic community. In the psychiatric hospital the art therapy department was in the old laundry building in the grounds. The day hospital was in a different part of town and housed in an old maternity centre. The images of cleaning and giving birth are apt as metaphors for therapy. The old laundry room in the hospital stood on its own in the grounds of a large psychiatric institution built in the 1900s. It was an oasis for the patients from the wards. The day hospital, housed in the old maternity centre, was a part of the community in a more integrated way. Where the private practice is located must have some effect on the work: whether it is in an urban setting, a residential area, a clinic, or a house which is or could be a home.

Using the Space, Using the Art Materials

To come back to the consulting room, it is not only what is said or not said; or with the images, what is made or not made. It is the feel of how you are together in the room. What are the little rituals, gestures, dances that you go through from the moment of walking into the room until the time someone has left? How free do they feel to make use of the space, using the couch, the chair, the floor and the art materials?

What I didn't say before was that my consulting room is carpeted. With my art therapy hat on, I think: how can you do art therapy in a room that is carpeted? What about being able to make objects, to use paint which might splatter or to make a mess? Since training as an art therapist I have trained as a Jungian analyst, and with this hat on, making images in a session could, by some, be seen as acting out or, more benignly, an enactment.

I have come to feel that whatever we offer in therapy, there are limits. What we bring to the table as therapists is defined not only by the tools of the trade but by who we are. When we qualify we go on to develop our skills. There are certain aspects of who I am that aren't going to change much, but over the years, and rather like my description of my consulting room, the 'furniture' has changed and developed. There is an internal equivalent in that I chuck out some ways of doing things and bring in new ways of working and thinking, and at times return to well-worn theories.

I do not offer a studio-type space where the art materials take front stage, but a room with the conventional two chairs and a couch of a psychotherapist. I have some degree of autonomy about how I look after the room but it has to take into account that the patient is safe, and as a practitioner I must make sure I'm insured to cover any accidents or complaints.

How patients use me, the space and the art materials is all part of the picture which is being built up between us.

Some patients make images outside of the session and then bring them to show me. Some of those who make them in the session sit on the chair opposite with a pad of paper on their laps and talk while they draw; some sit on the couch while they work on something; some sit on the floor and work on an image; some sit at the table, which means having their back to me.

The art materials: I provide paint, paper, brushes, water, clay, pastels, pencils, charcoal.

Patients have created sculptures out of paper; used a hole puncher to make images and used the punched-out circles to make images; sat on the couch moulding clay; dribbled ink down a piece of paper, changing direction until it nearly fell off the paper on to themselves and then my carpet, but never did.

How I Came to the Title for This Chapter

When I thought about the word 'private', I associated it with the private sector, which is about having a trade and exchange of goods which is not under direct government control. As a practitioner outside of an institution, the financial aspect is a direct exchange between the patient and myself, and I am under the regulations and ethics of my profession that, I hope, become internalised.

I also thought of 'The Privacy of the Self', famously captured in the title of Khan's (1974) book, and wanted to explore what privacy meant for both therapist and patient.

When I first set up in private practice it was against the regulations of the psychotherapy world to advertise. These days there is a mass of competing websites. As Dalley states in 'Where now? Looking at the future of art therapy', 'The Internet has transformed the social world of adolescents and adults by influencing communication, relationship patterns and social support systems' (Dalley 2014, p.7). She gives fascinating clinical examples of the use and meaning of chat rooms for adolescents, and use of iPads in art therapy sessions as being part of what art therapists are having to deal with and think about today.

There is the question of what a patient can access about you on the internet. Or you about them. I have caught myself googling someone's relative and then wondered what drove me to this, making me feel rather like a stalker. Why hadn't I relied on what was brought to a session? The information is there on the internet and it is tempting to use it. What can be accessed on the internet is about external privacy, which also relates to a sense of internal privacy. Of course this is true for therapist and patient wherever you work, but perhaps in private practice the field is less protected by an institution or a team of colleagues.

Privacy has to be respected and it needs to be nurtured. How much does the patient feel intruded on by our questions, attention or even looks? Winnicott (1982 [1963]) had an acute sense of the privacy of the self and understanding of the wish of a person to be both hidden but also to be found. In this quote he offers

> a picture of a child establishing a private self that is not communicating, and at the same time wanting to communicate and to be found. It is a sophisticated game of hide-and-seek in which it is a joy to be hidden but disaster not to be found. (p.186)

And how much do patients intrude psychically on the therapist as a way of communicating how they feel? Bion's (1993 [1967]) understanding of projective identification was as a form of non-verbal communication between a mother and a baby, used in later life in empathy and in therapeutic encounters.

The trust needed to foster respect and to be able to challenge defences when necessary depends, and is inextricably tied up with, the sense of privacy which is built up through containment (Bion 1993 [1970]; Winnicott 1971) and confidentiality (Bollas 2003). There needs to be a space in which the therapist and the patient can feel comfortable and safe so that the work of containing often unbearable feeling can be done.

The Internal Frame

Containment and reverie are concepts which Bion (1993 [1970]) wrote about in terms of mother/baby interactions where through the mother's reverie she helps her baby digest raw, overwhelming feeling. In a similar way a therapist receives undigested feeling from a patient, which Bion referred to as 'beta elements', and uses their 'alpha function' to help process the feelings, and feed them back in a more palatable way.

Internally, the therapist has work to do alongside what the patient is doing. A part of this work is holding the frame of what is happening in the sessions so that it is then possible to gauge and see what is significant in the work with the patient (Bleger 1967). This means how a patient will react to breaks and to fees, and also how a patient will use you, your room, the art materials and the surrounding environment.

All therapists will have examples of breaking a boundary in the face of what is demanded in a particular piece of work with someone. Sometimes it can be a mistake and have disastrous effects, but at other times it can be a turning point in the work. The work we do has its risks and wouldn't have the transformative potential without this.

I think there are times when we step out of our usual ways of working, and it is important to have confidence in the internal frame to do this, always gauging what is needed for each individual patient. Sometimes the way a patient uses the art materials can take them away from engaging in what may be too painful, and therefore is an autistic use rather than expressive use of images, and a defence. At other times the art work becomes the best possible expression of often unspeakable feelings. An embodied art work becomes alive with transferences (Schaverien 1992), reflecting the relationship, and being available for reference and further thinking as the work progresses, the symbols of the work offering up bridges to often unknown feelings.

This brings me to the painting done which had such qualities but was lost. I will think about the significance of it being lost and its relevance to this chapter later on, but now I want to write about the circumstances of when it was painted which, as I mentioned before, was the time when a dog came into my life. The fact that I had acquired one was 'picked up' by certain patients and meant something to them.

The Lost Picture

Clare, the patient who painted the picture, told me that she saw me in the park trying to control my 'wild' dog – obviously from her tone of voice I was not doing it very well. So she let me know she knew I had a dog. She had also encountered my dog one day trying to get to us through the connecting door that separates my consulting room from the rest of the house. We discovered her feelings of identification with the dog and were able to connect with other themes in our work together. They were to do with feeling trapped in my house/the mother's body; a wild/instinctual part of her which she perceives as not being allowed in my consulting room; but also the younger sibling brother who is being left outside of the consulting room just as she felt she was left out when he was born.

She is a painter, and around this time she did a painting, which she brought to a session, of a cat and dog. What was interesting, in my mind, was that the cat looked realistic but the dog took on a rather sentimental cartoon appearance. However, what was most striking about the picture was the painting of the dog's body and how she had captured that very particular phenomenon that you find on the fur of certain shorthaired black and white dogs – and which is the case with my dog. In places there is black pigmentation with white fur on top; the black skin shows through the fine, white, fur like a shadow. The dog was not quite real with its cartoon eyes but the body of the dog was more than real. She had perfectly captured the physical aspect of this observation, which only someone intimately involved with dogs could know – or did she know?

The intersubjective connections that occur between people are mysterious and in a therapeutic dyad they are under a spotlight. In Clare's image she was able to express an intimate knowledge of my dog through the observation of its fur, showing an acute awareness of something close to me. The effect of the accuracy of her painting had an effect on me. She could not express her wish to be close to me directly but did so in a painting and through my dog.

It goes beyond the scope of this chapter to go into detail about what may be occurring for this to have happened, but this quotation from Jung (1959) conveys a quality of our experience which goes beyond consciousness and factual knowledge – a place where there is

> a boundless expanse full of unprecedented uncertainty, with apparently no inside and no outside, no above and no below, no here and no there, no mine and no thine, no good and no bad. It is the world of water, where all life floats in suspension; where the realm of the sympathetic system, the soul of everything living, begins; where I am indivisibly this *and* that; where I experience the other in myself and the other-than-myself experiences me. (Vol. 9, para. 45)

In this passage he is describing the collective unconscious. In the discussion I will go into some thoughts as to the usefulness of Jung's idea of the collective unconscious, both for the thinking with this patient and how it might link to work in private practice. Jung's theory of the psychoid is also relevant to understanding the level of connection between patient and analyst expressed through the painting and will also be discussed.

The dog in Clare's picture looked rather submissive and easily cowed. The cat is on the left and the dog on the right. That is how I remember it since we no longer have the picture to refer to. Over the years that I have worked with Clare she has often brought art work to her sessions and sometimes left them with me and sometimes not. However, I am unable to find this picture and she also has been unable to find it. It is lost. In fact she remembers the cat being on the right and the dog on the left. We both know the picture that we are referring to, and the fact that it is lost means it has become a shared picture, rather like a dream which is returned to. Something in the material in a particular session recalls it to us. The other elements of the picture I remember are that the cat looks quite realistic, spiky and thin, whereas the dog has a fatter body and is lying down with paws outstretched in front of it, with the cat sitting up opposite it.

Clare remembers it differently. For her they are both quite cartoon-like and the cat is on the right rather than the left. We both agree that they are looking at each other, and her feeling about the dog's body was that it was breast-like, which connects it to a feeling of skin, of softness, of sensitivity.

In Clare's own words:

I remember it this way:

It was one of those works where the image seems to appear by itself and you just stand back and follow – for the dog bit.

The dog bit did feel exposing – it was sensual and full of feeling – a bit yucky, scary.

The cat I felt was like a 'key' – tall and thin – the opposite to the dog – like the cat was withered and had the feeling sucked out.

I remember the dog on the left and the top half of the picture being dark. I know I felt at the time that you were interested in it – more interested in it than in other things I'd brought. Somehow in the moment, that had the effect of me feeling angry and withholding so when you suggested leaving it I said no I'd take it home.

Now I feel that this was a shame – as it feels a bit like how I do tend to respond if there is interest from someone – i.e. not able to receive it – because in this case I guess I was feeling 'What about the rest of the things I've brought?'...anyway I feel sad now that I wasn't able to be more loving – but at the same time it's become this image shared, so maybe that's better...as if the rejection/withdrawal, incapacity to love on my part in fact is forgivable...the coldness in me has been accepted by you...understood...as difficulty not as coldness.

I think now the image has become symbolic of being 'held in mind' because of something shared – given/received (drawing to you, writing to me) and now after the writing I'm feeling more able to hold you in mind –

I imagine though the picture will turn up one day – although that doesn't matter.

Discussion

The painting being lost means it transcends boundaries and becomes like a dream image (Ogden 2007). It is lost but not forgotten. The object of the painting becomes part of the narrative of the therapy. Instead of blame about the loss there is a mutual sharing of the image. It has been witnessed and goes on offering meaning, as we 'play' with the elements of the image. The elements are two animals: a cat and a dog. Jung spoke of animals being closer to the unconscious and sublime.

In a letter to Marie Bonaparte a few years before his death, Freud commented, 'Dogs love their friends and bite their enemies, quite unlike people, who are incapable of pure love and always have to mix love and hate in their object-relations' (Sacks 2008, p.501). We know how much people can often express deep feelings of attachment for an animal, more often than not a dog or a cat, mourning their deaths more easily than for a person. In Clare's case, in her painting of a dog which so vividly and sensitively captured the skin of my dog, she more easily expressed an unconscious sensual closeness to me.

The depiction of the fur and skin: the soft, sensitive feel of it which seared into me, I see in terms of the psychoid, a term used by Jung to describe an area of the psyche where physical reality meets a spiritual, ethereal level of existence. It is unconscious and therefore can only be expressed indirectly and has been written about by various post-Jungian authors (Bright 1997; Clark 1996) who use the term to describe areas of therapeutic work where there is a muddle of feeling and even sensation in the analyst and patient, which is part of the work. In Giles Clark's (1996) paper 'The animating body: Psychoid substance as a mutual experience of psychosomatic disorder', he uses the term 'psychoid' as a metaphor for a 'dynamic, energetic, active vitalising process, which can be experienced imaginally, emotionally and sensuously' (p.367). He writes:

> …in regressed analytic relations this process can be necessarily sickening and near deadly, as well as erotic, healing and enlivening. Symbols and sensations are often similarly experienced; the analyst's dreams, fantasies and sensations belong equally to the patient and to the relationship, and so these contents feel simultaneously confusing, invasive and mutual, but demanding differentiation, interpretation and a real sense of autonomy. (p.367)

As Clark writes, when there is a muddle of experience on this level it can be 'confusing, invasive and mutual'. What Clare's painting produced in our work together was a confusion in that it had penetrated into a private part of my existence and my relationship with my dog. The fact that the painting was lost meant that the image in a sense became more 'mutual'. When for various reasons it re-emerged into a session it was our mutual memory of it that was being encountered rather than the actual painting, which was hers and had been executed by her. The necessity to differentiate this muddle and to be able to think about what this image meant was important in the work towards a more separate coexistence: a coexistence where metaphorically and in the transference we are still working out who is the cat and who the dog and whether there can be a modus vivendi that is more mutual and does not depend on one dominating the other. As the above quotes from Clark relate, the intersubjective field of the therapist and patient where there becomes a muddle between the two can be both invigorating as well as deadly and it is essential that the work is done to separate out in order for individuation to occur.

Jung wrote about individuation as being the lifelong work each of us does to become the person we are (Jung 1959). In order for this to happen, the shadow, all those aspects of oneself that we want to disavow, needs to be confronted and owned. The individual then enters into a different relationship with the collective unconscious, both being freer to 'play' in it but also not to be so driven by unconscious, collective forces.

I wrote earlier of the usefulness or not of Jung's concept of the collective unconscious. The quote I used to describe it I find particularly poetic and it has associations for me with Matte Blanco's concept of symmetry (Matte Blanco 1975) in understanding unconscious processes on a level where there is a lack of distinction between objects. I then talked of another Jungian concept, the psychoid, which is a further way of describing an area of our experience where subject and object, matter and psyche, meet. These are concepts that don't readily come to mind when I am sitting in the consulting room with a patient, but for the subject of this chapter I find they are a useful part of the bedrock of my thinking, on which I have built the structure of my practice. Jung, having worked in psychiatry, had a particular understanding of when the unconscious can burst through in psychosis, but also how it can be harnessed in creativity. He also was aware of the influence and importance of the social aspect of our lives. Here in this chapter are the extremes of unconscious activity and concrete realities of our world.

What goes on inter-psychically on an unconscious level cannot be controlled even though both therapist and patient will have their defences to try to protect themselves. There are the conscious elements of privacy which must be upheld to protect the work. A crucial aspect of this is to be aware of the context of the work. The context is being able to assess what the external pressures are, as well as being aware of what your own personal limits are. We have a sense, and get to know over time, what kinds of patients are in our capability to work with and which ones we are not so good with. But it is also about being able to assess what kinds of patients are suitable to be seen in the particular setting that is being offered. This of course can be aided by consultation and supervision, a subject covered elsewhere in this book (see the chapters by James D. West, David Edwards and Kate Rothwell). It is also about making sure that there are as few intrusions into the setting as possible. And it is about engaging ethically with the patient: another subject also covered in various sections of this book.

Clare, the painter of the picture, had found dealing with the world difficult and persecuting. It was important for her to feel a level of intimacy with me in the work, without feeling trapped, and the painting of the picture of the cat and the dog was part of the work towards achieving this. The painting held both a wish for sensory closeness and love as well as the aggression that can occur between a dog and a cat. It was Winnicott (1971) who wrote of the necessity of a person feeling that their expressions of love and aggression are accepted by an object in order for there to be a development of the spontaneous self and so that aggression can be used helpfully and not turned inwards. This can then lead to a greater ability to deal with the real world and the anxieties that life can bring.

Conclusion

Through describing my practice and also a painting made by one of my patients, I have attempted to point to some of the inner and outer realities of art therapy in private practice. Whatever the realities of the space that is offered, each aspect of that space becomes part of an inner reality both for the patient and the therapist.

Privacy for both the patient and the therapist is an essential part of the work. How it is achieved and maintained has to do with trust and confidence in both confidentiality and containment and it involves a dynamic which needs constant attention. The breaching of privacy can be protected against in thoughtful, concrete ways. Internal privacy, in the area of unconscious intersubjectivity, can be a potential area of play or a minefield. Whatever emerges is seen in terms of its meaning for the work with a patient: whether it is a communication, a seeking for an object, an attack. In the example of the painting where Clare expressed an extremely sensitive rendering of something close to me, it was a necessary part of the work.

There needs to be a strong enough container to be able to hold the extremes of what may be expressed. In order to do this there needs to be awareness of the context of the practice, where it is, how safe it is and how private it can be. It is this combined field of inner and outer privacy that has to be attended to, in order to do the work with whoever it is who has walked through your consulting room door.

References

Bion, W.R. (1993 [1967]) *Second Thoughts*. London: Karnac.

Bion, W.R. (1993, [1970]) *Attention and Interpretation*. London: Karnac.

Bleger, J. (1967) 'Psychoanalysis of the psychoanalytic frame.' *International Journal of Psychoanalysis 48*, 511–519.

Bollas, C. (2003) 'Confidentiality and professionalism in psychoanalysis.' *British Journal of Psychotherapy 20*, 2, 157–178.

Bright, G. (1997) 'Synchronicity as a basis of analytic attitude.' *Journal of Analytical Psychology 42*, 4, 613–635.

Clark, G. (1996) 'The animating body: Psychoid substance as a mutual experience of psychosomatic disorder.' *Journal of Analytical Psychology 41*, 3, 353–368.

Dalley, T. (2014) 'Where now? Looking at the future of art therapy.' *ATOL: Art Therapy Online 5*, 1, 1–14.

Jung, C.J. (1959) *Collected Works*. London: Routledge.

Khan, M.M.R. (1974) *The Privacy of the Self*. London: Hogarth Press.

Matte Blanco, I. (1975) *The Unconscious as Infinite Sets*. London: Duckworth.

Ogden, T. (2007) 'On talking-as-dreaming.' *International Journal of Psychoanalysis 88*, 575–589.

Sacks, A. (2008) 'The therapeutic use of pets in private practice.' *British Journal of Psychotherapy 24*, 4, 501–521.

Schaverien, J. (1992) *The Revealing Image*. London: Routledge.

Winnicott, D. (1971) *Playing and Reality*. London: Penguin.

Winnicott, D. (1982 [1963]) 'The Maturational Processes and the Facilitating Environment.' In J.D. Sutherland (ed.) *Studies in the Theory of Emotional Development*. The International Psycho-Analytical Library. London: The Hogarth Press and the Institute of Psycho-Analysis.

2

FROM PUBLIC TO PRIVATE AND BACK

Art Therapy in the NHS and in Private Practice

—— FRANCES WALTON ——

Introduction

This chapter comes from the perspective of having worked for over 20 years within the charitable and public sectors. Much of this time has been in the National Health Service (NHS) as an art therapist in mental health services. In the chapter I will explore my gradual and often tentative move into setting up a private practice as art therapist/supervisor as an adjunct to my ongoing NHS work. With a pull towards a more community-based focus I will question if this was a natural career progression for myself, encouraging greater autonomy and maturity for my clients, or a kind of complementary and necessary reframing of the work. I suggest that there may be something interesting in the interplay between dependency and the growth of personal responsibility for both the client and the therapist, offering fresh and dynamic insights.

As a profession we have always been creative, resourceful and adaptable in our approaches to the work, seeking out possibilities for sessional posts, taking on more generic roles and 'selling' the idea of art therapy to our colleagues and managers. Within the NHS traditional art therapy posts have come under threat as part of the devastating financial crisis. Posts and even teams have diminished or disappeared completely and there is a renewed need for us to evidence what we do and justify our roles through daily data collection, auditing and note writing. In the current and changing climate within primary and secondary mental health care, and a refocusing of resources, art therapists are needing to reappraise their areas and methods of practice. As an experienced therapist I find myself both weathering the change and managing the fallout. Recognising the need to preserve a thinking space, I also feel inspired to look outwards to reappraise my own practice. For trainees and newly qualified therapists this raises important questions and challenges of their trainings as they approach the start of their career.

To begin this chapter I will highlight where we are now as a profession and especially from the perspective of mental health care in the NHS, and how we move forward in the current climate. I will go on to give a historical context to the modern-day NHS, with a focus on the development of primary and secondary care and the shifts that have occurred in the commissioning bodies, leading to the idea of a more personalised care approach.

From a personal perspective I will show how I began my career in the NHS, what ideas and perspectives I brought with me and how the changing culture and environment impacted on my approaches to the work. Influenced by the concepts of change and the possibility of a 'care pathway' and the 'recovery' model of care for our clients, I will consider the paths I am now taking for my own personal and professional growth.

With the current legislation and shifts in funding of care, there has been a real impact on the demographic of patients that can be treated within Secondary Care. I will show how the introduction of Payment by Results (PbR) has impacted on the work that can be carried out within the NHS and also highlight opportunities in private practice.

In developing my private practice there is much that I have brought from my NHS work experience that has influenced my thinking and directed my approach. By choosing to 'manage' myself, the clientele and environment that I work in, I have been forced to reappraise some of the detail of the work that I am carrying out in both the public and private sector.

The Current Climate for Art Therapists in the NHS

In her key note speech at the AGM of the British Association of Art Therapists (BAAT) in 2015, Kate Pestel, head of arts therapies at NHS Lothian, reflected on the reduction of funding of art therapy in NHS services, and highlighted changes in the working environment as a starting point for discussion. She identified key concerns, including the governance of treatment offered when it is being outsourced, and the continued visibility and recognition of registered art therapists. She also recognised our strengths, including an increasingly powerful 'service user voice' of 'lived experience' to influence commissioning in a positive way. Overall she made an appeal for a united voice and a collective approach of working together with those in private practice and social enterprises. She emphasised the need to utilise skill sharing, making links with other arts therapists, support workers, general practitioners (GPs) and other professionals.

Themes that emerged from the day included the changing role of GPs as fund holders, which highlighted a different position to be taken up by allied health professionals. There was a recognition of the creative resources that we already have and utilise in our current work and a call to evidence this practice (Richardson 2015).

Art therapists are at a crucial point of development and transition and it is interesting to note that three recently published books focus on our resilience and creative adaptability to engage with other professionals, environments and ways of working. Susan Hogan offers a concise compendium of different art therapy theories and ways of working with a varied client group (Hogan 2016). Rose Hughes brings together the range of ways that therapists have adapted their work to the brief time frame required in the state sector (Hughes 2016). *Arts Therapists in Multidisciplinary Settings* (Miller 2016) targets the idea of 'working together for better outcomes', with an increased need to identify 'if' and 'how' we engage with the wider care teams.

There is also a wealth of research being carried out, and a burgeoning service user voice, offering much anecdotal evidence around the benefits of art therapy. The collective voice within social media is getting stronger and has been embraced by BAAT through the employment of a social media officer.

The energy needed for this galvanising and eclectic approach may feel difficult to find in a diminished and pressurised environment. With my head stuck in front of a computer for large parts of the day, entering data onto a system that does not seem to give anything meaningful back, it is easy to understand why long-serving therapists may consider leaving to set up private practice and it is also easy to understand why there are not so many opportunities for newly qualified therapists in the NHS at the moment. I also wonder how we sit with a certain reticence to let go of the identity of the artist in her garret. Like many of my patients there is a certain dependency on the system that exists with its hierarchical structure and medical model. We may still be holding on to a vestige of our role as the 'outsider', the 'misunderstood' artist within an organisation that just doesn't 'understand' what we are trying to do. And how does the call to adapt sit with our psychodynamic tradition of the slow client-led approach?

The Context of the NHS and the Development of Primary and Secondary Care and Commissioning Bodies

It may be helpful to consider that the NHS has been in a state of flux since its very conception, as well as a centre of political contention. Founded in 1948, the concept of the 'primary care team' soon followed in the 1950s, with GPs as autonomous contracted professionals. Over the next two decades patients started to have greater responsibility for their own care, with the right to choose different treatments and control of their own health (Petroni and Vaspe 2000).

The next two decades saw the development of more preventative aspects of health care and the closure of many mental health hospitals or asylums (Mental Health Act 1983; see Petroni and Vaspe 2000). With the development of new longitudinal frameworks for working with patients such as the care programme approach (CPA), there was the possibility of individualised care and joint working between service users and professionals with regular reviews, acknowledging the possibility of change and movement.

During the 1990s the Conservative government placed the Health Service within a market framework as part of the NHS and Community Care Act 1990. Hospital trusts and fundholding general practices provided a framework for costed episodes of care. It was the start of patients being seen as customers or consumers and the social workers, care workers and doctors as providers and purchasers. It also meant that NHS trusts and GP fund holders started looking for measurable outcomes (Petroni and Vaspe 2000).

The Health of the Nation

In 1991 and 1996, two white papers published by the Department of Health focused on services being 'user centred and needs based', with more transparency, access to information, public accountability, choice, opportunity and local flexibility being seen as important. In 1997 with a new Labour government came the primary care groups (PGIs): a collaboration with the local health authority and with multi-professional membership.

The National Institute for Health and Care Excellence (NICE) was founded in 1998 with the aim of monitoring evidence-based treatments and cost-effective methods for working with service users. By 2004 there was a push towards greater involvement from GP practices in the commissioning of health care services, and a refocus on the value of psychological therapies within the community.

The initiative Improving Access to Psychological Therapies (IAPT) began in 2008 based on a paper written by health economist Lord Richard Layard (2006), which suggested that some brief psychological interventions would enable people suffering from anxiety and depression to get back to work. With its focus on NICE-recommended therapies, IAPT has proven problematic for treatments such as art therapy. In 2012 the Centre for Social Justice (CSJ) published a paper that focused on the need for more accessible mental health services, offering greater choice to patients (Callan and Fry 2012). It highlighted the strong emphasis on evidence-based brief interventions such as cognitive behavioural therapy (CBT), for working with depression, which was seen as being value for money.

The CSJ also highlighted the limitations of choice offered for patients and suggested that the high numbers of patients with mental health problems turning up at GP surgeries did not suggest 'value for money'. They recommended a greater emphasis on preventative measures for wellbeing and also pointed out the apparent contradiction of IAPT training up a new workforce of mainly CBT therapists, when current existing NHS services (including arts therapies) were already satisfying equivalent NHS standards of clinical safety. A question about the validity of using randomised controlled trials as the 'gold standard' to prove the efficacy of therapies within mental health services was also raised.

The Personalisation Agenda

Since April 2009, the government has funded personal health budget pilots across 64 sites in England including physical and mental health treatment with some success. It has now been rolled out across the board since 2012 but still has a low profile. This may be in part due to the process of application and the pressure GPs find themselves under to treat many patients in a short space of time with too few resources. The Royal Society of General Practitioners recommends to its members that 'commissioners must put in place sufficient resources to support the care planning process, and to ensure that patients receive the assistance they need with managing their budgets and making arrangements to purchase care' (Mathers, Thomas and Patel 2012, p.6). It goes on to give advice on how to carry this out, stating that a care plan must be drawn up in conjunction with specially trained care brokers and specialty nurses, and links should be made with services in the community through the voluntary sector to signpost patients to locally available services.

Within the trust in which I work, the community-based Recovery Support Service (RSS) offers day services via personalised budgets. To access the service you must live within the borough, have been assessed as eligible for social care and go through the personalisation process, that is, have an approved personal budget which includes accessing this particular service.

My Role within the NHS and How I Got There: The Physical Environment and Approach

I have been lucky to have worked as part of a substantial and progressive arts therapy team in a large NHS trust. I have experienced instability as services have closed, relocated and been restructured, and supported patients facing these changes and losses. Survival of the profession within my trust has felt dependent on looking for ways of adapting to change and surviving as four arts therapy professions – art, music, drama and dance/movement therapy – as well as expanding the Arts in Health team. Through research, training, new initiatives and other forms of income generation, we have managed to hold on to many posts, though I understand that this may not be a typical scenario. I am also aware of how it is possible to feel isolated within a supportive team due to time constraints and the often fragmented and dispersed nature of our work settings. Creating and maintaining links and the development of one's own authority and self-management skills are essential components, as well as fostering reflective thinking within our teams.

Rehabilitation in Mental Health Services

I began my working life within the NHS in two brand new purposely built and conjoined residential mental health rehabilitation units. The typical resident suffered from enduring and complex mental health problems with a diagnosis of schizophrenia. Experiencing what is known as 'positive symptoms' such as psychosis and 'thought disorder', and 'negative symptoms' such as poor personal care, there can be a strong resistance to engage in any social activity including individual and group therapy. Residents can stay for up to three years and often have little family input. There can be a sense of deprivation and a need for a slow approach to the therapeutic 'work'.

I brought to the job ten years' experience of other residential settings, activity centres, special needs adult education and community clubs, and also of working with adults and children with different degrees of physical and learning disabilities as well as dual-diagnosis mental health problems. Much of this was within the charitable sector, embedded in the community and linked with a move towards rehousing, rehabilitating and mainstream integration and care in the community. I was familiar with the pace of engagement and the incremental changes that often felt like big steps.

On qualifying as an art therapist I had worked for three years in two residential drug and alcohol rehabs, before taking up the NHS post. The buildings were terraced houses in residential streets, and the closed art therapy groups were run in the sitting room or the kitchen, though it was run as a 'tight ship' with clear boundaries, rules and sanctions. As part of the treatment programme, residents were expected to attend the art therapy group and there was a tension between choice, freedom of expression and rules, which got enacted in the group and through the art making. This kind of residential treatment, offering a structured programme and with its base firmly in the community, seems to be a dying service provision. Like the therapeutic community, it straddles the hospital and the community, creating a secure base and a holistic approach to therapeutic work.

During his time working as a psychoanalyst with psychotic and borderline patients, Henri Rey would describe the Maudsley Hospital as the 'brick mother'. Fellow psychoanalyst John Steiner highlighted the importance of the hospital for Rey 'as a place of safety for patients who were afraid of breaking down...offering a kind of continuity and stability'. He suggested that Rey could also recognise that 'this kind of brick mother' could also be 'cold and unresponsive' (Rey 1994, p.ix).

I recognise something of this ambiguity or paradox for my clients and my own relationship with the institution, and have found the transition between the hospital and the community to be one that needs careful negotiation and recognition. This is also true of private practice and highlights the requirement to assess the level of containment needed by the client as well as support in stepping out of the institution.

There has been a tradition of art therapists working within mental health and drug and alcohol rehabilitation services. From the perspective of his work in the 1990s, Molloy suggested that the therapist must master the art of 'doublethink', with its philosophical basis of traditional rehabilitation as radically different to that of psychodynamic art psychotherapy. He recommended a robust approach to engaging and linking with the team to promote understanding (Molloy 1997).

There still exists quite a heavy focus on the medical model, with the term 'treatment resistant' often cited as a big factor in the referral of a patient to rehab. Though this seems to refer to medication, engagement of any kind can feel slow, fragmented or impossible. Hinshelwood talks helpfully about the struggle of the staff member's super-ego when working in such settings. He suggests that the anxiety felt by mental health staff can relate to a primitive fear of infection by the madness of the patients, including their meaninglessness. He also suggests that we can have infantile and unconscious motives that lead to omnipotent and unrealistic demands on what we can do and repair and suggests that an 'internal consultant' can be harnessed within ourselves with the aim of reflecting the reality of the situation and what is really possible (Hinshelwood 2004). In this sense the question arises as to whether 'rehabilitation' is a useful word to use or expect of our patients.

As my role has evolved I have been able to facilitate regular clinical review meetings, with the aim of bringing the views of the multi-disciplinary team together in our thinking about a client, and, it is hoped, some reality checks on what is actually possible. I hope to show how taking up that consultative stance has also influenced my need to take time out of the institution. Though this can feel at times a 'flight' from contagion and meaninglessness, there is also some hope that I can help the patients to do the same, to different degrees. I set up a bridging art therapy group in an adjacent community building. This was open to both units, with the aim of creating some transitional space for my clients between hospital and community, allowing an engagement to link with a life outside rehab, and one that they can continue to attend on leaving the rehab as a form of support. If the idea of rehabilitation suggests an idealised state of being with an end game and level of expectation for patient and therapist alike, does 'recovery' also allude to such ends? The concept of a service user becoming an 'expert in their own recovery' has become more familiar. It feels as though it may exist in the realms of Hinshelwood's 'infantile super-ego of staff members', though it has actually been defined by service users in a more realistic and useful way, opening up an opportunity for patients to be more involved in understanding and choosing the treatment available.

The Recovery Model

In mental health services 'recovery' has been defined as 'a process through which people find ways of living meaningful lives with or without ongoing symptoms of their condition'.

Key principles identified by service users include holding on to hope in seeking personal goals and ambitions and feeling a sense of control over one's symptoms. There is also a need to feel empowered by having opportunities to create a life beyond illness and gain control of one's life (NHS Confederation's Mental Health Network and the Centre for Mental Health, commissioned by the Department of Health).

The Financial Climate, Current Legislation and Implications within the NHS

Over the last ten years or so, there have been various new policies and practices that have impacted on the way that the NHS operates and therapies are funded, such as the introduction of mental health PbR:

> [This] is a major organizational change for both providers and commissioners. For the first time clinicians will have a direct impact on the funding that their organization receives through their work to

deliver high quality care and to achieve better outcomes. Commissioners will start to understand in detail how the services they are purchasing meet the needs of individual people, and how this directly affects the prospects for patient recovery. (Department of Health 2013, p.4)

With PbR comes the process of 'clustering' patients into brackets of diagnosis and of need which is directly linked to funding and a greater accountability of who can be treated and for how long. There is a considerable amount of literature and evidence that art therapists have historically worked with the most unwell or hard-to-treat patients within inpatient settings. Patients with a chronic or enduring psychosis, severe depression or risky borderline presentations would indicate the need for continued therapeutic and medical support. Those patients are unlikely to be affected directly, but there are many more who seem in danger of 'falling through the net'. With increased economic pressure and consequent restructuring of community mental health teams, including a single point of access for referrals, therapists offering community-based treatment are also feeling the impact.

Cost Centres

Cost centres are an essential but complex area of exploration when considering funding and the role of the Clinical Commissioning Groups (CCGs). The need for monitoring and researching projects appears to be a block in making funding available for pieces of work because any changes or variations in the services offered need to be stringently assessed and accounted for by the authorised signatories. It seems easier to conceptualise and control treatment when looking at the prescription of medication, but in the less concrete areas of relational therapeutic interventions this all looks a lot less straightforward to measure and assess.

Within the realms of private health care insurance provision there is also a blurry area, where currently Health and Care Professions Council (HCPC)-registered practitioners are not yet sufficiently recognised to be contracted as private practitioners within health care insurance cover. This is an area that the BAAT Private Practice Special Interest Group (PPSIG) is exploring and pushing forward.

Community, Work and a Different Role

With a link to the community, my own work expanded into running more community-based groups with three strands. One was the bridging group for inpatient and community rehab clients: all members experience psychosis and are clustered to a degree that they are care-managed, though this feels increasingly fractured as care teams restructure, staff leave and new staff arrive. The other two are for people with mixed diagnoses: severe depression, bipolar disorder or other personality disorders as well as post-traumatic stress disorder (PTSD). One runs in the north of the borough and is based in a non-clinical environment in the basement of a large terraced house, with access to a garden that members can utilise. Tea and coffee are available, and both my co-therapist and I engage in art making with a reflective period at the end. The other is in the south of the borough, embedded within a community mental health centre. Sometimes group members are care-managed by community teams, but increasingly I am called upon to be a lead professional for service users no longer care-managed, but still complex enough to be 'clustered' within a working remit. My liaison is predominantly with the GP and mostly through letters, and I am conscious of a real shift in my role and how it impacts on the therapeutic work that can be done. In many ways these groups feel more complex than the bridging group, where more holding of the patient by care teams still exists.

Issues brought to the mixed diagnosis group include struggles with addictions, eating disorders, displacement and trauma from country of origin, the challenges of managing prescribed medication, suicidal thoughts, loss, and family and housing difficulties. The backdrop to these groups is the uncertain financial and political climate, changing care teams, instability in terms of benefits, and the closure of specialist community services that limit the aftercare available. Added to this is an instability and uncertainty of tenure of the buildings being used for these groups.

Though few of my group members remain with the community recovery team in the south of the borough, once accepted for art therapy, my physical presence within the communal office and input into clinical thinking feels an essential element of my work. I need to straddle being an autonomous therapist and also representing part of the thinking process in these challenging times. As a team we have to adapt to a different way of working that can feel akin to that of a social worker. Complex patients can feel like hot potatoes passed around from team to team, and a good and thorough assessment has never felt more important. Service users used to a more containing and supportive structure are also having to adapt to a less secure hold, which is challenging their own sense of dependency upon the system, and having to deal with this loss. I am also conscious that I may become more concrete in my thinking as I hold different roles for different patients.

Despite these challenges, or maybe because of them, creative therapies feel more important than ever and artists particularly have the capacity to respond and adapt to the changing climate. My own need to look outwards for new or different stimulation feels essential for building new ways of working from within.

Filling Gaps, Making Bridges and a Collective Approach

Within my trust there has been the introduction of a 'single point of access' (SPA) for patients. The idea is to streamline the process of referrals both for the referrers and the patient, and to simplify the experience of assessment and transition to treatment for the patient. It still feels early days to get a sense of how this will work but there is an understanding that many more patients will be directed back to their primary care teams and will not be eligible for secondary care. This highlights the importance of more community-based services such as IAPT and the Recovery College, which offers a range of courses, workshops and resources accessible to service users both as participants and co-creators. The Arts in Health team certainly has a part to play in working towards a more inclusive presence in colleges and galleries.

Within certain boroughs initiatives such as the Health and Wellbeing Programme and more specifically the GP Exercise Referral Programme offer an opportunity for people to gain financial support with accessing local gyms as well as guidance and support in doing this. Within my capacity as lead professional I have been able to support several clients in accessing this service. I am not sure that this would have been so readily responded to if I had not been proactive in supporting the client to fill out the form and in making contact with the GP as a prompt for them to complete and sign the form. Not surprisingly this engagement with physical health needs has proven to be beneficial in supporting clients in their mental health. I feel a more holistic approach is one to explore further as well as considering the possibilities to translate this type of scheme into arts therapy services.

It seems essential at this time that private practice finds its place within primary care teams and has a presence in negotiating personalisation budgets for this client group. Already arts therapy departments will be looking to build greater links with primary care teams and GPs and finding ways forward for collaborative working.

At the time of writing, the health trust I am working in has just introduced arts psychotherapy evening therapy clinics, offering NHS space to be rented by private practitioners from GP referrals, with the possibility of a sliding pay scale for clients. London Arts Therapy Centre also had some success in GP-funded referrals, as well as funding via other statutory organisations. At the outset this has tended to be time limited, but on seeking additional funding to extend the interventions, as long as the outcomes and reports have been positive, funding has been extended for some clients. This is surely an area of growth and one to be taken seriously by new graduates and trainings.

From the NHS to Private Practice

As I have become more experienced as a clinician in the NHS and developed reflective roles as supervisor and facilitator for clinical thinking, I have also sought to create the space to develop my own resources and capacity to think outside of the institution. Through further study at the Tavistock and Portman Clinic I gained a master's in 'Working with Groups – A Psychodynamic and Systemic Approach' and the opportunity to practise and learn from other professionals holding different roles and perspectives. Observational studies and group relations offered an opportunity to stand back from the chaos and take a look at how it functions and then play with these ideas and roles. All of this has helped me tolerate, adapt and even appreciate the changing state of my NHS work: closures and reorganisations of teams, and the challenges of working with people experiencing serious mental health difficulties. With greater confidence and through taking up a more self-managerial stance I have also felt able to take a step out of the institution, reframe the work and explore something new.

In this book practitioners are showing the breadth of their work and the broad range of the clients that they see. For me this has included an interest in addressing the balance of art therapy offered for art therapists in training (see Dave Rogers in Chapter 8). My own personal experience when training 15 years ago suggested an emphasis towards students receiving personal therapy with a verbal psychotherapist, rather than an art therapist. This raises important questions about how we perceive and value what we do as a profession and our own emotional relationship with and understanding of our own creative process. With the potential for a 'cold' climate of data collection, generic working and evidencing of our work with limited thinking space, maybe we should ensure that our own creative expression is given the air to breathe and grow through 'lived experience' of exploring our emotional lives through art therapy.

Private Practice Community Art Therapy Group

Part of my hope for creating a private practice art therapy group was to be able to offer a sustainable and affordable therapy that could evolve at a more organic pace than the increasingly time-constrained groups within NHS practice, though I should add that there has been a certain amount of thinking around this within my particular arts therapy department, where we have sought to explore realistic and flexible options for our clients. I also hoped for the experience and the contrast of working with a client group with greater 'ego strength' and hoped to challenge my own relationship with the dependency of the institution.

Having made two attempts at setting up a private art therapy group with two different collaborators, we were confronted by the challenges of getting enough referrals, finding a suitable space and keeping hold of it whilst building and assessing referrals, which of course also involved a financial investment and commitment. Other challenges were to do with gaining an understanding of business, not an immediately comfortable fit for many a creative brain with a certain amount of resistance to the less organic aspects of the therapeutic process. We also needed to identify our client group, seek funding via GPs, or even make the initial contacts with GPs, and making sense of how funding may work. There was plenty to take from my NHS work with the exception of the more direct financial transaction, but psychologically it felt a challenging and tentative move.

A year or so after the second of these attempts, and having established individual therapy at an art therapy centre, I agreed to facilitate an art therapy group there and started the process of assessment all over again. This was different, and I was collaborating with the centre but running it on my own, and I was able to establish a base through my individual work.

The aims of this group were/are to offer a creative space for people considered to be in recovery: based on a therapeutic community model, members may typically experience isolation, have issues around self-worth and have anxieties around prescribed medication. Presentations of depression, bipolar disorder, eating disorders and addiction have been typical. Though members have often received treatment within the NHS as inpatients or day services, there is an understanding that they will be able to contain themselves and manage a group such as this now. It does highlight the need for an ongoing awareness and assessment of the client's fluctuating state of mind whilst in therapy in private practice, and the potential for linking with GPs or other mental health professionals remains important. Mutual understanding, trust and a certain amount of transparency must be harnessed in this more private space.

The group has highlighted some key points in looking at the links between the different sectors, and also what I may bring from my NHS role and take back to it. Within a private practice the financial and contractual transactions become concrete and significant symbolic aspects of the therapy, allowing a greater exploration of the issues of value, responsibility and intimacy. Finance may dictate the length of therapy offered and is an area that needs further exploration and is currently directing me to a more brief therapy approach. One of my group members secured funding from an NHS trust for ten sessions. She sought out the art therapy group on the internet and requested this via her GP, who sent her to a panel that assessed her and granted her ten weeks of funding. I feel that this process facilitated a more dynamic investment in her own wellbeing, though highlighted the limitations of what may currently be paid for.

Another member gained a Personal Independence Payment (PIP). This has replaced the Disability Living Allowance (DLA) and was offered in response to her experiencing isolation through her mental health difficulties. She was able to personally advocate for her need to integrate with people in a manageable way via an art therapy group.

In the process of the group she has been able to make an assessment of her own needs with the support of the group and how she spends this money. Having completed ten sessions, she decided to test out a renewed sense of her own creative drive, confidence and resilience, dipping her toe back into previously realised musical pursuits. Choosing to miss the next block of five sessions, which would enable her to afford this, she also tested out her own resources to cope, with the understanding that she could return to the group. My holding on to her art work during this time also added to this sense of both containment and a door being left open for her return.

This financial aspect of the fee in private practice is a different type of transaction where the exchange of money, be it funded or the client's own personal expense, creates a conversation grounded in reality and meaningful decision making. It also makes me question a culture within the NHS of our own dependency on keeping the patient/service user within treatment and where the whole process of assessment and case management can feel so extensive. In the health service we also have a real dependency on a measure of 'successes' in terms of duration and consistency of attendance of patients in relation to PbR. How much focus can we really give to the changing needs of our clients? How much do our choices depend on feeding our professional and organisational super-egos?

Another self-funding group member, who had been diagnosed with bipolar disorder, had previously been proactive in developing a communicative relationship with her consultant. She used the group to consider ongoing treatment, and also as a creative thinking space removed from family members and her contacts with medically orientated professionals. I feel that a removal from the system allowed her some perspective on this and the treatment offered and received. She described a sense of freedom in her use of the art materials and the reconnection with her drive and creative self. My position was one of support and holding, but also my understanding and appreciation of the treatment she has had, and may continue to receive via her consultant, meant that it was possible to explore her treatment in a transparent way. It felt important to recognise and name these splits within herself and the potential enactment between the different places of support – between private and public.

All members seem to have made considered decisions when choosing to attend a private art therapy group. Reasons given were that 'It felt important that I found out about the centre myself' or 'I attended an inpatient art therapy group, which was helpful at the time – now I want to be in a group that is less part of the hospital setting.' A common concern amongst those locked into the trials and management of anti-depressant or antipsychotic medication is the side-effects such as lethargy, memory loss, or a sense of remove from one's self, including creativity and libido. There is obviously a balance to be reached between what is gained and what is taken away through the use of these medications, and whilst I am not advocating that these medications should not be used, it is important that these issues can be explored in the group through the process of creativity, the finished work and the reflective space, and it is certainly something that is discussed with my patients within my NHS work. In my experience this can involve a profound sense of loss, grieving and anger as well as hope for some sense of recovery.

I feel that my work in the NHS highlights the need for a solid assessment and a clear understanding of the ground rules, working with breaks, beginnings and endings, how to manage a group and the importance and storage of art work. These aspects are of course not exclusive to NHS work and should be a fundamental aspect of our basic training, but I am often struck by how many trainees have had little previous experience of carrying out assessments by the time they reach their final placement in the NHS. It remains a solid and thorough aspect of NHS work and is equally important in private practice.

Conclusion

It does feel that we are in a crucial time of change in the provision of art therapy within the private sector and to those who may have the need and desire but do not have the means. I would like to see the possibility within my own practice to offer a sliding scale of fees, but I also see that there needs to be a greater engagement and understanding of commissioning and the funding bodies. Through some enquiries I have made into current provisions I have received quite negative responses from art therapists in private practice – that 'NHS funding is unheard of'. At best it seems small pockets of funding for brief pieces of work may be found, as is currently my own experience. I have been heartened by the few examples of funded referrals that I have received for my group and how interestingly these have often come about through the clients themselves being proactive about finding the art therapy and making enquiries within existing care teams to get funding. A more direct link with GP practices may be a way of building the understanding of the value of art therapy. I am aware that work is already being carried out by therapists working in private practice to make these links, offering short presentations to teams within GP practices and building on changing the culture of understanding. Hephzibah Kaplan, director of London Art Therapy Centre, is one such therapist. She has also run 'introduction to art therapy' events for health professionals, medical and psychology students and carers.

ICAPT (the International Centre for Arts Psychotherapy Training) is also exploring these potential links within Central and North West London NHS Trust. The evening clinic is facilitated by arts therapies private practitioners, who also have NHS experience of working within mental health services. It aims to bridge the gap created by decreased resources within the NHS whereby GPs can now refer patients not eligible for secondary care within the NHS.

Studies of art therapists who have worked within GP practices, such as Turnball and Omay (2002), reported positive outcomes – that is, a decrease in visits to the GP whilst engaging in art therapy. Wilson (2002) also notes an interest from GPs in her brief work with patients presenting with somatic types of illnesses. Exploration of this area of mind/body relationship is certainly important and appears increasingly in my community NHS work. I feel that the link between physical and mental health is one that needs further exploration at this time of depleted resources. Certain illnesses may be explained as 'somatic' or stem from the inherent understanding by the patient that physical health problems are generally taken more seriously than mental health problems and therefore provided with greater resources, or it may simply be a physical response to a body subjected to a lifetime of stress and neglect, further impacted by the current harsh economic climate.

In terms of funding and referrals both within the NHS and within private practice it seems that much depends on the relationship that the patient is able to make with their GP. Supporting and educating patients to understand that a more holistic approach is open to them feels important.

It feels essential to be aware of what exists outside of the system as well as within. By offering private supervision it has been necessary to keep in touch with different areas of work, on a systemic level. It has also enabled me to tap into my skills, knowledge and experience that exist outside of my usual frame of reference.

I have found something restorative about my private work, reconnecting me with the essence of my own creative art therapy practice and my knowledge and experience. It can feel hard at times to hold on to my identity as an art therapist within the NHS, whilst recognising that creative therapies are needed more than ever within a depleted and restrictive system.

Within my private practice I welcome being able to recognise my own authority to choose the 'team' that I work with and feels fit for the specific purpose, recognising also that my support needs may vary and change. Business becomes much more essential to the task, and gaining a business head has been a learning curve for me. The contract between my client and me can feel very meaningful and the sense of responsibility for both therapist and client heightened.

Though my path into private practice has been a slow and tentative one, with many stumbles, blind alleys and ambivalence, the self-managerial aspect feels significant and operates on many different levels, from developing skills as a business woman, appraising boundaries and risk, to the emotional and reflective aspects of the work. Each involves creating real and virtual 'teams' and raises questions about the essential aspects of the work, be it private or public. There may well be a perception of private practice that engages the 'worried well' and there is of course a reality to the accessibility or usefulness of a service outside the institution for more people suffering from acute or enduring mental health problems. The 'brick mother' may always be necessary in some form, but I have also now appreciated the contrast in my work across all the sectors, where different depths of therapeutic work may be possible and one sector may inform and enhance the other.

References

Callan, S. and Fry, B. (2012) *Completing the Revolution: Commissioning Effective Talking Therapies.* London: The Centre for Social Justice.

Department of Health (1991) *White Paper: The Health of the Nation. A Consultative Document for Health in England.* London: HMSO.

Department of Health (1996) *White Paper: Choice and Opportunity.* London: HMSO.

Department of Health (2013) *Mental Health Payment by Results Guidance for 2013–14.* Accessed on 18 May 2017 at www.gov.uk/government/uploads/system/uploads/attachment_data/file/232162/Mental_Health_PbR_Guidance_for_2013-14.pdf.

Hinshelwood, R.D. (2004) *Suffering Insanity.* Hove: Brunner-Routledge.

Hogan, S. (2016) *Art Therapy Theories: A Critical Introduction.* London: Routledge.

Hughes, R. (ed.) (2016) *Time-Limited Art Psychotherapy: Developments in Theory and Practice.* London: Routledge.

Layard, R. (2006) *The Depression Report: A New Deal for Depression and Anxiety Disorders.* Report by the Centre for Economic Performance's Mental Health Policy Group. London: London School of Economics and Political Science.

Mathers, N., Thomas, M. and Patel, V. (2012) *RCGP Position Statement: Personal Health Budgets.* London: Royal College of General Practitioners.

Miller, C. (ed.) (2016) *Arts Therapists in Multidisciplinary Settings: Working Together for Better Outcomes.* London: Jessica Kingsley Publishers.

Molloy, T. (1997) 'Art Psychotherapy and Psychiatric Rehabilitation.' In K. Killick and J. Schaverien (eds) *Art, Psychotherapy and Psychosis.* London: Brunner-Routledge.

NHS Confederation's Mental Health Network and the Centre for Mental Health, Commissioned by the Department of Health – website.

Petroni, M. and Vaspe, A. (2000) *Understanding Counselling in Primary Care: Voices from the Inner City.* London: Churchill Livingstone.

Rey, H. (1994) *Universals of Psychoanalysis in the Treatment of Psychotic and Borderline States (J. Magagna ed.).* London: Free Association Books Ltd.

Richardson, S. (2015) 'The role of art therapists within a changing environment – professionalism, ethics and identity.' *BAAT AGM – Newsbriefing.* London: BAAT.

Turnbull, J. and Omay, F. (2002) 'GPs' and clients' views of art therapy in an Edinburgh practice.' *Inscape 7,* 1, 26–29.

Wilson, C. (2002) 'A time-limited model of art therapy in general practice.' *Inscape 7,* 1, 16–26.

3

SEARCHING FOR SPACE

Reflections on the Work of a Collaborative
Arts Project in Private Practice

—— ANDREA HEATH AND CATHERINE STEVENS ——

We do not deny reality. We affirm that there are experiences and people
who wrong-foot us with their reasoning and behaviour. These are
people and experiences we want to have a relationship with, coexist with
and share the meaning with.

Bucalo 2014, p.18

Introduction

In so many ways it can be a challenge to accept the human condition as it is and to respond to its mystery with responsibility. This is a concern that artists and philosophers have addressed for centuries. We (the authors) have collaborated on this chapter to give a glimpse into our experience and involvement with a working arts studio, which aimed to run along the lines of a democratic arts community. It came into being through the collective desire and involvement of professionals, volunteers and artists, many who through exile, illness and oppression had come to lose a sense of their place in the world. As a group, we shared a belief in the therapeutic benefits of art and community. Over the years, alongside studio practice and workshops, we organised many events to engage people in discussions about the politics of mental health, stigma and inequality. We decided not to name the charity in this chapter, as it can only be an account of our experience. Our intention is to show the possibilities of collaborative work as applied to governance and facilitation of therapeutic arts provision outside statutory services. With this in mind we have focused our attention on the project once it became a registered charity. Our account includes several anonymised quotes from members involved.

Beginnings

The biggest danger, that of losing oneself, can pass off in the world as quietly as if it were nothing: every other loss, an arm, a leg, five dollars, a wife, etc. – is bound to be noticed.

Kierkegaard 1989 [1849], pp.62–63

Before the recent government austerity cuts, day centre drop-ins were available in most areas for people using mental health services. They were places of few demands, small oases. They offered an opportunity for professionals and users of mental health services to come together informally or find a sense of solidarity with others also trying to find their way through the ever-changing complex systems and structures. It was through conversations in a drop-in that the idea for this project came about. Inspired by the service user vision of 'recovery', user participation in the governance and delivery of services was at the heart of our collaboration.

Context

A keynote speaker from the Mental Health Resistance Network spoke about changes in mental health provision at the 2015 'historic' conference (see Watts 2015) entitled 'Welfare Reforms and Mental Health – Resisting Sanctions, Assessments and Psychological Coercion':

I want to take you back to the early 1990s when I first became involved in the survivor movement after a few unhelpful admissions to psychiatric wards. As you might know, the survivor movement opposes the medical model of mental distress and has been campaigning for decades for care to be provided from the perspective of a social model. We have also been fighting the power imbalance between healthcare provider and service user, an imbalance that is enshrined in law; I'm referring to the Mental Health Act. Soon, the user group was closed down and user involvement was controlled by managers at the hospital which was now a Foundation Trust. Over time day centres closed while the press were going crazy demonising us for being scroungers and liars and we were still being pumped full of powerful drugs. Loads of people were discharged from secondary care and left without support. People were isolated and in 2008 many started losing their benefits. (McKenna 2016)

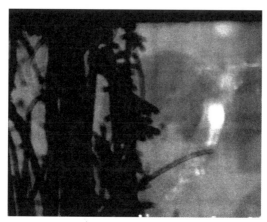

From 'The Ghost Series'

What the medical model and the recovery model have in common is that both are a process of reducing the social and political down to the individual, blaming them for their distress while ignoring the material realities of their lives.

Recovery in the Bin 2016 – Mental Health
Survivors and Supporters Group

There are critical thinkers who have added much to the discourse and understanding of 'mental health', famously Franco Basaglia, Franz Fanon, Erving Goffman, David Smail, Karen Horney, and R.D. Laing. However, credit must also be given to the persistence and developing networks of survivor groups such as the Hearing Voices Network and the Mental Health Resistance Network, to name a few who have challenged the structures and mechanisms of social control. Although they continue to be influential, their work invariably becomes marginal within the economics and practice of mainstream psychiatry.

Laing summed up an anti-institutional argument way back in 1964 in the preface of *The Divided Self*:

Psychiatry could be, and some psychiatrists are, on the side of transcendence, of genuine freedom, and of true human growth. But psychiatry can so easily be a technique of brainwashing, of inducing behaviour that is adjusted, by (preferably) non-injurious torture... Thus, I would wish to emphasise that our 'normal' 'adjusted' state is too often the abdication of ecstasy, the betrayal of our true potentialities, that many of us are only too successful in acquiring a false self to adapt to false realities. (p.12)

Laing wrote about people who had lost their standing in the world. He used the term 'ontologically insecure' to speak of individuals existing within the margins of society, who after seeking help experienced further alienation through their conduct being understood as a sign of 'illness' and treated biologically.

There is well-publicised research into the negative effects of psychotropic medicines (see Healy 2003; Moncrieff 2003), but structural inequality and the increasingly punishing welfare system continue to devalue human experience and contribute to psychiatric disability. In recent years the 'evidence-based' IAPT (Improving Access to Psychological Therapies) programme of short-term psychotherapy has cost the client, who is economically reliant on NHS resources, time and space to be taken seriously. In 2015 plans for IAPT services to be put into 350 job centres linking welfare benefits to state therapy led to protests from health care professionals, therapists and survivors.

Campaigning against a lack of choice of models of therapies available, they highlighted the ethics of coercive short-term interventions in a target-driven culture (see Atkinson 2014; Friedli and Stearn 2016; Gadsby 2015; Leader 2008; Samuels 2012; Scott 2016; Watts 2015). According to the Mental Wealth Foundation, 'The top-down nature of policymaking causes alienation and distrust of government workfare policies with a reliance on expert think-tank research, "evidence-based" reports, and a reluctance to engage in any real collaboration with either service users or practitioners' (Alliance for Counselling and Psychotherapy 2016).

Professor Peter Beresford, a British academic, writer, researcher and activist known for his work in the field of citizen participation and user involvement, has written extensively on developing new approaches to epistemology which highlight the role of service users' lived experience as a knowledge source to influence practice, policy and research. He stated, 'Findings highlighted the complexity of service users' views, their reluctance to impose monolithic interpretations on their experiences and desire to take account of both personal and social issues.' Calling for more of mental health funding to be redistributed to smaller user-led community-based initiatives, he explains, 'They want to see a different approach to welfare reform based on supporting people to make the most of their lives, rather than having to demonstrate incapacity. They offer a blueprint for truly modernising mental health thinking and policy' (Beresford 2016).

The Psychiatric Hospital

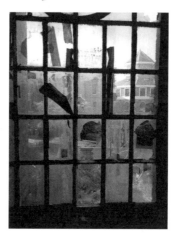

True, in the enterprise of psychotherapy there are regularities, even institutional structures, pervading the sequence, rhythm and tempo of the therapeutic situation viewed as a process... But the really decisive moments in psychotherapy, as every patient or therapist who has ever experienced them knows, are unpredictable, unique, unforgettable, always unrepeatable, and often indescribable.

Laing 1967, p.47

Alongside the lack of actual studio spaces for providing arts therapies, the hospital environment is compromised by the growing proliferation of rules which impinge into various aspects of its life, mostly in the guise of health and safety and risk management. The manner in which the environment becomes controlled could be seen as an attempt to manage anxiety through indiscriminate generalisations. A way of distancing and disassociating from the source of anxiety and displacing this onto those using the services can lead to the loss of capacity for reflection. For example, after a single incident involving a plastic bag within an NHS hospital, plastic bags were banned from all Trust-wide premises. The speed of the response without wider discussion could be seen as another oversight, which more time for reflection may have prevented. It was not long before the brown paper bin liners, which had replaced the plastic ones, posed a risk of their own, this time as a fire hazard, causing another wave of restrictive procedures to be put in place. From this point onwards, everyday items such as plastic and paper could no longer be used in a way that was not laden with anxiety, anxiety that closed down the creative space of the art studio. Keeping clay moist became difficult, and considering the expressive range of the medium of clay as a vehicle of artistic expression, this was a significant loss to patients' art practice. The reduction in clay's plasticity can be seen as a metaphor for an increasing rigidity of thinking leading to fear-driven decision making.

'Wisdom is sold in the desolate market place where none come to buy, And in the withered field where the farmer ploughs for bread in vain.'

Blake 2004 [1797]

Whilst funding cuts undermined psychological therapies, money was being spent on the demolition and redevelopment of NHS sites (Russell 2012). Centres were being closed and buildings left empty whilst community services struggled to continue because of a lack of affordable premises. This created a puzzling picture with many contradictions.

The arts project began with no clear direction but collectively there was a strong desire to create a self-organised community arts provision framed within the arts rather than health, with systems of governance: democratic, visible and legible. Initially as an unincorporated group, we shared a studio space in a local arts collective targeted for refugees. In exchange we collaborated with a lead artist from the collective on funding bids, contributing to its charitable aims through our work. This arrangement worked well for five years, but as the project grew, there was discontent from our host that we were competing for resources. It became clear that we needed to find an affordable alternative to maintain our independence.

Once we began to define our aims we found individuals with experience in the private and voluntary sector who helped us find alternative approaches to organisational governance, systems for accounts and protocols for volunteers. Applying for charity status seemed our best option. Several members met with a 'user involvement consultant' to write our objectives and decided who was willing and able to take on the obligatory roles of responsibility.[1]

Once registered as a charity we secured funds from the local council for core funding and grants for specific projects. With agreed charitable objectives we found it easier to engage with other organisations on our own terms, offering skills from our membership in exchange for studio space. This provided us with an opportunity to learn from each other.

For people able to contribute to the programme but also dependent on welfare benefits, there was concern that their involvement might lead to disability benefit sanctions. In response to advice on this we set up a number of supported permitted earnings posts so that we were able to pay people for their contributions at a rate not less than the minimum wage but that did not compromise their basic income.

Collaboration

For people who find the frustrations of isolation easier to bear than the struggles of negotiating relationships, working in a shared space can become a minefield. This dynamic was particularly alive around issues to do with space, leadership, authority and responsibility. To be in the dual role of both service user and service provider highlighted conflicts and sensitivities about how people inhabited their roles. We frequently came together to discuss and untangle some of the assumptions we were holding onto around power and responsibility. Not everyone could find their voice in our meetings. To work together and tolerate each other's limitations and differences without relying on codes of conduct for safety, balanced against the demands of responsibility and the limits of authority, was a dynamic and ongoing process. That we were art therapists, working within health services that some of our members might subsequently become patients of, added to the complex dynamics. Identified as 'the professionals', there was often an expectation for us to take up the position of authority and to 'know what to do' and sort out difficulties when they occurred and be left to do the jobs no one else wanted to do.

---

1   Charity Commission website: www.charity-registration.com.

The Arts Warehouse

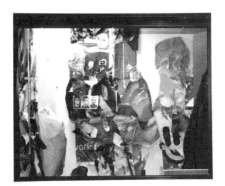 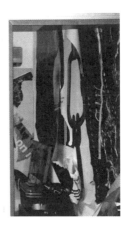

I can't tell you what art does and how it does it, but I know that art has often judged the judges, pleaded revenge to the innocent and shown to the future what the past has suffered, so that it has never been forgotten... Art when it functions like this becomes a meeting place of the invisible, the irreducible, the enduring, guts and honour.

Berger 2006

Everyone had their own space and other rooms where we could share our different concepts. No one person was really in charge. We were in charge for looking after our own spaces, no labels just artists. We came together to create things. (John, a studio member)

In our eighth year we were offered the use of a large warehouse as part of a vacant space management scheme. This was welcome because for a small charity like ours inner-city property rentals were impossibly high. The warehouse had stood vacant for a number of years and as an unused industrial space offered the opportunity for our project to attempt to reflect fully our ethos. Despite it being run down we were able to see the potential of the space. The warehouse became a fitting metaphor for what many of us were addressing in our own lives, exiling certain kinds of intense emotional distress. It was these kinds of experiences we wished to house. Society's discarded materials, both physical and psychological, became a source of inspiration, giving rise to new ideas and a wish to incorporate these materials into the fabric of new artworks. The creative use of the building enabled us to capitalise on the differing qualities of its various spaces for individual and shared studio use. There was a real sense of team effort in furnishing the warehouse. We reclaimed furniture from skips or from outside houses, and this kind of resourceful recycling was a good way of getting by on our meagre finances.

We were a diverse group which included individuals who had never managed the move away from the parental home, others who had lived on the streets for periods of their lives or had spent time in psychiatric institutions, and those who lived isolated lives alone in flats on estates in deprived inner-city areas. Some came from very different countries, and had experienced exile or lived as refugees, others were second-generation UK citizens. All of us were living with the increasing pressures of loss of public and community space, and the ongoing fragmentation of communities. We had a wide range of experiences of occupying or feeling unable to occupy space. All this had an impact on how we each negotiated working alongside each other.

The size of the warehouse facilitated each of us having our own space and choosing studios according to what conditions were conducive to our own creative processes. There were larger communal spaces for workshops and guests. There was much discussion and negotiation about space. Some sought isolation, and were very sensitive about having others in close proximity to them, whilst others sought the company of a shared studio. One artist consistently couldn't find any space at all, and when she finally did, it became a frustration for her as she experienced others intruding into it. One artist chose his space close to where people leading projects would meet on certain days. He hung mobiles from the ceiling of the studio and over time it became an obstacle course, dodging sharp hanging web-like objects.

A very different way of being with others could be seen with the artist who took up residence in a more isolated, deteriorated area. She was adamant that she was not able to work if anyone worked near her. She would work early in the mornings, and as soon as others began arriving she would promptly prepare to depart. She remained something of an outsider.

How we each used space helped us to get to know each other. It emerged that one artist was quite a hoarder and she attempted to empty the excess contents of her flat into her studio.

Our oldest member, a man in his 80s, occupied a small room for himself. He furnished his studio with his possessions and furniture. He invited people to his room to drink coffee and talk whilst he painted their portraits. He filled the walls from floor to ceiling with portraits of friends, famous political activists and others from his homeland, which he had fled. He enjoyed telling stories about his past and the situations he had lived through and explained how after years of resettling in various places due to war and conflict it had been difficult to 'home' possessions. He became a kind of grandfather figure in the project, sharing his wisdom when people needed advice.

One studio doubled as a passageway because of its location between the front and the middle of the building. It was chosen as the studio space of an artist who lived on the streets. He was comfortable to work on the floor surrounded by his lunch, drying paintings, water pots, tubes of paint and other useful equipment he'd scavenged on his journey in.

There was at times rivalry between artists over space. A resident artist who in his home country had built his own rural studio seized the opportunity to have a large studio once again. He chose the biggest space in the building, and was well able to fill it. Prior to having this space his paintings were crammed three to four layers deep in every room of the small flat that he shared with his family. It seemed that the studio space offered him the hope of regaining his lost status as a recognised and respected professional artist in his home country. The perceived atmosphere of grandiosity around him seemed to amplify feelings of inferiority in others and at times he was the object of much envy. This dynamic threatened to destroy the whole project. Fortunately there was enough trust and familiarity amongst us to come together to discuss and transform this potentially damaging and volatile situation towards a more integrated solution.

Our different tolerances for mess and wastage was a recurring theme. There was a regular need to sensitively negotiate limits around food when 'food to share' threatened to overtake the whole communal space. Food alienated one particular member who felt that as a group we were colluding with her being force-fed generosity, when she did not feel generous to the person bringing the food. Not knowing whether to eat it, she was left burdened with feelings of guilt. The dynamics of ordinary encounters between us amplified confusion about what as individuals we were or were not responsible for.

Inhabiting Life Creatively

There were benefits and value to combining skills, and we were fortunate enough to find local artists who were willing to contribute their expertise in exchange for the studio space we could offer. Roles included resident artist caretakers, key holders, project supervisors and workshop facilitators.

After submitting a successful bid to Arts Council England we were able to offer a series of workshops under the title 'Inhabiting Life Creatively'. Resident artists and members co-facilitated a series of five six-week workshops in their chosen medium. This included portrait drawing, animation, collage, clay sculptures and film. We advertised the workshops widely and they were well attended. Through this project we developed links with the Early Intervention Service, forensic services and other voluntary groups.

Roles were clearly defined, but there was flexibility as to which role someone took up at any one time so that an individual could be in a position of leading or supervising a project whilst being a participant in another. Workshops were supervised by an art therapist who offered a space to explore the issues that came up for the facilitators. Member co-facilitators were able to learn about workshop planning and teaching from the artists, which supported them setting up their own satellite groups. In turn they advised the artists about the possible sensitivities and difficulties faced by the people attending workshops.

Individuals volunteered to set up the studio, make lunch and welcome visitors, and between us we were able to manage the project. This project in particular showed us what we could achieve working together. Importantly we saw how others benefited from what we offered through the workshops and through the conversations that took place.

Warehouse Opening

A man knows he has no power when he cannot inhabit the walls he lives in.

Marco, a studio member

Anyone who has organised an exhibition will have some idea of the task involved and we exhibited twice yearly over the period of ten years. There was a strong sense of solidarity amongst us when organising an exhibition, showing the public and at times funders our work. They were also occasions when we invited friends and family who helped to organise private views and film the occasions.

To celebrate the arts warehouse we organised an open day, transforming the whole warehouse into a gallery. One artist used the corridor behind the main warehouse space to exhibit her three-dimensional work in the form of an installation that the viewer walked through. This narrow corridor set the scene and formed a dramatic spatial backdrop for showing her artwork, which hung from the ceiling and walls of the corridor, adding dramatic expression to her work.

A darkened space easily lent itself to being transformed into a small cinema where we showed short films and slides. We were able to use an ex-boiler room, where the artist covered the walls with creepy illustrations of faces and gothic-styled comic script narratives. Visitors were handed a lantern when entering to illuminate this cavern-like space.

In the airy high-ceilinged main body of the warehouse hung large-scale (3.6m by 4m; 12ft by 14ft) colourful canvases. Many viewers commented on how this gave the space a cathedral-like elegance, the large colourful canvases giving an impression of stained glass windows. Below this space was another unusual exhibit by a different artist of a vintage car covered in rust and yellow lichen.

Going Green

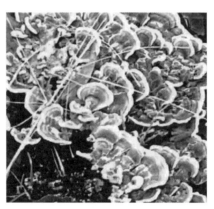

A garden is the purest of human pleasures. It is the greatest refreshment to the spirits of man [or woman], without which buildings and palaces are but gross handiworks.

Bacon 1928, pp.529–531

I understood more from tending gardens about my life than from the years I spent in psychiatric systems.

James, a studio member

We were invited by one of our members to share his allotment as he was struggling to maintain it. This outside space offered us new possibilities and we were able to create a neighbourhood gardening role and horticultural supervision after a successful funding bid. This led to a partnership arrangement with a local supported housing charity which saw two of our members design a six-month project with residents of a hostel to create an attractive outside space. Another member designed a programme of 'therapeutic walks', researching the history of the sites we visited. Both the gardening and walks provided inspiration for paintings made at the studio. In these ways we worked together to deepen our observational skills and enhance our understanding and connection to the local environment. Walking and gardening offered both a space for contemplation, dropping in and out of conversation, and working with the land. It was a very different experience from gatherings in the art studio.

Borrowing a metaphor from the realm of ecology and organic gardening, what we observed in the art studio and gardening was that the more complex the systems, the more stable and resilient they are. This could be said of both organic gardening and social systems like a community group, where the complexities of reciprocal relationships and the finely tuned sense of balance enable them to be sustainable. In both these contexts, oversimplification damages resilience, creativity and sustainability.

Afterthoughts

So we need a space for thought and reflection and this to me is what therapy is about [...] a space that stands apart from the rush, the now, the results, evidence based culture – a space where people may...let their mountains be mountains and not pretend they are molehills.

Gordon 2011

In *Where in the Waste Is the Wisdom?* Paul Gordon (2011) considers the ethical space of therapy to stand for the place of freethinking and conversation; a space protected from the results, evidence-based culture or adherence to theoretical dogma. He speaks of the space for people to come 'to their own positions through their own reflection and most important in conversation'.

The warehouse experience showed us that, for people who struggle to find a creative space in their lives, coming together in an ordinary way allows a cross-fertilisation of experience and ideas that can both house differences and extend creative therapeutic provision. Despite operating on a meagre budget and managing feelings of dissonance between us, benefits flowed from having a space to give attention to each other and what went on between us. There are possibilities that emerge through the work in the studio and open-ended therapy. With the loss of these spaces in statutory services, private practice could offer more and new possibilities to develop and extend this work through experimental communities outside the psychiatric institution.

In times of financial hardship, giving can seem philanthropic or an option available only to the privileged. Lewis Hyde's 1992 book *The Gift* asks us to consider the commerce of art as a 'gift exchange'. To quote from *The Gift*, 'the spirit of market forces destroys the gift' (2007 [1992], p.158). Hyde asserts that art must reach beyond its point of origin in order to form ties between people and groups, for 'it is when a part of the self is given away that community appears' (p.94). Alongside sharing creative practice there were many gift exchanges between us, the gift of being there, sharing diverse life experiences, and through them finding our own voice and stories. There was also the creation of good memories: celebrating occasions together.

The value of the work can best be judged by the testimonies and long-term involvement and commitment of our membership. The sense of comradeship and self-awareness gained from what we created together was a framework able to withstand any ongoing tensions arising from our individual sensitivities and differences. We feel it is fitting to leave the last word to our most senior member:

> After leaving Iran I found myself in a place of despair, but hospital for me was 100 percent worse than the Iranian prison. Someone with my history cannot tolerate a hierarchical or oppressive system. I had already escaped that and what I needed was compassion and friendship, an opportunity to give and receive. (Quoted in Heath 2014)

References

Alliance for Counselling and Psychotherapy (2016) *Jobcentre Therapy: MWF Exchange Letters with the Big Psy-Organisations*. Accessed on 18 May 2017 at https://allianceblogs.wordpress.com/tag/jobcentre-therapy.

Atkinson, P. (2014) *The Sorry State of NHS Provision of Psychological Therapy*. The Free Psychotherapy Network. Accessed on 17 May 2017 at https://freepsychotherapynetwork.com/2014/03/09/the-sorry-story-of-state-provision-of-psychological-therapy.

Bacon, F. (1928) 'Of Gardens.' *Elizabethan Verse and Prose* (ed. George Reuben Potter). New York: H. Holt and Company.

Beresford, P. (2016) 'What service users want to change in mental health policy.' *The Guardian Social Care Network*, 9 June. Accessed on 1 July 2017 at www.theguardian.com/social-care-network/2016/jun/09/what-service-users-change-mental-health-policy.

Berger, J. (2006) *Here Is Where We Meet*. Accessed on 17 May 2017 at www.johnberger.org/home.htm.

Blake, W. (2004 [1797]) 'The Four Zoas.' In *The Complete Works* (p.319). London: Penguin Books Ltd.

Bucalo, G. (2014) *Mental Illness Does Not Exist. Antipsychiatry: Basic Operating Instructions* (trans. Emilio Florio and Laura Mazzatenta). Charleston, SC: Createspace.

Friedli, L. and Stearn, R. (2016) 'Positive affect as coercive strategy: Conditionality, activation and the role of psychology in UK government workfare programmes.' *Medical Humanities 41*, 1, 40–47.

Gadsby, J. (2015) *Mad Old Vic – Issue 1*. Mental Health Resistance Network. Accessed on 17 May 2017 at http://mentalhealthresistance.org/2016/05/03/mad-old-vic-issue-1.

Gordon, P. (2011) *Where in the Waste Is the Wisdom?* Philadelphia Association Occasional Papers. Accessed on 17 May 2017 at http://media.wix.com/ugd/dab2b7_a0862ed3fa8f477780a7d7c5f1ed154e.pdf.

Healy, D. (2003) 'Lines of evidence on the risks of suicide with selective serotonin reuptake inhibitors.' *Psychotherapy and Psychosomatics 72*, 71–79.

Heath, A. (2014) 'Sage community arts.' *Asylum 21*, 1. Accessed on 18 May 2017 at www.asylumonline.net/portfolio/21-1-spring-2014.

Hyde, L. (2007 [1992]) *The Gift*. Edinburgh: Canongate Books.

Kierkegaard, S. (1989 [1849]) *The Sickness Unto Death* (trans. Alastair Hannay). Harmondsworth: Penguin.

Laing, R.D. (1964) *The Divided Self*. Harmondsworth: Penguin Psychology.

Laing, R.D. (1967) *The Politics of Experience and The Bird of Paradise*. Harmondsworth: Penguin.

Leader, D. (2008) 'A quick fix for the soul.' *The Guardian*, 9 September. Accessed on 18 May 2017 at www.theguardian.com/science/2008/sep/09/psychology.humanbehaviour.

McKenna, D. (2016) *Welfare Reforms and Mental Health*. Accessed on 18 May 2017 at https://recoveryinthebin.org/2016/03/10/welfare-reforms-and-mental-health-resisting-sanctions-assessments-and-psychological-coercion-by-denise-mckenna-mental-health-resistance-network-mhrn.

Moncrieff, J. (2003) 'A comparison of antidepressant trials using active and inert placebos.' *International Journal of Medicine 12*, 117–127.

Recovery in the Bin (2016) *Mental Illness and UnRecovery*. Accessed on 18 May 2017 at https://recoveryinthebin.org/2016/03/05/mental-illness-and-unrecovery.

Russell, M. (2012) 'Mental health services will be lost in relocation.' *Ealing Gazette*, 16 March.

Samuels, A. (2012) 'Cut-price therapy and the trauma underlying mental ill health.' *The Guardian*, 7 November. Accessed on 18 May 2017 at www.theguardian.com/society/2012/nov/07/cut-price-therapy-mental-ill-health.

Scott, B. (2016) *The Cultural Hegemony of 'Mental Health'*. Bella Caledonia. Accessed on 18 May 2017 at http://bellacaledonia.org.uk/2016/09/22/the-cultural-hegemony-of-mental-health.

Watts, J. (2015) *Welfare Reforms and Mental Health – Resisting Sanctions, Assessments and Psychological Coercion. Conference Report – Part Three*. Alliance for Counselling and Psychotherapy. Accessed on 18 May 2017 at https://allianceblogs.wordpress.com/category/jay-watts.

4

FAITH, CULTURE AND DIVERSITY IN A LONDON PRIVATE PRACTICE

—— HEPHZIBAH KAPLAN ——

Art therapy has always been a socially conscious practice. We aim to work sensitively with anyone who may be facing difficulties and hardships. At first glance private practice art therapy may seem at odds with this approach in that clients need to be able to pay for it themselves and this may exclude many for whom private health care is simply unaffordable. However, since starting private practice in 1998 I have been privileged to encounter people from many faiths, cultures and socio-economic groups disproving the view that private practitioners only work with an exclusive segment of society.

While most clients in private practice tend to self-fund, there are also clients whose art therapy is paid for by their employer, education or health service. Thus I have met clients from all sectors of society, from all races and religions, from different countries and contexts. I have also run art therapy workshops in the varied cultural environments of Germany, Greece, Israel, India, Japan and South Africa, each place offering new insights into cultural diversity, cultural uniformity and differing socio-political circumstances.

In our diverse society in the UK where we strive to be non-racist, non-sexist, non-homophobic and more, there can be a tendency to homogenise all people in order not to articulate any differences between cultures. Paradoxically there have also been movements against cultural appropriation and for cultural exclusivity. Yet in the course of therapy we usually focus on the internal world of feelings and processes which tend to operate in similar ways with whomever we work.

Despite the inner world of these conscious and unconscious processes, there are also subjective experiences of different cultures, as well as the observable differences between people, often maintained by different cultural mores, beliefs and attitudes. This suggests that we cannot allow ourselves to be caught up in what Cross *et al.* (1989, in Van Servellen 2009) called 'cultural blindness', where practitioners embrace an ethnocentric view and assume that traditional treatment approaches are universally applicable. 'Advanced cultural competence' requires the therapist to value diversity, manage the dynamics of difference and acquire cultural knowledge.

The culture of the therapist too has bearing on the work, specifically its influence on the subtle transference and projective identification processes. Like many therapists I am a white middle-class heterosexual woman. I am also Jewish, have a very unusual name and a bit of a London–South African hybrid accent. From the outset new clients are intrigued by my name and curious about my background. I do not share anything about myself, though am often asked where I am from, in particular by non-English-born clients. This is often the first moment when I need to consider adapting my classical training in psychodynamic art therapy. Does the standard protocol of non-disclosure, the very culture of psychodynamic psychotherapy, offend clients from a different culture? If I am inscrutable in the service of developing the transference processes, can this be perceived as 'being English' – as suggested once by an overseas client – or perhaps rather cold and distant? Will it perhaps alienate a client and make it feel unsafe? When working with people from different cultures, perhaps additional bridges need to be crossed in order to develop a stable therapeutic alliance. In this chapter I will share some of my clinical experiences and challenges around the themes of faith, culture and diversity in private practice.

Much has been written about race, gender and class in therapy. In particular Carter and Qureshi (1995, cited in Doby-Copeland 2006) outlined

> the philosophical assumptions undergirding multicultural training programs into five categories: **Universal** – The Etic approach that assumes all people are basically the same as human beings. Universal constructs are used to affirm human similarities and therapists should transcend the construct of race. Special attention must be paid when using an Emic (culture specific) approach so as not to stereotype or to develop separate standards for particular populations. **Ubiquitous** – A liberal position that assumes any human difference can be considered cultural. People can belong to multiple cultures, which are

situationally determined. **Traditional** – An anthropological approach that assumes culture means country and is determined by birth, upbringing, and environment and is defined by common experience of socialization. **Race-Based** – An approach that assumes that the experience of belonging to a racial group transcends/supersedes all other experiences. **Pan-National** – This approach allows for the broad and global understanding of race as it relates to oppression, imperialism and colonialism throughout the world. (p.257)

While these are significant discourses in and of themselves and may be explored in many permutations, ultimately the therapeutic encounter is about the coming together of two people, one working to aid and support the other in their personal and creative journey.

Establishing the Framework

Most private practice clients have not previously been patients in the health services so they usually arrive for the first visit without the art therapist knowing much about them. Clients contact the therapist directly to book an initial session and they may let you know over the phone or email some information in regard to any cultural-specific issue. Equally there may be no clue at all as to what may emerge in the therapy. At this stage, although I always ask if the potential client has had any previous experiences of therapy, it is never certain if they even have an understanding of what art therapy is or entails. The first assessment session addresses these questions and will raise thoughts about any significant cultural hegemony.

The contractual format in private practice is that the client and therapist meet to discuss the possibility of working together. There is no hierarchical structure or potential splitting between other professionals in the organisation, so client and therapist develop a self-governing arrangement. The length and frequency of sessions, cancellation and illness protocol, holiday and work arrangements, as well as remuneration method, will be discussed and agreed between, usually, two adults alone. At the initial meeting we also discuss making and reviewing the art, as well as confidentiality, care and ownership of the artworks. The client asks the therapist to provide a service, and if the service is not helping, for whatever reason, the customer-client will terminate therapy. Establishing these protocols is an introduction to boundaries for some clients and sets up the container for the work.

A further consideration in private practice art therapy is how to pace the intervention. When a client is an art therapy trainee, this tends to be fairly straightforward. A two- or three-year training is the frame for the work, with some trainees opting to end therapy when the training is over. Other trainee-clients may want to extend the therapy either to address something that may have come up, or to hold them for a bit longer after the training is over. Yet most clients are not art therapy trainees and there are various unknowns as to how long the client will engage, how they will manage breaks, what happens when they 'break-down' or 'break-through' and what happens if they can no longer afford to continue ongoing work.

Each intervention seems to have a beginning, middle and end and this often follows a developmental continuum. Initially the client can be committed, enjoy the work and love the therapist. This is like the dependent stage of the infant. Then as the work progresses we hit the adolescent stage. The client will turn up late or abscond, with very good reasons of course, or may challenge the work and the therapist. The client may also drop out of therapy at this critical point. It is not that the therapy or therapist are above being challenged or criticised, it is what this may represent at the time. Can the client trust the therapist to endure and survive the criticism? Will the client prefer to abscond rather than articulate any symbolic or real grievance? Can the therapist take the new negative projections? Will the two of us be able to manage some difficult conversations and nudge the work into a more adult realm? When we do this right the client is taken into the third stage of therapy, into a place where maturity and mutual respect is fostered.

Being aware of the developmental stages of therapy may imply that therapists need to pace the work accordingly; however, the progression may not follow a developmental sequence. Sometimes a new client may present as mature, capable and reflective but then needs to regress. Hence we are usually working with the different personae or sub-personalities of adult, adolescent and child all at the same time.

I believe it necessary to hold the framework for the developmental continuum in whichever order it appears throughout the intervention. Although it is helpful when we know the approximate length of the intervention, this does not mean that we can direct the pace or the unfolding of the material. In holding the parallel narratives in our minds this can be an unconscious communication to the client that we are holding their different parts and will work to support them through this process.

Phases of Therapy

During the initial stage of the art therapy intervention the therapist concentrates on the symptomatic presentation of the client as well as what the client would like to explore in words and images, be it the depression, the trauma, the anxiety, the difficult relationships and so on. Clients come from diverse cultures, and in the initial recounting of their stories they may talk about the cultural context and sometimes spiritual beliefs or practice. I hear about the various cultural expectations and obligations as well as the joys and celebrations.

As the cycle of the year turns, there are traditional festivals, births, marriages and deaths – each with their own social codes and rituals. Some clients may experience a bereavement during the course of therapy, some clients get married and all sorts of family issues can surface during these significant life events. The scope of the therapy may include identifying core beliefs and values which the client has held or been influenced by and in particular when there is a significant life event to manage.

Religion and Faith

The Pew Research Center's Forum on Religion and Public Life (2012) states, 'There are 5.8 billion religiously affiliated adults and children around the globe, representing 84 percent of the 2010 world population of 6.9 billion.' This would suggest that most clients coming to art therapy will have some relationship with religion, be it about faith, active observance or rejection, offering very rich material where the persona may be formed, anti-authoritarianism established, sexuality determined, family culture forged, beliefs rooted and so much more. Religions offer stories, metaphors, symbols, traditions, ethics, laws and lifestyles; they also offer prohibitions and edicts; and they stimulate an ebb and flow of seekers, rejectionists and reconstructionists.

Some clients have let me know early on in the work that they actively observe a particular religion and that this adherence is unquestionably part of their core identity and culture. Some clients have found converting to a particular faith a supportive move. Other clients may be struggling with an existential crisis or seeking guidance from a 'higher authority' or moving away from religious obligations. There are also clients who have grown up with no allegiance to any religion and they may have quite strong feelings about this too.

On occasion I have worked with clients who have held unwavering religious beliefs or who have been stuck in unyielding relationships and situations which seem to be culturally or religiously bound to a set of rigid rules. This creates a conflict in that for many clients art therapy offers an opportunity to resolve past wounds, develop new resources and foster autonomy, and this may conflict with observing their faith.

An example is the female client whose husband kept asking her why she wore the hijab. She decided to put on the hijab aged 17 and some of her friends followed suit. When she married someone less observant than her, although also a Muslim, he was keen on questioning everything, challenging his wife for her lack of curiosity about why she made this decision. Whether this difficult issue was symptomatic of other relationship difficulties displaced onto the hijab question, or in itself was worth exploring, was discussed in depth. The young woman wanted to understand her general lack of curiosity. Was this about acceptance or submission or something split off in herself? If she really started to question she might have to make difficult changes and face potential losses.

If there is a pre-requisite to therapy it is to be curious about oneself; the art-making process, taking this client into the unknown, encouraged her innate curiosity to emerge, allowing for the development of symbolic thinking, understanding of metaphor and the co-existence of multiple narratives. Eventually the client was able to hold onto the symbolic meanings of her choices and appreciate that some conflicting positions may remain unresolved.

For nearly two years I worked with a client who, amongst his other explorations and issues, was contemplating becoming a Catholic priest. He had had a strong religious upbringing and this may have been an obvious path for him in furthering his spiritual development. Equally I thought it important to consider a potential life choice of abstinence. Did I have the right to discuss this spiritual journey with him? Was this about my 'protection' of his future, or identifying any unresolved issues, avoidance or denial? Had we sufficiently explored his difficult sexual history? What about his ambivalence about the potential loss of *not* becoming a father or family man? There were several parallel dialogues, and as we know, language that makes sense is usually sequential and linear. Yet the art-making allowed all the simultaneous narratives to be expressed at the same time, in juxtaposition to one another, within the same painting. In the artwork co-existing stories that contradict in language may offer resolution as representational dominance and preference emerge. One that belonged to a strong and evolving faith in that ordaining as a priest was a legitimate and natural path; the other was potentially born out of unresolved trauma and could bring about painful loss. For his own authentic journey the client needed to test the extent of his faith and, in parallel, perhaps this was also a test of my faith in him?

When faith becomes a theme in the process, at some point my own identity may be referred to. Some clients have wanted to know if I was Jewish – a combination of my name and my stereotypical 'Jewish looks' I imagine – and it would seem churlish, if not impolite to some cultures, not to nod in reply as it is clearly self-evident. At the same time I try to be acutely aware of the transference and counter-transference processes and to remain very still in the moment, curious about their courage or trepidation in asking me about my own culture or faith.

When reflecting on the family history of a client born in Germany, the client seemed tentative and shameful. The client was keen to let me know that she did not share the anti-Semitism of her birth family and that some of her best friends were Jews. There were a multitude of projections that needed to be untangled. What did I think of her? What did I think of her family? Would I shame or punish her? Who was the real victim? Did we have a shared second-generation experience? Was I meant to 'forgive' her? Could she forgive her family? I believe that in exploring all these themes together we allowed something to become resolved in her story. She may not have consciously chosen a Jewish therapist but perhaps unconsciously she needed to broach these subjects in a personal context where she hoped there would be unconditional positive regard. In the intimacy of private practice, the therapeutic relationship can become more than the container, it can develop into both the metaphor as well as the conduit for change.

Culture and Diversity

In the early days of developing my practice, I left an information flyer about the slow-open art therapy group on a noticeboard at the

Africa Cultural Centre in London. Someone contacted me and booked a one-to-one session. The client told me she had been 'transracially adopted', from a black birth family into a white family. We had a good first session but the client felt she wanted to work with a black therapist. It seemed that the therapist-mother she was seeking needed to resemble her own forgotten birth mother and I could not visually fit that description. Sometimes the client's therapeutic objectives, conscious and unconscious, conflict with the standard protocol about racial discrimination. In the counter-transference I felt the not-good-enough mother as the client spoke of her being the not-good-enough daughter who was given away.

Clients whose cultural and ancestral roots are African, Afro-Caribbean or Asian, whether they were born and brought up in the UK or not, may have a shared experience of colour prejudice and racism. In an attempt to be sensitive to these issues, therapists may avoid naming discrimination directly and at the same time may project assumed grievances and suffering onto the client. I have found that sooner or later experiences of racism are brought up by the client him/herself and it is always important to engage directly and with ease.

The inexperienced therapist may feel defensive, as if s/he has to protect or justify him/herself, as well as society, against the assumed or real projections of racism when the issue is far larger and systemic than the individual. Sometimes the therapist has to survive the phase of being the 'bad object' even though to be the 'racist', 'perpetrator', 'abandoner' and so on is deeply unpleasant. This can be explored in supervision to ascertain proportionality as well as any mirroring of personal narratives. As we know, therapists do not have to have had the same experiences as their clients to understand them but they do need to show authentic empathy in regard to these issues.

In the spirit of humanity, not omnipotence, we should be able to work with all cultures, religions and races regardless of our own ancestral and cultural heritage. A benefit of private practice is that clients can choose their own therapist and may choose to work with a therapist whose own culture, religion or race matches their own. Equally we need to be attentive not to conflate empathy with over-identification and even collusion.

What happens when the beliefs of therapists and clients are possibly in conflict? How does the therapist work with the spoken and unspoken prejudices in the clients? How are these dynamics expressed through the artwork and the therapeutic relationship? In private practice I have not shied away from addressing these issues, in some cases facing prejudice head on.

A lady from Saudi Arabia asked if she could see me while on a trip to the UK. She told me she was a health care professional and wanted several sessions of art therapy (nine sessions over a three-week visit) to enable her to be creative in a safe space. As she entered the art therapy studio she asked if there were any men in the building and then removed her hijab. Very quickly I heard a devastating story of abuse and betrayal. She disclosed the sexual abuse her daughter had endured from the father and decided she could no longer live with this 'vile man'. In order to divorce her husband, she explained she was culturally obligated to explain to *his* family the reasons for the separation.

Her young teenage daughter was furious with her mother, as exposing her was akin to a public shaming and would cast her as a tainted woman for life. According to Saudi and Moslem law, the husband kept custody of their children. He told her that if she re-married she would never see her children again. She eventually moved to another city, found a new partner and, despite the risk of possibly never seeing her children again, decided that her own happiness was equally important – and so she agreed to become a second wife to her new man. She explained to me that men can take up to four wives and each wife has her own status with various requirements and understandings.

The client's story was difficult to take in, being bound up in multiple cultural mores or perhaps regulations, as well as my own clinical concerns to assess the issues as well as limitations in this very short-term intervention. It would have been a further betrayal, if not rude, to let this nice lady know that her story was too complex to process within nine sessions; the themes of grief, loss, shock and anger were substantial enough. I explained her story needed a longer intervention to address all the issues and suggested that the art therapy sessions could offer a safe place to focus on her creative expression. We agreed that I would show her a way to use art-making as a resource for self-help and stress release, while bearing her painful story in mind. I also encouraged her to find ongoing psychological support in her home city and some for her daughter too. She engaged well with the creative process, and the art-making allowed her to express some of her sadness and rage at what had happened. My own equanimity was being tested. I was concerned about her daughter and their relationship and, furthermore, the idea of voluntarily becoming a second wife was antithetical to all those influential feminist writers of my youth.

When the cultural and religious variants seem to flood the clinical material it is supremely important to rise above any personal indignation, judgement or confusion and try to identify the main psychological themes that unite us as human beings. Identifying shared human experience is enriched via the art-making where both client and therapist hold the artwork together and honour its meaning.

Another story from my practice put me in a memorable difficult predicament. Salma had been attending weekly art therapy for about three years, paid for by her employer. She found it a useful place to be herself and not have to attend to the needs of the many people she looked after. She often came late, explaining that this or that person needed some food, flowers or a hospital visit, and told me the art therapy sessions were the only space she had to be herself. I supported her in recognising that her one hour per week was indeed the only place she gave to herself and encouraged her to ring-fence her own time more often.

Salma and her family had run from Iran in the 1980s and there was a lot of unresolved grief as well as ongoing concerns with serious family health issues. Salma described herself as Shia Moslem and prayed throughout the day. In sessions she often looked up to the skylight imploring God to look favourably upon her and answer her prayers. She was also scornful of fundamentalists and intolerant of the burka.

In the summer of 2013, two weeks before the long break, she announced she wanted to end therapy immediately. I suggested that the impending break was anxiety-provoking and, as she did not want to be abandoned by me, she decided to discard me first. We spent the session reflecting on why she would terminate so precipitously, and towards the end of the session she suddenly declared, 'I don't want to work with you because you are a *Jew*!' I remained silent. Then she asked, 'How do you feel about *that?*' I gathered my thoughts and, redirecting the focus, said that hearing words like that was not unfamiliar to me but wondered how *she* felt about holding that point of view? As she was a teacher and may encounter children from other cultures, perhaps she may want to think about some of her beliefs?

I was also acutely aware of the concomitant renewed warfare between Hamas in Gaza and Israel and wondered if Salma, or her family members, felt she was compromised by having a Jewish therapist? Of course Salma and I never spoke about politics but she often referred to me as her Jewish therapist whom she revered for just 'being Jewish'. In this intervention I was juggling multiple projections that went beyond faith, religion and culture, although my own culture was the named container for her antagonistic challenges.

We decided to have the summer break and reconvene in the autumn to discuss what had happened and to reassess our ongoing work. Privately I was reeling from the attack and needed a break to reflect on the work and its meanings.

We met in the autumn and Salma said she had thought more about it and decided she would like to address some of her prejudices. She then said, 'I did think about leaving and working with a Christian or Moslem therapist but they would only agree with me.' Again I was rather dumbfounded by her views and wondered if the role of the therapist in her mind was to be the adversary and perhaps in going with a Jewish therapist this was possibly an acting out with some deep-seated historical purpose.

When such entrenched material arises in the work, the private practitioner has to evaluate the pace, depth and direction of the therapy. I didn't want the work to end prematurely or for the wrong reasons and I felt we both needed time to complete the process – however, in private practice the client can leave at any point and there is little the therapist can do to insist on continued attendance. Tenuously, Salma agreed to continue our weekly sessions. The work needed resolution and we pushed through the pain barrier together. It has been a useful, if not mutually painful, story in the work and she is indeed far less prejudiced now than she used to be.

Art therapy in private practice is an ongoing evaluation and negotiation between the client and therapist where we both decide on what would be useful to work with and for how long. When new material arises, which may open an extra narrative chapter, there may be a temptation to keep the process work ongoing regardless, but we need to be ethical about the ultimate purpose of the work. It would be easy to push for continuation, to the therapist's financial benefit, and one needs to be super-vigilant around consistency regarding the agreed therapeutic work.

Fees

Professional fees are agreed at the outset and on occasion there may be a financial crisis where austerity is called for and the client asks if a fee reduction is possible. I am always prepared to discuss this and see what might work, preferring to keep ongoing weekly sessions for a shorter time frame rather than fortnightly for longer, for example.

As a general rule we are mindful not to touch our clients and to be very respectful when touching their artwork; however, there may be inadvertent or perhaps even deliberate touch with clients when they pay for their sessions. The fee may be left on the table or handed over in person in the form of cash or a cheque or, increasingly, online payments may be arranged. Whether it is from the back pocket of the jeans or the depths of the handbag, scrumpled notes or a scribbled cheque, it is transferred from one to the other. In that split second when the fee is being handed over, both client and therapist may be touching this same valuable piece of paper which bridges the connection and can represent a symbolic currency in the relationship in addition to its fiscal value.

People's affinity with money often gets played out in their relationships. Therapists may not even have considered their own relationship to money and may find that when starting out in private practice there can be an awkwardness in the fee exchange. Clearly this should be processed in supervision so that it can also be explored in the art therapy sessions.

From a cultural perspective I have not encountered any significant cultural variations in the fee exchange, although people will use money to assert power or manipulate the therapist and more. For example, one client asked for a discounted session fee at the initial session, then whipped out her cheque book from Coutts, a private bank, to pay the fee. This action signposted potential manipulation which did get played out on one occasion when the client said she wanted to pay for eight sessions in advance so that she wouldn't lose time at the end of the session writing her cheque. Knowing her story, I offered an interpretation that she wanted to write a big advance cheque as a way of punishing her husband who funded the work, signalling to him that she was very much in need – and perhaps she felt he could only recognise the scale of her need if she paid a lot of money for it.

Psychosis, Religion and Neuroscience

As a sole practitioner in private practice it is inadvisable to work with people who are psychotic or schizophrenic as they generally need a much greater level of therapeutic support. However, I want to briefly mention these clients, as some people suffering enduring mental health problems may well profess strong religious beliefs or have a relationship with God. There may be beliefs about being sacrificed, crucified or having specific messianic roles. There may be beliefs about salvation and redemption. In my previous work in adult mental health I have even been 'accused' that I, the Jewish therapist, killed Jesus Christ. Identification with the victim may take on a psychotic form, and in the artwork the client may depict themselves with stigmata, on a crucifix, with a halo, or a ring of thorns (see Figure 4.1). This is potentially very disturbing for the observant Christian therapist and may well be experienced as a severe 'attack' on the therapeutic container.

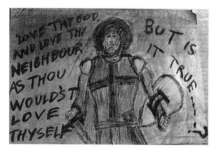

Figure 4.1

Psychotic thoughts, words and images can be full of religious iconography. The role of the art therapist is not to untangle what may be a belief attributed to an observance of a particular faith or religion from what may be a psychotic 'belief', but to focus on the nature of the distress the client brings to the session. Do these 'beliefs' bring respite or further agitation? How does following a faith or practice enhance one's life? Or perhaps in some clients it merely forges complexes, grievances and guilt?

Sigmund Freud considered believing in a single god to be a delusion, which is an extension of his comments of 1907 that religion is the indication of obsessional neurosis (Freud 2010 [1939]). However, he too was largely conflicted, having been a neurologist and scientist and then venturing towards beliefs in the unknown. In his fascinating book *The Hidden Freud*, Joseph H. Berke writes, 'But Freud, the scientist, also believed it was important to keep an open mind. ...he refused to dismiss events like telepathy just because they could not be rationally explained or understood. He thought it was important to respect the unknown' (Berke 2015, p.35).

In recent times there have been scientific attempts to explain religious experience and behaviour. Studies in neurotheology – using neuroscience to prove the existence of consciousness, universal consciousness, transcendence and even the God-gene – have suggested that practising some religious observance is beneficial to long-term cognitive functioning. Belief in 'the other' or a higher power seems to be processed in the pre-frontal cortex, and when this is damaged, the beliefs no longer exist.

What of the client who is a non-believer or even a secular fundamentalist? The philosopher and psychiatrist Dr Eric Ledermann writes that 'existential philosophers express the dilemma of the modern person who has lost his faith in God and who has to make his own laws of conduct' (1984, p.xiii), and suggests that the goal of psychotherapy is to make the unconscious conscience conscious. Ledermann suggests that all psychotherapy is essentially a quest for morality, to act according to one's conscience.

While I was working at the Arbours Crisis Centre (2005–2011) where the guests (resident patients) were often going through difficult psychotic episodes, the art therapist would paint during the group art therapy sessions as part of the therapeutic community approach. There were two facilitators and, at the time of this painting, two group members. One of the participants would, on occasion, attempt to split the therapists along sectarian lines. She would talk of being a second-generation Holocaust survivor and try to draw me into a special alliance against the other group member, as well as my secular co-facilitator.

Figure 4.2 shows something of my struggle to show how the group of four needed to work together to understand persecution, pain and humanity, above divisiveness and separation.

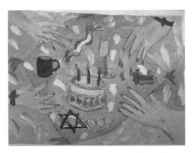

Figure 4.2 (See colour plate 2)

Some clients will even engage in quite fringe practices. I have had clients speak of visits to spirit mediums and trying to make contact with deceased family members. One spoke of her addiction to 'spiritual guidance online'. Clients often say something hopeful and quickly search for something made of wood to 'touch wood' – a symbolic gesture invested with hope, prayer and good luck. This happens with sufficient frequency that I've placed a wooden tree next to the tissue box as even the secularists can be superstitious at times! (See Figure 4.3.)

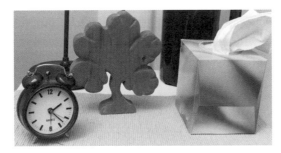

Figure 4.3 (See colour plate 3)

One does not have to be unwell in order to pursue what people over the millennia have done in an attempt to make sense of the world by finding answers outside of oneself, in an external framework or lodged with an external 'authority'. We should also not underestimate belief as an agent of change. Enough has been written about the power and influence of will, intention, conviction, visualisation and meditation to suggest that concentrated focus can and does support internal and external changes. We need to notice our own reactions to the various safety anchors people may develop and give them due respect as being part of the client's narrative, as opposed to pathologising them.

Towards the end of the intervention, some clients may bring the big existential questions in the form of some potentially new material to explore. Just like an impending death when faced with the unknown, questions of uncertainty, survival and after-life are raised consciously and unconsciously. It seems right to ponder on the big questions, though this may also be a way of fuelling the therapeutic relationship, rather than ending it. I encourage the clients to explore the themes further and independently so that this material may become a transitional bridge to life-after-therapy.

While finding a way to be culturally sensitive within the art therapy culture, there can be cultural differences that go directly against the training. Overseas clients often want to bring gifts at the end of the process. It can be impolite, if not damaging, to refuse. I usually nod in appreciation and explain that therapists don't normally take gifts but I would put the flowers in a vase or the chocolates in a bowl for everyone at the group practice to share and enjoy. These awkward but human moments always feel compromising to the traditional dynamics in therapy, though I think that preserving the good of the therapeutic relationship overrides this occasional discomfiture.

I could not complete a brief chapter on faith, culture and diversity in art therapy without mentioning the artwork. I have never seen any artwork that was exclusive to a particular culture. Just as our internal worlds work in similar ways, so the artwork coming from the inside place is universally consistent. Authentic human expression in art is alike across different cultures and faiths, although different cultures will have varying relationships and rules about religious iconography.

All the experiences of conflicting cultural challenges that arose in my practice have left me in awe of the connectedness of people, while at the same time acutely aware of the diverse range of faiths and cultures. This has necessitated being receptive to seeing and hearing unusual situations and responding with equanimity and authenticity. The symbolic and real pursuits in spiritual development are often brought to art therapy as art therapy honours the symbolic, as well as the unknown, and the art therapist may have to support the client in finding his or her authentic self in the process.

Ultimately we remember the stories of people's lives and their hopes and struggles to make sense of the world; we remember how the art therapy process opens something up and encourages the clients to continue a life-long creative journey, with, it is hoped, an increased sense of purpose, as well as understanding. If therapists can be more at ease in articulating difference it will lead to an increase in understanding of personal process work. When we are open to the questions, it opens it up for the clients, helping them connect to their inner resources and perhaps with renewed thoughtfulness and insight about their true conscience.

References

Berke, J.H. (2015) *The Hidden Freud: His Hassidic Roots.* London: Karnac Books Ltd.

Doby-Copeland, C. (2006) 'Cultural diversity curriculum design: An art therapist's perspective.' *Journal of the American Art Therapy Association 23*, 4, 172–180.

Freud, S. (2010 [1939]) *Moses and Monotheism.* Eastford, CT: Martino Fine Books.

Ledermann, E.K. (1984) *Mental Health and Human Conscience.* Farnham: Ashgate.

Pew Research Center (2012) 'The global religious landscape.' Accessed on 19 May 2017 at www.pewforum.org/2012/12/18/global-religious-landscape-exec.

Van Servellen, G. (2009) *Communication Skills for the Health Care Professional: Concepts, Practice and Evidence.* Burlington, MA: Jones and Bartlett Publishers.

Part II

WORKING WITH CHILDREN, FAMILIES AND THE CHILD IN THE ADULT

5

'MY PARENTS SAY THAT EVERY MINUTE HERE COSTS MONEY!'

Working with Children and Adolescents in Private Practice

—— NILI SIGAL ——

This chapter is based on my experiences of working with children, parents, the wider family unit and the professional team around the child, with clinical examples from my own work and the work of colleagues. Additionally, I interviewed the mother of a child I saw in private practice for four years. I have been very fortunate to offer sessions in a bespoke art therapy environment, where mess-making and containment could be achieved and where the setting supported and facilitated the clinical work.

This chapter offers only a small window into a topic which is so broad and complex it could easily expand into an entire book; therefore many areas will remain unexplored, while others will be considered only briefly. The writing is divided into four parts, which are: assessment and boundaries; therapeutic contract and ethical considerations; the parallel relationships, different ways of working and evaluating the work; and a brief case study including a parent's perspective. I hope to illustrate that private art therapy with children is far more likely to be successful if therapists communicate with parents about the work and try to ensure that the work is supported at home. The parents, who pay for the intervention and often bring the child to the sessions, are the private therapist's customers – but they are not the client. They may feel desperate and vulnerable by the time they bring their child to see a professional and are (in most cases) keen to help their child engage with the support on offer. Yet their own unconscious difficulties around attachment, anxiety or envy, and their ambivalence or shame about asking for help, have the potential to sabotage the work if not sensitively handled. The relationship with the parents needs to be conducted with empathy and thoughtfulness, in ways that differ from working with children in the educational or voluntary sectors.

General Considerations

For ease of writing I use 'parent' when referring to the 'primary caregiver' involved in supporting the intervention. This could be an adoptive parent, a relative or a family friend. Yet in most scenarios it will be parents who bring the child to private art therapy sessions and who pay for the intervention.

There are some clear differences between working with children and with adolescents, both in terms of the work itself and the level of parental involvement that is appropriate. Adolescents are more autonomous and have some legal rights to make decisions regarding their health and wellbeing (see Unicef's United Nations Convention on the Rights of the Child (1990) and NSPCC (2017) on the legal rights of the child in the UK). Adolescents may also attend sessions and communicate with the therapist independently. However, the issues around the 'commissioning' of the work in private practice and the need for a systemic focus still apply.

The examples and suggestions in this chapter do not refer to cases where the family environment is unsafe, where there are safeguarding issues or if the child must be removed from the family home. It is also beyond the scope of this chapter to explore the vitally important area of safeguarding children. I would strongly encourage practitioners who work privately with children to have safeguarding training and to ensure they know who to contact if they become concerned about the wellbeing of a child or if a disclosure has been made.

It is important to ensure there are robust support systems in place if working privately with children who have been removed from their family environments, to liaise with designated social workers and to have direct contact with reliable adults who can ensure the child is supported at home. It is also crucial to ensure that the child can attend sessions regularly and consistently, in order to avoid a re-enactment of traumatic experiences which can happen if the work ends abruptly.

Children who attend private art therapy might (but certainly do not always) belong to a middle-class demographic and typically suffer from less economic deprivation than some clients in the statutory or education sector. It is important that the therapist is aware of his/her own potential prejudices around class and monetary issues, so that clients are not seen as being less 'in need' or deserving of less help than those who cannot afford to pay for therapy. There can be stigma or reluctance for some art therapists to work with the so-called 'worried well', so it is necessary to reflect on such issues to ensure this does not affect the therapist's attitude towards the family and child.

Groundwork – Assessment, Space and Boundaries: Father in the Waiting Room, Sister Wants to Come in, and Who Owns the Artwork Anyway?

Assessing children for private work is a complex process. When a child starts attending therapy there might be multiple people involved including parents, siblings, grandparents and other agencies. Assessment is crucial in establishing the direction of the therapy and unearthing any gaps between the wishes and needs of the referrer, the parents and the client. The therapist must consider in advance whether to meet with the parents before meeting the child, whether to meet the child together with the parents, and what to do if the child insists on having a parent in the room when therapy commences. In her book on counselling children in private practice, Kirkbride (2016) writes about the importance of assessment and notes that 'developmental stages will influence the form that therapy takes and this is of particular importance at assessment' (p.5). She expands on this throughout the book, which is a useful manual for private practitioners. *Art Therapy with Children: From Infancy to Adolescence* (Case and Dalley 2008) also highlights the different developmental stages and their therapeutic considerations. However, the concept of a 'normal' or 'neurotypical' trajectory of development can be contentious: Timimi (Timimi and Leo 2009; Timimi, Gardner and McCabe 2010), a consultant child and adolescent psychiatrist, has questioned the concept and diagnosis of autistic spectrum disorder (ASD) and attention deficit hyperactivity disorder (ADHD), while Saul (2014), a behavioural neurologist, has called into question the existence of ADHD. Each therapist should therefore ensure they are informed about current debates around diagnosis and are led by their understanding of the child's needs.

Private art therapists may see clients in the therapist's home, a generic counselling room or in a bespoke art therapy environment, which is where I worked with the majority of my clients. Parents or carers often need to be provided with a parallel space to the client – physically, psychologically and symbolically. For example, Welsby (1998) writes about the groundwork she put in place when she started working with an adolescent girl who had a fused relationship with her mother, as the therapist was aware the mother could become envious of the work or find it threatening. Case (1998) wrote the following about parents:

> Therapy arouses anxieties: two common ones are a sense of failure as parents on seeking therapy, and ambivalence because the parents are unconsciously using the child's difficulties to disguise their own troubled relationship. Both of these situations can lead to the therapy being sabotaged. (p.27)

Parents might be in the waiting room for the duration of the intervention, or have siblings in tow. Some clients express themselves loudly and parents or siblings may hear aspects of the session, or they might try to find reasons to enter the room. Envy or jealousy can be powerful unconscious motivators, as other family members might resent the child for receiving 'special treatment' and wish to have access to their own support. As Segal (1988 [1973]) writes about Klein's conceptualisation of envy, 'Envy aims at being as good as the object, but, when this is felt as impossible, it aims at spoiling the goodness of the object, to remove the source of envious feelings. It is this spoiling aspect of envy that is so destructive' (p.40). The gaze of the parents, and the child's fantasy of what parents or others might think about their images, can be a powerful part of the transference. Parents might see which materials were used when collecting clients by looking at hands or clothes; I ask them to be sensitive and to discuss this with the child only if the child chooses to bring it up.

I have found that negotiating boundaries with families can provide useful insight into family dynamics, which might not be possible to access in other settings. In one case, I was working with a child who wanted her younger sister to attend the session with her. This led us to explore her relationship with her sister and the way she feels protective and responsible for her, which made it difficult for the client to focus on her own needs. The proximity of the waiting room to the clinical space can also lead to other intrusions on the therapeutic space – for example, parents speaking loudly on the phone while the child is in the session, which provides some insight into the way the child's psychological space may or may not be considered in the home environment.

Part of the assessment process involves establishing risk and client safety, which can be a separate issue from safeguarding and might be present even in the most supportive family units. In the absence of the detailed background and context provided in institutional settings, the private art therapist should remain alert to any warning signs or indications that it might not be in the best interest of the child to undertake the work. In one case, a colleague was asked to work privately with a girl who had anorexia nervosa. The colleague, concerned that her condition seemed serious, asked about her body mass index (BMI) and discovered that her BMI was low enough to warrant hospital treatment in keeping with clinical guidelines. The therapist refused to work with the client until she engaged with medical treatment with appropriate health services, and made future work contingent on regular liaison with her parents, a psychiatrist and a dietician to ensure her safety. The family agreed to the conditions, and an assessment by a psychiatrist led to an immediate period of hospitalisation, after which the art therapist commenced private work with the client. Other warning signs can be parental ambivalence to commit to therapy, or, conversely, parental over-investment in the child attending therapy when the child does not seem to want the intervention. The child might then feel obliged to engage because s/he knows it is important for the parents, leading to the parents' needs being prioritised over the client's and making it difficult to establish a direct therapeutic relationship between client and therapist.

Once the private therapist establishes that art therapy can be offered safely and is appropriate for the client, other issues may involve payment, handling of money and over-involving the child in the financial side of the transaction. This can bring up either feelings of guilt about the costs involved, or feelings of entitlement and seeking to gain from the session in a material way. The client quoted in the title of this chapter was overly involved with family finances and especially the cost of therapy; he therefore felt he had to make dozens of images in a session to get 'value for money'. As a child who had many difficulties including physical health problems, it seemed he felt a need to justify his parents' investment in him becoming well or 'normal' – that he needed to be 'value for money' as a child. This gave me an indication of the way he was taking on responsibilities for the impact of his difficulties on the adults in his life, which caused him a great deal of anxiety. The parents were very supportive of the intervention and changed their behaviour after this was reflected to them, which was helpful for the child.

As the monetary side of private art therapy (and the private therapist's awareness of the cost of art materials, room rental and other expenses) is a factor in the work, it is useful to note any financial considerations which might impact clinical decision making. An interesting perspective on the financial transaction was provided by a mother of a previous client who was interviewed for this chapter (see the section '"Beware Rigidity": A Brief Case Study and a Parent's Feedback' below). She described meeting a psychotherapist who had worked with the family in the National Health Service (NHS) for a private consultation. He told her, 'I can't cope with giving you a bill when you're sitting here with me, I will send it in the post.' She pointed out, 'I'd have been fine if he gave me the bill because I actually wanted to pay him… I felt uncomfortable *not* paying!'

A major difference between private art therapy and working in the education sector is that, typically, there are no long breaks during school holidays. This provides the opportunity to offer more consistent sessions; however, it can also lead to tensions when negotiating with parents who assume there would be no therapy on school holidays or half-term, so it is important to communicate this clearly from the start. It can also bring up issues in the transference if the child does not wish to have therapy during school holidays, which offers an opportunity to explore the meaning of the sessions and the therapeutic relationship for the child.

Another dilemma can arise around the ownership of the artwork, as younger children often want to take their work home to show their parents. I have found that children are less reluctant to leave their artwork in the room when working in a school, since taking the work with them could lead to it being seen by peers and teachers. But in private art therapy they are often collected directly by parents, which makes it more complicated. In one case, a client refused to carry on with art therapy because I asked him to keep his artwork in the room, despite him saying he wanted to take it home. Unfortunately he had made up his mind to end therapy and only agreed to attend a final session to say goodbye and collect his work, which meant we could not resolve this issue in the therapeutic relationship. Looking back, he had been trying to tell me that he found this aspect of the therapy difficult and I should have been more willing to negotiate and work flexibly, rather than rigidly maintaining the boundary.

Getting Started – The Therapeutic Contract and Ethical Considerations: Diplomatic Negotiations, Missed Sessions, Liaison and Referrals

Once art therapy commences, certain issues can emerge, such as parents not bringing children to sessions on time or being late to collect them at the end of the session, late or missed payments, and parental anger or disapproval (sometimes directed towards the child) about personal issues arising in therapy or even about mess-making. In one case, I had a client who was often collected late from sessions, sometimes by cab; I did not address this issue directly with the family until, one day, I stood outside with him in the rain waiting for a car that failed to arrive for nearly 30 minutes. I remember sensing his disappointment and abandonment but being unable to help him to process his feelings, as we were outside the safe therapy space and he was due to leave at any moment. Consequently I now tackle such issues as early in the therapy as appropriate. Where possible, I use the relationship I established with parents during the assessment process to help me discuss the real reasons parents might 'forget' sessions, bring or collect the child late, or cancel at the last moment.

Another area of concern is 'splitting' – either between the parents about the therapy, or between the parents and therapist (for example, parents who denigrate the therapy in front of the child but do not discuss any concerns with the therapist directly). Segal (1988 [1973]) writes that, according to Klein, splitting is a defence mechanism which separates others 'into a good and bad object' (p.35) and is 'linked with increasing idealisation of the ideal object, in order to keep it apart from the persecutory object and make it impervious to harm' (p.27). In such cases, parents might consider others in the family unit, or the therapist who is challenging family dynamics, to be the 'bad object'. This helps them to maintain their own stance as the 'good object' and to defend themselves from the painful process of change. Finally, any indication of parents using therapy as a 'reward' for good behaviour or cancelling sessions as 'punishment' for bad behaviour is a major concern and can damage the therapeutic process.

Private art therapists often differ in their approaches towards working with a child if the therapy is not being fully supported by the parents, or if there is implicit or explicit sabotage of the therapeutic work. Some therapists advocate that the intervention can focus on helping the child 'survive' the family environment and focus on creative expression, confidence building or relationship skills; however, in this case, the goals of therapy might be different. This needs to be carefully considered before committing to the work and before the child develops an attachment to the therapist. In one case, I worked with a child who had suffered a traumatic experience which seemed to be the cause of many of his emotional difficulties. The parents were very ambivalent about their commitment to therapy – paying late, cancelling sessions at short notice, and initiating long breaks in the therapy despite the fact that the child wanted to attend regularly and formed a good attachment. The work entered a state of limbo; due to the parents' inconsistency I could not safely address the trauma with the client and help him to process it, as they might end the therapy with very little notice. Explaining this to the parents, and asking for some clarification, only led them to disengage further and eventually they ended the intervention. The client still had a positive and beneficial experience of art therapy as a space where he could express himself and be understood. However, had we started trauma-focused work, the abrupt ending could have been re-traumatising. I therefore proceed with caution and review the goals of the intervention if it is unclear whether parents are going to commit to the therapeutic contract, before opening up issues in therapy I might not be able to contain.

Multiagency work to ensure children's wellbeing is recommended in the government's Every Child Matters initiative (DfES 2003) and can help the practitioner to develop a more holistic picture of the client's difficulties. I usually ask for permission from parents to liaise with schools and other agencies working with the child. Refusal to do so from parents can have different meanings: for example, a colleague shared a case where parents declined to use a school's counselling provision when serious concerns were raised about their child's impulsive and aggressive behaviour, seeking a private therapist instead. They did not consent for the private art therapist to liaise with the school. After a few sessions it became apparent that they were mostly trying to 'tick the box' by doing as the school had asked, in the hope that the child would 'play with some colours' in art therapy, but did not in fact acknowledge or accept there was a problem. When the full extent of the child's difficulties was discussed with them they terminated therapy immediately. On the other hand, it is also important to remember that parents may have other reasons to be reluctant to allow the therapist to liaise with statutory services. These may include negative previous experiences, shame, cultural issues, mistrust of services, anxiety about other children or family members finding out about the intervention, feeling unsupported by the child's school or worry about the client's medical records.

Another area of difficulty involves situations where it is clinically advisable to recommend an assessment (for example, if the therapist suspects that the client might be on the autistic spectrum or has ADHD, or to exclude physical health conditions) and the art therapist needs to find ways to discuss this delicate issue with parents in a sensitive, gentle and compassionate way. I have found that some Child and Adolescent Mental Health Services (CAMHS) will consider referrals initiated by private or sessional art therapists if they are supported by the child's school, general practitioner (GP) or other agencies and I have had some beneficial collaborative working relationships with CAMHS. Establishing a network of other private practitioners for parents who prefer to have fully private care – be it psychiatrists, psychologists, occupational therapists or speech and language therapists – can also be an important resource, especially in more complex cases.

It is sometimes apparent that family units can be avoidant about acknowledging deeper areas of difficulty. If there is a sense that parents are seeking a private art therapist to collude with this, it is important that the therapist does not compromise his/her own integrity in an attempt to keep the client. In such cases, collusion with the family's avoidance or refusal to have the child assessed could do more harm than good. I have found good supervision to be vital when making such difficult ethical decisions.

The private art therapist is ultimately responsible for paperwork, liaison with external agencies, storage of confidential artwork and the production of reports about the work. I write reports about clients' progress when asked by parents or other agencies, end-of-therapy reports as standard when finishing the intervention, and annual reports when working with long-term clients. In my personal experience, I have found that these reports and other reports by private professionals are usually acknowledged and taken on board by statutory services. Kirkbride (2016) writes about the administrative and record-keeping aspect of the work, as well as referring on and working with other agencies in the UK, including CAMHS.

It is increasingly common for therapists to write reports in a collaborative style and address them 'to' the client (rather than being 'about' the client). However, my priority when writing about children is to help the adults involved develop a better understanding of the child's difficulties. I seek to explain the way these difficulties are communicated non-verbally, in order to encourage compassionate and holistic thinking about behaviours which can be difficult to manage or contain, and to offer a different perspective on the client's emotional expression. A well-considered and well-written report can impact on a child's life and improve aspects of their home or school environment. If a practitioner produces a collaborative report addressed to the client in a language accessible to children, it might therefore be useful to write an additional report which is accessible to 'grown-ups', for other service providers and the adults involved in his/her care.

During and After Therapy – Navigating the Parallel Relationship, the Tricky Subject of 'Parenting Advice', and Evaluating the Work

Working with parents or the family unit can be an important part of the intervention in private art therapy with children. CAMHS teams sometimes offer systemic therapies, sibling group work or work with parents, while some art therapists work with parents and children together in the sessions or offer dyadic therapy for mothers and children, but the situation seems to be different in the voluntary and education sectors. Karkou's (1999) findings from a UK nationwide survey of arts therapists working in education shows that none of the respondents working in schools mentioned parental involvement. Case and Dalley (2003 [1990]) suggest that most art therapists in the education sector do not work with parents due to the culture of schools, where children are mainly viewed as individuals. In most UK art therapy literature before the turn of the century, direct contact with parents is mentioned in only a few articles about working with children, although it is difficult to ascertain how common it is in practice. Some publications from the 1990s which mention the client's parents include Murphy (1998), who writes about groups for parents of sexually abused children, Welsby (1998), on working with a mother and other agencies in a collaborative way, and Reddick (1999), who described his work with a child who had a merged relationship with her mother and the way this was played out in the countertransference.

More recent art therapy literature on working with parents and caregivers includes Case's (2003) article on working with children in chaos, which describes a meeting with a mother whose own vulnerability and history of trauma was key to the therapist's understanding of the client's reality at home. In several chapters in Case and Dalley (2008), working with parents and caregivers is considered part of the therapeutic work, perhaps indicating that this is becoming increasingly common practice: O'Brien writes about parallel work with a child and a grandparent (see also O'Brien 2003), Welsby describes a meeting with her client's mother, Hall writes about her work with mothers and infants, Meyerowitz-Katz describes contracting and communicating with the parents of a private client with Asperger's syndrome, and Dalley writes about multi-family work with a client who has anorexia nervosa.

When a child starts art therapy, parents may feel anxious about the impact of their own behaviour, personal history or family dynamics on the child's wellbeing. The client's everyday reality is shaped and dictated by their home and school environments, and therapists should not work with the children as though they are 'miniature adults', able to effect change in their lives or to control their external circumstances. Children are dependent on their parents, whose support of the therapeutic process (or lack of) can have a major impact on the outcome of the intervention. In a family system, the child can represent the family unit's dysfunction, especially if the child is the 'symptom bearer' and is showing the behaviour and the distress for the family unit or for unresolved difficulties which belong to the parents. In her book *Treating Troubled Children and Their Families*, Wachtel (2004) discusses a range of perspectives, including systemic approaches, for working with such complex dynamics. Systemic therapy can certainly provide a useful perspective on the child client's difficulties and experiences.

I usually meet with parents to discuss the client's progress at different stages in the therapy and tend to have such meetings without the child present. I always tell clients about these meetings in advance, explore their feelings and fantasies about them, ask clearly what they would like me to discuss with their parents and clarify what is going to be kept confidential. I aim to be transparent about the process and give feedback to the child afterwards. I charge for such consultations at the same rate as a standard session – although some therapists offer such meetings for free, as part of the therapy 'package', and factor this additional time into their rate. The potential advantage of this approach is that parents are more likely to engage with such meetings, which can be a crucial part of the work, if they do not incur extra costs for attending.

It is not uncommon for parents to seek concrete advice on ways to manage their own emotions in relation to the child's behaviour and levels of distress. While being placed in the 'expert' position is certainly seductive and plays to the therapist's own fantasy of omnipotence, I proceed with caution if asked for parenting advice. In contrast with clinical decisions such as recommending a specialist referral, I consider 'parenting advice' to be the provision of behavioural guidelines about interacting with the child, or a response to a parental query about ways to deal with a child's distress. For example, when working with a six-year-old client who tried to behave like the 'head of the family' and struggled to acknowledge any vulnerability, in an attempt to mask and over-compensate for areas of difficulties and gaps in his understanding, it emerged that in fact he wanted more time with his mother and found it difficult that he didn't have 'special' one-to-one time with her, without his younger brother present. With his permission, I raised this with both parents and suggested ten minutes of individual time daily with his mother, which would be unconditional (e.g. not to be cancelled or reduced as punishment). His mother was surprised to hear this, as she was under the impression that he was very independent and did not need her attention. She was pleased to hear that he wanted to spend time with her and was happy to accommodate his request. This was beneficial for the client, as it showed him that vulnerability does not have to be hidden and that sharing his emotions and anxieties can lead to his needs being met.

In such situations I see my role as being an advocate or 'interpreter' for the child, with his/her consent, while reflecting in supervision before giving such directive advice to parents. It is important to stay attuned to family dynamics and not to collude with the child or split between the child and parents, which can happen if the therapist's frustration about parental behaviour becomes in any way apparent in the sessions.

In their interactions with parents, therapists might feel compelled to answer when asked if they have children – which can place us as therapists in a tricky position; if we say no, parents may conclude that we have no understanding of their experience and become dismissive of the work. If we say yes, parents might fantasise about the therapist's children being perfectly behaved and feel envious and angry, or use this information to try to find out more about the therapist's parenting style. Personally I do not answer questions about myself and gently explain that we need to think together about their family and their child, and that any information about me would only muddy the water – although many therapists do talk about their own experiences of parenting, especially in the context of problem-solving, and have found it helpful in forming an alliance with parents.

Despite the inherent complexity of private work with children, there is also a great deal of freedom and creative potential in private practice. One therapist working from home found herself running sessions in the kitchen and cooking together with a client who would not engage in other ways, as a starting point towards establishing a therapeutic alliance. Another therapist had an adolescent client who would regularly arrive over 30 minutes late (if at all), swearing and 'acting out' in various ways, but the therapist was able to establish trust with the client as he was able to contain behaviours the school or other institution would not have allowed. During one of my sessions, a child client stormed out of the room in a rage, but I was able to contain and interact with him in the waiting area until he agreed to return to the room before the end of the session. This allowed us to begin to understand his anger and find ways we could think about it together.

Other creative ways of working I've experienced in private practice have included parallel treatments (where parents are offered a therapeutic or complementary treatment while the child is being seen) and dyadic work. Containing 'challenging' behaviour and risk in private settings is always an important area for clinicians and will be considered in more depth by Kate Rothwell in Chapter 9 and Colleen Steiner Westling in Chapter 10.

Despite the lack of constraints and institutional pressures to 'justify' private art therapy or to meet targets, private practitioners should constantly seek to evaluate and question the way we understand and undertake our work. I use outcome assessment tools where appropriate and have, at points, designed custom-made questionnaires and feedback forms to evaluate specific outcomes or to monitor progress against the reason/s for referral. For outcomes related to general functioning, standardised outcome questionnaires such as the Strengths and Difficulties Questionnaire (SDQ) can be appropriate. During private interventions, I regularly explore with clients their thoughts about therapy, have regular review sessions and request feedback from carers, parents or other agencies. I use the processes of transference and countertransference, and the processes that happen in the therapeutic relationship and during art-making, as tools to reflect on and understand the client's way of relating to him/herself and others. I also consider the client's capacity to use the art materials, the changes in his/her artwork over the course of the therapy and the styles of art-making as another way to gain an understanding of the client's internal world – especially, as is the nature of art therapy, into processes which are non-verbal in nature.

'Beware Rigidity': A Brief Case Study and a Parent's Feedback

When looking through art therapy literature I have found that the parent's perspective is often unrepresented, and so for this chapter I interviewed 'Linda', a mother of an autistic child I worked with for four years in private practice (all names have been changed to protect client confidentiality). Her son, 'Henry', had applied behavioural analysis (ABA) at home, alongside a range of other interventions. He had good verbal ability, speaking mostly in short sentences or to express his needs, and had access to a varied range of activities and social interactions at home and in the community. It was, however, felt that he could benefit from a creative outlet to express his feelings of frustration and anxiety. Henry gave verbal consent when I asked him if I could use some of his artwork in the book. Linda agreed to be interviewed for this chapter, sharing her perspective and experiences as a parent whose child had private art therapy.

I would like to describe my work with Henry and the different manifestations it took over the years, in order to illustrate the flexible and collaborative interventions which are possible in private practice.

Henry was 12 years old when we started working together and was engaging well with his ABA programme, despite having difficulties and frustrations which sometimes took the form of aggressive or repetitive behaviour. His ABA programme focused on improving his communication skills, reading comprehension and maths and help him with socialising, affect regulation, managing anxiety and learning everyday skills. He seemed emotionally vulnerable at the time; he would oscillate between being disconnected and in his own 'internal world' and engaging with intense interactions, which he seemed to crave but which he also found frightening. Henry had a difficult early life which left him highly anxious about any form of conflict (in addition to the anxiety that is often seen in children on the autistic spectrum). He was surrounded by loving and supportive family and a caring and skilled team, which meant that the therapeutic work was well supported. I met with Linda and the team regularly during my work with Henry.

I initially worked with Henry at home – something many art therapists would probably avoid, but which provided us with a good foundation of trust and familiarity. His early work was regressive and reminiscent of the work of very young children. He enjoyed mixing all the colours together, which would often result in a brown liquid substance which he would smear with his hands on the paper. The sessions had a similar structure each week and would last as long as he found the activity soothing or absorbing. Over time, he seemed to be increasingly in charge of the process and tolerated longer sessions without fearing the loss of control. Figure 5.1 is an example of this earlier work.

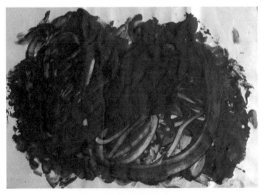

Figure 5.1 (See colour plate 4)

After about six months of working at home, I started seeing Henry at the London Art Therapy Centre. I felt that he would benefit from the move away from his home environment into a separate space as part of his emotional development, which might facilitate a separation from the family unit and help him feel more autonomous. As he was emotionally working from a raw, anxious and early place in his development, I chose a small room which had, alongside a wide range of art materials and art media, the opportunity to use a wet and dry sand tray and a large collection of objects and miniatures. Initially Henry seemed to find the freedom somewhat confusing and often constructed 'tunnels' from tarpaulin to hide in, as though being in a confined, interactive space with me was too difficult to manage. He had a strong emotional response to the 'Sad Story of Henry' from the children's TV show *Thomas the Tank Engine* and at times re-enacted it in the sessions; the narrative, of an engine who becomes stuck in a tunnel, abandoned and unable to get out, seemed to resonate with him and I felt it symbolised his internal experiences and his autism. I chose 'Henry' as the pseudonym for this client because it was a character he identified with so strongly.

Once he became more comfortable, Henry seemed to thrive in the room – alternating between art-making, working with water, using sand play and toys to create special environments, including 'rivers' with different animals he liked, and using stories and engaging in increasingly symbolic play. During this time, Linda was offered a parallel treatment and had reflexology in the room next door while he worked with me. This seemed to help both of them to manage a separation process which was becoming more poignant and difficult as Henry was growing up; Linda later reflected on the way it made it easier for her to 'let go', as she could overhear some of the sounds from the room and knew he was fine and contained. Henry became distressed occasionally in the sessions but was able to self-regulate, and we never had to ask Linda to enter the room. At the same time, it seemed to me that he found it reassuring to know she was not far away.

It was approximately after 18 months of working in the small room that I suggested to Henry we move to the bigger room at the centre. He seemed increasingly constricted in the small room as he grew taller and older, and I wondered if the larger space would help him to grow and 'expand' in his therapeutic process; he was increasingly moving away from play into painting and using bigger sheets of paper, which the larger room was more suitable for. Additionally, parallel treatment had come to an end and he was no longer being brought in exclusively by Linda. As his frustration and his separation anxiety lessened, it seemed appropriate to move into a room which was physically further away from the waiting area, where he would not be overheard. Henry agreed to the move and, despite some initial anxiety, adapted to the space quickly and used it fully. His artwork at that stage encompassed writing, drawing and painting, sometimes at the same time. In Figure 5.2 he used paint and wrote 'The Sad Story of Henry', which he talked about during the session – a theme which by that point had become less frequent in his artwork. I wanted to include this image as a way to depict his move from the regressive, smeary paintings he made at the start, followed by the non-symbolic construction of actual tunnels and 'rivers' during the next stage of the therapy, into being able to write and paint his ideas and feelings.

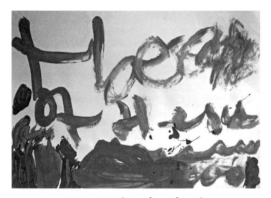

Figure 5.2 (See colour plate 5)

Over time, he started making more creative, colourful and emotionally expressive images (such as Figure 5.3), using vibrant colours and shapes and often including elements of water and motion which he would talk about. These were symbolic rather than concrete in their representation, using the 'as if' quality of paint to represent water. By this point in the therapy Henry would often verbalise what he was doing as he worked, sometimes naming the colours he was using, and had a clear idea of what the images meant to him. When asked at a later date about such painting he said, 'We're swimming in the sea, trees under the sea...' His images also increased in size. In a painting which he made several months before art therapy came to an end (Figure 5.4) he drew arches – perhaps again representing a tunnel, but using symbolic artistic depiction rather than writing or making physical tunnels. The image is more complex, involves different styles of mark-making and has a more carefully considered composition.

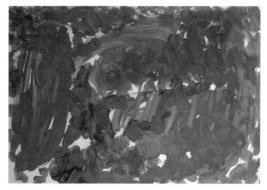

Figure 5.3 (See colour plate 6)

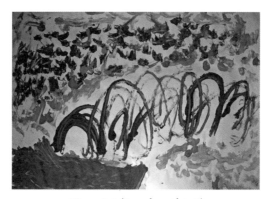

Figure 5.4 (See colour plate 7)

I hope that this brief case study demonstrates the potential therapeutic benefits of working independently and being able to adapt the practice – seeing the client at home, offering parallel treatments, using elements of play therapy, and changing the therapeutic spaces to match the developmental needs of the client.

In my interview with Linda about the work with Henry, she explained that she had found it difficult to find a private art therapist who was willing to work systemically and communicate with the team of practitioners working with Henry: 'It really horrified me – that people were all claiming that they had the truth... I just felt that his needs were multifaceted... If anyone had the answer we'd all be at the door.' After I worked with Henry for a couple of years, I devised with Linda a 'five-minute handover' at the start of each session, where she would inform me if anything had happened at home or if there was anything I needed to be aware of. Henry was present and, at times, involved in this conversation. We both agreed that this was very helpful. She said, 'The anxiety that a child with autism brings... It's so important to then identify to the therapist the things he might be thinking about.' She pointed out the potential advantage of keeping the parents in the loop: 'If there's something [being opened up in therapy] that is extremely delicate, the parents would like to know as well, you know, because there may be repercussions later, anxieties...' which parents can be prepared for and support the child with.

She felt that the therapeutic relationship was at the heart of the intervention and that Henry developed a 'secure' relationship and felt safe in the room. 'I think he was able to exhibit things that perhaps he didn't exhibit here because he had a different medium, and I think he did express a lot through his art... I think that the relationship strengthened the therapy, the efficacy of the therapy.' I asked Linda what advice she might give art therapists who would like to work with children in private practice: 'Beware rigidity. Within your discipline and your code of practice and ethics, try to move with the parents, try to be receptive to the parents, and to work with them rather than separately in isolation...to develop a relationship with the family as a whole, so you're not just reporting in, you're having a conversation.'

Conclusion

In this chapter I tried to demonstrate that working with children and adolescents in private practice can be a complex undertaking requiring systemic and dynamic thinking, clear boundaries, good liaison and communication skills and, at times, diplomatic negotiations and willingness to work in less than ideal circumstances. Yet the work can also be joyous, playful, rewarding and creative. Communicating clearly with parents and carers, other professionals or family members, sharing practices and explaining the process of art therapy can be key to engendering real change, by working collaboratively with the system around the child to support the therapeutic work in the room. Private art therapists should remain reflective and flexible in their practice, hold in mind the parallel relationship as well as the child's dependency on caregivers, and not treat the client as a 'miniature adult'. When working with children there is scope for a meaningful, positive change affecting not only the child but sometimes the entire family unit. It is always worth bearing in mind that, as Linda said at the end of our interview, 'No therapist is an island; no therapy is an island.'

References

Case, C. (1998) 'Brief encounters: Thinking about images in assessment.' *Inscape 3*, 1, 26–33.

Case, C. (2003) 'Authenticity and survival: Working with children in chaos.' *Inscape 8*, 1, 17–28.

Case, C. and Dalley, T. (eds) (2003 [1990]) *Working with Children in Art Therapy.* Hove: Brunner-Routledge.

Case, C. and Dalley, T. (eds) (2008) *Art Therapy with Children: From Infancy to Adolescence.* Hove: Routledge.

DfES (2003) *Every Child Matters.* London: Stationery Office. Accessed on 19 May 2017 at www.education.gov.uk/consultations/downloadableDocs/EveryChildMatters.pdf.

Karkou, V. (1999) 'Art therapy in education: Findings from a nationwide survey in arts therapies.' *Inscape 4*, 2, 62–70.

Kirkbride, R. (2016) *Counselling Children and Young People in Private Practice: A Practical Guide.* London: Karnac Books.

Murphy, J. (1998) 'Art therapy with sexually abused children and young people.' *Inscape 3*, 1, 10–16.

NSPCC (2017) *A Child's Legal Rights: Gillick Competency and Fraser Guidelines.* Accessed on 19 May 2017 at www.nspcc.org.uk/preventing-abuse/child-protection-system/legal-definition-child-rights-law/gillick-competency-fraser-guidelines.

O'Brien, F. (2003) 'Bella and the white water rapids.' *Inscape 8*, 1, 29–41.

Reddick, D. (1999) 'Baby-bear monster.' *Inscape 4*, 1, 20–28.

Saul, R. (2014) *ADHD Does Not Exist: The Truth About Attention Deficit and Hyperactivity Disorder.* New York: HarperWave.

Segal, H. (1988 [1973]) *Introduction to the Work of Melanie Klein.* London: Karnac Classics.

Timimi, S. and Leo, J. (2009) *Rethinking ADHD: From Brain to Culture. International Perspectives.* Basingstoke: Palgrave Macmillan.

Timimi, S., Gardner, N. and McCabe, B. (2010) *The Myth of Autism: Medicalising Men's and Boys' Social and Emotional Competence.* Basingstoke: Palgrave Macmillan.

Unicef (1990) *The United Nations Convention on the Rights of the Child.* London: Unicef. Accessed on 19 May 2017 at https://downloads.unicef.org.uk/wp-content/uploads/2010/05/UNCRC_united_nations_convention_on_the_rights_of_the_child.pdf?_ga=2.157921726.52158113.1495198657-652534151.1495198342.

Wachtel, E. (2004) *Treating Troubled Children and Their Families.* New York: The Guilford Press.

Welsby, C. (1998) 'A part of the whole: Art therapy in a girls' comprehensive school.' *Inscape 3*, 1, 33–40.

6

THE CONTRIBUTION OF INFANT OBSERVATION TO ART THERAPY IN PRIVATE PRACTICE

—— STEPHEN RADLEY ——

In the 1960s, infant observation was introduced as a requirement of psychoanalytic training. Its aim is to enrich the understanding of infancy, the parent–infant relationship and 'the infant in the older patient'. This academic component is largely absent in art therapy training; however, the experience could contribute to private practice. It offers art therapists a means to understand infantile projections, observational skills and to bear pain, uncertainty and confusion from the 'intense emotional impact' of being within a family with a baby (Bick 1964; Harris Williams 2011). The sessions are conducted once a week for one hour in a family home from the baby's first few weeks to his or her first or second birthday. Students learn to concentrate on the minute detail of the baby's appearance and movements. They record observations from memory for a small seminar group of other observers supervised by a senior child psychotherapist.

In this contribution, I would like to explore the aesthetic experience of infant observation and its applications to art therapy in private practice. Caroline Case (1996) writes eloquently about the 'aesthetic moment' of sacred beauty and awe shared between mother and baby. She observed moments of 'conversational love' in the interactions between the nursing couple. She compares these fleeting moments of wonder with those when client and art therapist share a sense of 'oneness'. On another level, Donald Meltzer (Meltzer and Harris Williams 1998) adopts the term 'apprehension of beauty' to indicate both the understanding and the anxiety of being in the presence of a beautiful object. Gregorio Kohon (2015) similarly conveys the ambiguity of the aesthetic experience, which oscillates between the strange and the familiar in the presence of the object.

In this chapter, I would like to explore the aesthetic experience in the caregiver–baby relationship and the 'infant in the adult' client in art therapy. I wish to invite the reader to explore my experience of infant observation, which has contributed significantly to the development of my private practice.

Infant Observation

I carried out observations for two years with a family in London. The mother, 'Anna', a university English lecturer, had been married to 'James', a psychologist, for six years. They were in their early thirties and had a three-year-old son, 'Will'. Anna was keen to have an observation for a new learning experience with her second baby, 'Charlie'. She found that she struggled with conflicting views from her family and friends on caring for Will. She felt anxious and confused, which resulted in a lack of production of breast milk for him. She wanted greater clarity and attunement with her newborn. Anna's early life had been traumatic after escaping with her family from a war. James came from a reportedly relatively stable middle-class English family. I wondered if she had selected James as a container for her anxieties. Anna decided to engage in observations in order to 'give something back to the UK' for the help in this country. She wanted to take two years off work to look after her children.

The observations began when Charlie was three weeks old in March. In retrospect, the first session provided themes that seemed to have recurred throughout the two-year period. It commenced as follows:

> I walked into their home and witnessed a peaceful scene of mother and baby on the couch. After congratulating Anna I sat down. She told me that she hoped to train Charlie to sleep more regular hours and in his own bed eventually. She said that she wanted to allow him to cry and settle himself. She added that she felt guilty and anxious when her sons cried but she knew that she was supposed to allow them to express these feelings. Occasionally I could hear Charlie breathing though he was still for most of the session. All the while he lay blissfully at her breast as she supported him under his bottom with her hand. I couldn't see his face, though at times I saw a fraction of his right side. From time to time she gazed at him calmly.

Anna told me that she felt more relaxed with her second child. She added that she had received conflicting information on how to care for Charlie. I asked her if she had a health visitor. She started to complain that the health visitor was uneducated, unskilled and simply provided by the NHS to 'tick boxes' for the government. She said that the health visitor came once and took an interest in one of the accessories for the baby. The lady asked if she could have the accessory and Anna gave it to her. She said the experience was very bizarre with a stranger coming in and taking something of theirs.

The observations begin with a beautiful scene reminiscent of Meltzer's description of the aesthetic moment between mother and infant:

> No flower or bird of gorgeous plumage imposes upon us the mystery of the aesthetic experience like the sight of a young mother with her baby at the breast. We enter such a nursery as we would a cathedral or the great forests of the Pacific coast, noiselessly bareheaded. (Meltzer and Harris Williams 1998, p.15)

At the same time, there appears to be a mystery beneath the surface: Anna is worried that Charlie will become dependent on her. She has carried him for nine months and might feel anxious that he will continue to weigh her down. She has received conflicting information from others and wants to think independently to care for her newborn. In spite of her worries, Charlie looked at peace at her breast.

Anna recounted an odd experience with a health visitor who seemed more interested in taking from her rather than giving caring support. I felt 'nudged' by Anna into colluding with her to exclude a figure who may exploit her. However, I was aware of the risk of collapse of the 'analytic frame' (Milner 1987) into something simpler. Marion Milner suggests that the frame is conceptualised as a boundary marking off external reality from the internal world. The frame is constructed by regular slots for sessions, protection from interruptions and intrusions and the consistency of the therapist's (or observer's) attitude (Ruszczynski 1993). I was aware that I needed to be resilient in order to maintain my observer role.

In the first few weeks, Anna appeared to attune to Charlie's needs. I watched her method of soothing him, which seemed to help manage their dread. The following example when he was four weeks old might illustrate this:

> Charlie was crying after having been startled by his brother. It felt like his cry was diffused panic or terror out into the world. Anna placed him on the changing table. She undressed Charlie and started cleaning him. He continued to wail. She spoke rapidly and moved her hands quickly to clean and dress him. She looked around for a change of clothes and alternated this with checking how clean he was. She seemed to be wiping vigorously while speaking rapidly. While she was putting fresh clothes on Charlie, she scratched his belly a few times, and other times held her palm on his belly as she moved around looking for clothes. When she settled her palm on to his stomach, his crying seemed to change from a diffused scream to a more focused cry. I wondered at that point if he was screaming at her rather than at the universe.

Initially Anna appeared startled and desperate to change him. The scene underwent a dramatic shift when she rested her palm on to his stomach. His screams transformed from terror to a focused cry for her. Case (1996) suggests that the aesthetic experience allows for transformation when fragmentation can be contained. Anna seems to tolerate Charlie's state of mind and feed back to him that she was there. He was comforted once returned to the safety of her loving embrace and breast.

In the first few months, I occasionally wondered if Anna's interest in Charlie bordered on a sense of intrusion for him. A couple of times, she brought her face a few centimetres from his face to look into his eyes while he was on his back. As she approached closely, he would stiffen his arms at his side and look up and away from her. It appeared he was recoiling from her gaze. In a similar fashion, Anna sometimes asked me questions about childcare. However, I was aware that I needed to invite her to return her attention to her baby and the mysteries within their relationship.

The love between Anna and Charlie seemed clear from the first few weeks. She gave him plenty of physical contact such as stroking his face as he fed. He appeared relaxed with her, resting his hand on her leg when together. While changing him she engaged him with songs and the animal mobiles above. She would nibble at his feet, conveying his deliciousness for both of them. I wondered if this had set up a kind of 'aesthetic reciprocity' for the mother and infant (Meltzer and Harris Williams 1998). The nursing couple reciprocated precious and beautiful moments with each other. Meltzer suggests this experience could commence before birth. He writes that 'proto-aesthetic experiences can well be imagined to have commenced in utero: "rocked in the cradle of the deep" of his mother's graceful walk; lulled by the music of her voice set against the syncopation of his own heartbeat and hers' (Meltzer and Harris Williams 1998, p.17).

Anna was very tactile with Charlie and did not seem to mind mess. She asked if I was fine with his evacuations of poo. This could have been a way of managing a potential persecutory aspect of the observation. By two months, she sought to invite me into Charlie's world. Charlie would smile at me, bounce and kick his legs like a frog. He started watching me watching him as I followed them around the house. I also observed that her relationship with Will appeared more distant. The older brother seemed to resent the new configuration. He often removed Charlie's toys or drew Anna's or my attention away from the baby.

Over the summer Anna took the boys back to her country. Returning from the break she was late, suggesting that she had forgotten the time, though added sweetly, 'Charlie misses you.' I wondered if the separation had indeed been difficult for her. During the break, she also stopped breastfeeding, which may have been painful for him. While he was teething, he sometimes looked at me suspiciously at the beginning of the observation as if I was an unwelcome intruder. Over the course of the hour I felt that he was 'piecing me together' and beginning to remember me.

From six to twelve months, Anna tried teaching Charlie motor skills by presenting toys just slightly out of his grasp. He appeared to contain his feelings in her absence. He chatted to himself while she was not visible to him. I wondered if he was learning to hold her in mind. With growing independence, Charlie started to stand and would crawl 'like a soldier', using his elbows to push himself across the floor. At 11 months, he took his first few steps. Interestingly, he began to watch Anna and me as a type of couple. A triangular relationship between Anna, Charlie and me seemed to emerge, which the following sequence at 11 months old might convey:

> While we were in Charlie's bedroom Anna placed his hands on a pushcart. He pushed it back and forth and she expressed delight. He seemed pleased and he looked at me watching him. She then returned to the kitchen. He lifted himself up by his bed rails, stood up and

moved over to an adjacent shelf. He then went under the shelf and found that he was in difficulty. He only had the sides of the crawl space to hold on to. After a couple of moments he let out a worried moan and found himself stuck under the shelf. His legs gave way and he collapsed on to the floor and cried. Anna came around and picked him up and kissed him on the forehead. She commiserated with him and took him out of the room to the hallway.

She held him up and he turned to me and smiled. Anna then faced him and Charlie attempted to grab at her glasses. She twisted her head away, telling him off. He then latched on to her hair. She grabbed on to his hands and managed to release his grip on her. She then lowered him to the floor to prepare for him to climb the stairs. She made sure that he didn't topple backwards by gently helping him up the steps. On the landing by the parents' bedroom, he held on to the baby gate and manoeuvred his way behind it. This led to what seemed like a game, which involved Charlie opening and closing the gate, allowing us in and keeping us out. I wondered if he was taking us in as a couple, looking from one to the other. He opened the gate and then closed it with a triumphant smile. It felt like we were all in this game together and the message was clear that Charlie was the master.

Charlie appeared to accept me as a benign observer, tracking my response while he walked proudly with the cart. He then felt possibly trapped in an enclosed space, from which his mother freed him. He seemed to counteract his fear by grabbing on to her hair and glasses. He then shut us out with the gate, possibly reversing what had happened to him. I wondered if he felt in charge of who could come and go into his world at that point.

When Charlie was a year old, Anna expressed a desire to return to work. I wondered how this was worked out between the couple. James was present in a handful of observations but often retreated to their bedroom to do work. Charlie seemed to pick up on the couple's anxiety. He would panic when Anna was out of sight. He started giving toys to me, a possible expression of his gratitude towards me for being there. In the face of uncertainty, however, he became a sturdy toddler. At 15 months old Anna felt reassured that she could 'leave him on his own' and called him 'an intrepid explorer'. The following vignette at 14 months could illustrate the love that Charlie may have introjected from her:

In their garden, Anna and I watched Charlie dig his hands into a potted plant. He moved his fingers around the pot to feel the earth's texture. He picked up the soil, squeezed and inspected it and returned it to the pot, sifting through the earth. He removed a pebble and presented it to me as a gift. He handed it to me and I thanked him and looked at it briefly and smiled. I returned the pebble to him and he continued to work with the soil, speaking to himself, saying 'Mamama'. He fished out a twig and a clump of roots and brought them over to Anna. She returned the roots to the pot and twig to him. He held on to it and grabbed the pebble again from the pot.

Anna offered a doll's pram to Charlie. He placed the twig and pebble on the seat. He reached for the chair's handles and pushed it towards the gate. The stick and pebble were like babies about to be taken out for a walk into the courtyard. As we followed him, Charlie occasionally struggled with the paving stones but persisted. He came to the steps that led to the car park below. He then launched the pram down the steps, causing the twig and stone to fly out. Anna groaned and picked Charlie up and retrieved the buggy. She told him that this area was dangerous. She pointed around the car park and he listened attentively. She started to return to the courtyard; however, Charlie turned his head around towards the stick and pebble on the ground. Anna picked up the objects that she had perhaps absent-mindedly left behind. She returned them to the pram, which he pushed towards the other corner of the courtyard.

Charlie appears to convey the special relationship with his mother through exploratory play. Meltzer and Harris Williams (1998) suggest that 'every baby "knows" from experience that his mother has an "inside world", a world where he has dwelled and from when he has been expelled or escaped, depending on his point of view' (p.21). When Charlie discovered babies (the pebble and twig) in his mother's belly (the soil), he seemed to show that he was a precious baby in his mummy's tummy. He had learned what it could mean to take care of a baby, and Anna seemed to be in touch with his fantasy. Tossing the objects into the abyss of the car park could have been an attempt to articulate the pitfalls of being a dependent baby. Watching Charlie search for babies in his mummy's tummy and take care of them was deeply moving for me. I suspect that, as the one being observed, he was becoming attuned to his feelings and desires.

From 16 months, Charlie started to use two objects together (two cars, trains, etc.) in his play. He would hold on to two cars, for example, and push them along the arm of the sofa. He would attach a couple of figures to a car seat. I wondered if he was attempting to hold on to the idea of a loving couple in his mind. Charlie played with a fantasy of a baby made from two united objects.

At 20 months, Anna decided to return to work full time and hired a nanny. She found a carer to work four days a week. In the session that she told me this, the following exchange took place:

> Anna was seated by Charlie on his bedroom floor and he went towards his Noah's Ark game. He lifted out a toy man and then covered him again with the lid of the boat. Anna said, 'Bye bye Daddy.' He lifted the man out again and placed him on the ship that was beside the ark. He returned to the ark and lifted out animal pairs and placed them on the floor. He discovered a lion and Anna said, 'What's that?', and he roared and she roared back. She then took the lid and said that the reverse side acts as stairs for the animals to climb on to the boat. She demonstrated a rhino climbing the stairs. He took the rhino and looked a bit perplexed and turned to me for a response. He then paraded the rhino around the deck of the ark and returned it to the animals' sleeping quarters below deck.
>
> Anna went on to tell me about her new job. She described having an argument with James about her return to work. As she said this, Charlie took a lion and a tiger and made them kiss. He pressed their lips together and smacked his lips. He smiled after he did this and made the big cats kiss once more.

Anna conveyed the idea of a couple splitting. I wondered if she either reversed the focus on her by saying 'Bye bye Daddy', or displayed my eventual departure. Charlie seemed to deny this reality by bringing the lion and tiger together. Rather than fighting with each other, as one would expect from these big cats, the opposites embraced. He showed a loving experience between mother and father, and participated in their union by being directly involved in their kiss. He appeared to recognise the three-dimensional space of a couple and baby. The Noah's Ark was a powerful message about couples rescued from the apocalypse.

The loss of his mother and replacement by a nanny appeared particularly difficult for Charlie. For several weeks he had little appetite and his sleep was disturbed. He often asked me where Mummy was as though I knew something he didn't. His play seemed to reflect his distress: he often threw toys on to the ground, tore up railway tracks and hid cars behind the television or under the sofa. He would appeal to me to help him find them. I watched him turn his nose up at some toast that the nanny had made. In those instances, I wondered if he had experienced her presence initially as an unwelcome intrusion into his world.

The last quarter of the observation made for some painful moments for me. Privately, I felt saddened by Charlie's loss. There was one particularly moving visit at 23 months when James left for work and Charlie threw himself on to the floor by the front door, wailing. Will picked his baby brother up and carried him to the living room. I felt a sense of loss for Anna's departure as well. The seminar group allowed for me to remain curious about what was unfolding and acknowledge the despair faced by this family. The group helped me draw the observations to a close by counting down the visits.

Discussion

Melanie Klein (1926) suggests that children possess an epistemophilic instinct based on their desire to learn and know about the world. Their innate curiosity is first expressed through an interest in the mother's body as an internal space. Here, the caregiver provides a container for the infant's thoughts to come into being. Charlie developed rich symbolic thinking and an intense appetite to explore the world. He appeared to recover from upset relatively quickly. He used two objects in his play; placed pots inside of each other, figures in containers, linking together railroad tracks and making puzzles. He acquired a sense of wonder of his mother's mysterious interior, possibly seeing her as 'other'.

When Anna returned to work, the pain of separation threatened Charlie's images of a beautiful baby and a loving couple. This could reflect the aesthetic conflict faced by the infant:

> ...the meaning of his mother's behaviour, of the appearance and disappearance of the breast and of the light in her eyes, of a face over which emotions pass like the shadows of clouds over the landscape, are unknown to [the baby]. He has, after all, come into a strange country where he knows neither the language nor the customary non-verbal cues and communications. The mother is enigmatic to him; she wears the Gioconda smile most of the time and the music of her voice keeps shifting from major to minor key. (Meltzer and Harris Williams 1998, p.21)

The aesthetic conflict appeared to be Charlie's confusions with his mother. Underneath her loving gaze, Anna may have feared a dependent relationship with him. Her return to full-time employment appeared to leave him in a state of confusion and mourning. Anna's departure before the end of the observation clouded my sense of the significance of the separation for her.

The other participants of the observation, notably James and Will, occupied a minor presence. James was home a few times in the two years. I wondered if he felt self-conscious by being observed by another male. He was proud of Charlie and commented that he expected him to outgrow his older brother. Charlie clearly adored his father and would launch himself into James's lap, climb on top of him or herald his return with joy. Will was also largely absent as his paternal grandfather took him out for swimming during the visits. Initially Will referred to me as 'Mr Poo'; however, he soon tried to engage me in play, drawing my attention away from Charlie. On the whole, the boys seemed very close. They would bundle together in a heap on Anna's lap. Occasionally Will would take toys from his brother; however, this was offset by the abundance of laughter and excitement shared in their play.

The Aesthetic Conflict in Private Practice

In *The Apprehension of Beauty* Meltzer and Harris Williams (1998) radically situate the experience of the object's beauty as primary in infancy. They write, 'The depressive position would be primary for development, and the paranoid-schizoid secondary – the consequence of his closing down his perceptual apertures against the dazzle of the sunrise. In Plato's terms he would hasten back into the cave' (p.28). They argue that Klein's (1946) depressive position (feeling guilt towards one's internal objects) precedes the paranoid-schizoid position (persecutory anxieties). Art therapy, then, aims to recover the precious object from this angle. It involves working through the fragility of the enigmatic object to recapture depressive feelings in the transference (Begoin 2000; Williams 2000).

I shall now turn to a case study of a woman who tried to overcome the terror and horror within her internal world to recover a loving experience.

Clinical Illustration: Rachel

Towards the end of the summer Rachel contacted me through an online directory. Her email was brief, stating that she was interested in exploring a career change to become an expressive therapist. At the initial consultation, I met a small and spirited woman in jeans and a jumper. Rachel offered a weak smile and entered, scanning the office and commenting on the books and toys for play therapy. As she settled in the chair opposite me, she was surprised that I was a male therapist. She dismissed this with a joke and suggested that it would be 'good to work with a male'. To date she had worked with female counsellors and therapists.

Rachel had worked in education for several years, and felt irritated with the 'stresses and traumas' of her colleagues whom she regularly watched argue. She grew up in an area rife with gang culture. She described her mother as self-righteous and highly controlling of both her and her father. Her parents frequently quarrelled and her father flew into sudden rages. Following a very turbulent early childhood, she was bullied quite badly at secondary school. She withdrew into her own world from the danger outside.

Rachel told me about her stormy relationship with her boyfriend. On one occasion, she threw at knife at him 'to make a point', and added that she was 'cut off' from her emotions. I felt that she attached little importance to her stories. At the end of the session, she reflected, 'I decided to contact you because you have my father's smile.' I picked up on this contrast with her earlier statement. I wondered if Rachel found this new experience too much to bear, from which she recoiled. Meltzer and Williams (1998) write, 'How, then, may the bombardment of colour, form and patterned sound of such augmented intensity as greets the newborn, impinge upon [her] mind?' (p.107). Rachel had remarkable curiosity about the material interior of the consulting room. She turned her gaze away from the thought that I was a male. Towards the end of the session she recovered a loving memory of her father to fit into her image of me.

In the second month of our work, there was one occasion that the consulting room had been double booked. This was a rare and unfortunate event. Unable to return to our space, we were placed into a position to move to another room. She sat down and began telling me that she felt sorry for her father; he was not educated and was often criticised by her mother. She recalled her parents' deeply hostile relationship. I attempted to explore her feelings and suggested links with the double booking. Rachel was familiar with the transference but denied any concern for the move and reiterated that she did not have a problem. She complained about my use of interpretation and recommended that I use other methods in art therapy. I felt pressured by her. I saw her wish for exploration of this issue to be closed down.

In the following session, Rachel started off by saying that I reminded her of her first boyfriend who had taken his own life. She spoke with sadness as she remembered a series of traumatic deaths in her family. She loosely drew three toadstools in red and white framed by jagged strokes or flashes of lightning (Figure 6.1). My eye travelled diagonally across the paper towards a trap. She jotted down terms like 'Holding', 'Too much for others', 'Seeing not being seen' and 'Efforts of containment' in pencil after surveying the scene. She told me that she has spent too much time crying about her ex-boyfriend and was now happy. She spoke warmly that she felt at one with me and knew me in a past life. I reflected on her confusion and the grief that she had been carrying. I added that she wanted to hold her feelings together in this space. She continued to use the language of containment for the rest of the session.

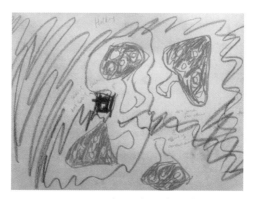

Figure 6.1 (See colour plate 8)

Helen Greenwood (2000) presents a powerful illustration of surviving attacks on the three-dimensional mental space with a particular group of art therapy clients. She describes the transference of a failed object who could not understand the patient. I sometimes found myself 'ousted' from Rachel's internal world when I attempted to interpret her images. I realised that my reflections had possibly caused Rachel to retreat. The sessions were at risk of becoming stagnant and repetitive. Her images started to include a number of geometric shapes inside one another and eyes inside of bellies. She drew walls, a prison, a well and a rabbit hole. In one session, I wondered if dependency was difficult for her and she wanted to show me that everything was fine. She responded that she became anxious once when her colleague held her face in an exercise at work. She described feeling angry when people enter her personal space 'when they don't know what they're doing'.

Case (2005) and Dalley (2000) describe the unconscious fantasies that children may have about being inside the mother's body. They draw upon Meltzer (1992), who introduced the concept of a *claustrum* for the infant's omnipotent intrusion into parts of the mother's body. Getting inside of the mother's head could allow the baby to experience her thoughts; intruding into her genitals reflects a desire for erotic activity, and her rectum could provoke a claustrophobic state of mind where escape and transformation seem impossible. I found this notion of the enclosed space was important for understanding Rachel's dilemma. She wanted to retreat from contact with me and yet was left feeling trapped and alone within herself.

Over time, I began to invite Rachel to think about my thinking. By the eighth month, she began to mourn the loss of her father. He died of cancer several years ago, before which she had returned home to care for him. The image in Figure 6.2 emerged from a memory of watching him in the shadows from her bed as a child. He is trying to find his way in the dark. She spoke about his loneliness though suggested that, at the time, she did not know how he was feeling. She wanted me to convey my understanding of her to feel understood. The session reflected a turning point where we recognised that we were trying to find a way in the dark. In the following session, she made the image in Figure 6.3, which included the words to her father, 'I'm sorry, please forgive me and I love you.' The heart looks as though it is being held by a loving presence.

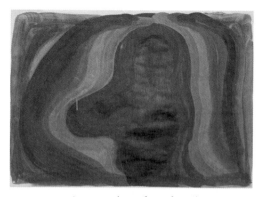

Figure 6.2 (See colour plate 9)

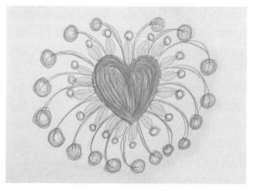

Figure 6.3 (See colour plate 10)

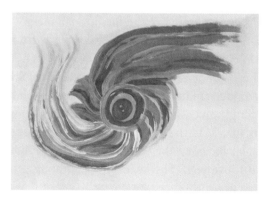

Figure 6.4 (See colour plate 11)

After a year of art therapy, Rachel decided to withdraw her application to train as a therapist and return home. Figure 6.4 was painted the session prior to telling me of her decision. Her image depicted 'turbulence and energy, coming from inside, it's a dragon or a bird or a person'. She compared the figure to herself; it had one eye on her internal world and the other 'on God'. Throughout our work, Rachel conveyed loose associations about her images. I wondered if she felt estranged by her creations. Before the summer break, Rachel sketched a snowflake and then changed her mind and said that it was a spaceship instead, returning to its planetary source. In the final session she drew Figure 6.5, from an earlier dream she had about the 'butterfly effect' or the notion that small changes in one area could generate a dramatic impact in a different state. In this image, this butterfly was outside the world before returning to its alien home.

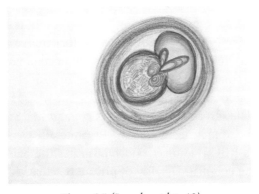

Figure 6.5 (See colour plate 12)

Discussion

In a letter to her sister in 1908, Virginia Woolf wrote, 'The world is a dangerous place. I felt like a happy animal in its own burrow – weathertight and safe' (quoted in Kohon 2015). Rachel recoiled from my curiosity and retreated to a hideout, possibly confusing my interest with intrusion. The sessions were at risk of becoming stagnant. When I adapted my approach, she started to become more present and engaged. I wonder if this dynamic could shed light on the aesthetic conflict for many of our clients. When the environmental conditions are hostile or depriving for the child, recapturing primary love requires more time as, without love and beauty, we may only encounter horror or terror.

The work with Rachel taught me the precarious nature of the aesthetic object in private practice. Case sees these fleeting moments of beauty in art therapy:

Other aesthetic experiences in the world explode like a firework filling our minds, only to go out to leave a dark sky. The memory and feelings are intense, but in our apprehension we split off that other mother who does not satisfy and she lurks like a ghost in the wings to take the place of the aesthetically pleasing mother. In an aesthetic moment, the unsatisfying mother, split off, and the absent mother, who cannot always be there, lurk as shadows. (1996, pp.44–45)

Meltzer and Harris Williams illuminate the complexity of the aesthetic object. They write, 'The tragic element in the aesthetic experience resides, not in the transience, but in the enigmatic quality of the object, "Joy, whose hand is ever at his lips/Bidding adieu"' (1998, p.27). In my mind, the infant observation and case illustration show aspects of the familiar and unknown, visible and invisible, and the external and interior. In private practice the aesthetic conflict resides in the privacy of the space and the minds of art therapist and client. For the outsider, private practice could be greeted with intrigue or suspicion. Those in the dark might wonder or make assumptions about what happens behind closed doors. The success of the TV series *In Treatment*, Stephen Grosz's *The Examined Life*, public lectures at the Institute of Psychoanalysis, and Suzie Orbach's BBC Radio series demonstrates the public appetite to get to know the enigmatic quality of private practice.

Within the confines of this intimate space, clients may have fantasies about the art therapist's own art making, opinions, holidays, boundaries and other clients. Some clients might wish to work through their issues outside the session. It is as if sharing their space is too novel or daunting for them. The art-making process also contains an aesthetic conflict, eliciting awe or fear. It 'entails a complex participation, full of potential ambiguity, irony, pain, memories, logical relations, emotions, revelations, anxieties and confusion' (Kohon 2015, p.3). Within the trusted space, aesthetic reciprocity might unfold between art therapist and client.

The case material with Rachel could illustrate the value of remaining committed to learning in art therapy. She ended her sessions after a year. One wonders when could be the right time for clients to 'leave home'. In 'Talking Nonsense and Knowing When to Stop' Phillips (2006) suggests that therapeutic endings are what full stops are to punctuation: they indicate or arrange a transition. He cites the oft-quoted, 'An analysis is never finished, it is only abandoned' (p.23).

Private practice could offer the time required to work through the retreats and resistances to treat unique and complex problems. This seems urgent when the provision of long-term therapy in the public sector is under threat. The shared privacy, commitment, patience and sacrifice to engage in private art therapy could thus allow for aesthetic moments between client and art therapist to endure.

Contribution of Infant Observation to Private Practice

In 1965, Wilfred Bion introduced a metaphysical concept to psychoanalysis simply called 'O'. It represents omega, the last letter of the Greek alphabet and final building block in Bion's model of thinking. It characterises a state of mind that allows for contact with the 'unknown, unknowable, ineffable, inscrutable, ontological experience of ultimate being' (Grotstein 2007, p.121). The aesthetic nature within O rests in the beauty of the unknowable 'beyond'. Anna tried to provide a container for Charlie's symbolic thoughts to come into being. Similarly, the art therapist strives to create a space for the art work to be explored, to expand the field of understanding and to manage turbulence for the transformation in O.

The art therapist attempts to bear pain and uncertainty in the face of the clients' deepest, infantile projections. Martha Harris (2011) conveys these states of mind clearly:

> The observer may learn from his own experience and from watching the mother's reactions to the first few weeks of the baby's life, how painful it is to stay with the recognition that something as helpless as a young infant [has] to suffer the pain of waiting until help comes. Their pain is relieved not only by their bodily needs being met, but through understanding, social contact, love. (p.123)

The infant observation has allowed for me to appreciate the 'infant in the adult' more fully. Clients' unintegrated mental states may be concealed or avoided in words, actions or art making. They could be played out in 'the giving-withholding-organising, receptive-comforting-indulgent qualities of the primary object' (p.123) in art making and the transference. Within the trusted space of the analytic frame (Milner 1987), clients could begin to gain insight into these early experiences.

An infant observation could allow for art therapists to turn towards further exploration of preverbal mental states and symbolic thinking, containment, the transference and the tolerance of uncertainty, to name a few. Given the pressures within the public sector, private practitioners are possibly best placed to develop this field of enquiry. Exploring the links between infant observation and private practice could therefore help restore deep connections between art therapy and psychoanalysis.

References

Begoin, J. (2000) 'Love and Destructivity: From the Aesthetic Conflict to a Revision of the Concept of Destructivity in the Psyche.' In M. Cohen and A. Hahn (eds) *Exploring the Work of Donald Meltzer*. London: Karnac.

Bick, E. (1964) 'Notes on infant observation in psycho-analytic training.' *International Journal of Psychoanalysis 45*, 558–566.

Bion, W.R. (1965) *Transformations*. London: Karnac.

Case, C. (1996) 'On the aesthetic moment in the transference.' *Inscape 1*, 2, 39–45.

Case, C. (2005) *Imagining Animals: Art, Psychotherapy and Primitive States of Mind*. Abingdon: Taylor and Francis.

Dalley, T. (2000) 'Back to the Future: Thinking About Theoretical Developments in Art Therapy.' In A. Gilroy and G. McNeilly (eds) *The Changing Shape of Art Therapy: New Developments in Theory and Practice*. London: Jessica Kingsley Publishers.

Greenwood, H. (2000). 'Captivity and terror in the therapeutic relationship.' *Inscape 5*, 2, 53–61.

Grotstein, J.S. (2007) *A Beam of Intense Darkness: Wilfred Bion's Legacy to Psychoanalysis*. London: Karnac.

Harris, M. (2011) 'The Contribution of Observation of Mother–Infant Interaction and Development to the Equipment of a Psychoanalyst or Psychoanalytic Psychotherapist.' In M. Harris, M H Williams and E. Bick, *The Tavistock Model: Papers on Child Development and Psychoanalytic Training*. London: Karnac.

Harris Williams, M. (ed.) (2011) *The Tavistock Model : Papers in Child Development and Psychoanalytic Training by Martha Harris and Esther Bick*. London: Karnac.

Klein, M. (1926) 'Infant analysis.' *International Journal of Psychoanalysis 7*, 31–63.

Klein, M. (1946) 'Some notes on schizoid mechanisms.' *International Journal of Psychoanalysis 27*, 99–110.

Kohon, G. (2015) *Reflections on the Aesthetic Experience: Psychoanalysis and the Uncanny*. Hove: Routledge.

Meltzer, D. (1992) *The Claustrum: An Investigation of Claustrophobic Phenomena*. London: Karnac.

Meltzer, D. and Harris Williams, M. (1998) *The Apprehension of Beauty: The Role of Aesthetic Conflict in Development, Art and Violence*. London: Karnac.

Milner, M. (1987) 'The Role of Illusion in Symbol Formation.' In *The Suppressed Madness of Sane Men: Forty-Four Years of Exploring Psychoanalysis*. Hove: Psychology Press.

Phillips, A. (2006) 'Talking Nonsense and Knowing When to Stop.' In *Side Effects*. London: Penguin Books.

Ruszczynski, S. (1993) *Psychotherapy with Couples: Theory and Practice at the Tavistock Institute of Marital Studies*. London: Karnac.

Williams, G. (2000) 'Reflections on "Aesthetic Reciprocity".' In M. Cohen and A. Hahn (eds) *Exploring the Work of Donald Meltzer*. London: Karnac.

Part III

TRAINING AND TRANSMISSION

7

TOWARDS PRIVATE PRACTICE

Aspects of Training and the Cycle of Learning

——— THEMIS KYRIAKIDOU ———

Introduction

Art therapists, like most other professionals, are experiencing the effects of the current financial crisis. Since the early part of this century financial restrictions and budget cuts have been part of the landscape for social and health care providers (Campbell and Meikle 2011). Workers are often pressured and as a result at risk, there are redundancies, and services are closing due to limited funding and resources. The need for social and health care provision has not decreased; in fact, as a result of the economic situation, needs for services have increased, but funding is often contested and difficult to find.

Staff members who are lucky enough to hold a paid job are often under enormous stress to deliver quality services and deliver 'more for less'. Under these stressful and worrying conditions it is not surprising that art therapy, like every other profession, has suffered. Services are limiting their resources mainly to professions promoted by National Institute for Health and Care Excellence (NICE) guidance, such as psychologists and cognitive behavioural therapy (CBT) therapists, which offer clear assessments and measurable evidence of effectiveness. It is also worth remembering that the arts therapies are still recommended by NICE for adults, children and young people experiencing certain mental health issues (NICE 2009–10, 2013, 2014) and although it is often the service users who are asking for more creative interventions, rather than commissioners, service-user voices are sometimes heard (Glover 2016). There are nonetheless occasions when their wishes cannot be realised.

Consequently, finding contractual art therapy employment within the National Health Service (NHS), or any other private or public service provider, is difficult. This is a daunting reality. Newly qualified art therapists who are eager to practise their skills and knowledge as soon as they obtain their registration are often left disappointed when they realise the limited *conventional* work opportunities. Of course, this news is not new to them, but the reality of this, as well as the financial pressures after completing their studies, leaves some newly qualified art therapists apprehensive about their career prospects.

Early Developments

As a BAAT (British Association of Art Therapists) regional coordinator (for BAAT region 11, Yorkshire and Humber) for the years 2009–2013, I came into contact with many art therapists from my local area. Anxiety about employment and future careers was often expressed. Some art therapists managed to secure employment in generic mental health roles, some had to change their career direction completely and a few gained employment under the job title of art therapist.

In my experience, newly qualified art therapists often have as their initial career choice the wish to work in a permanent position within an organisation such as the NHS, to ensure financial and professional stability. Nevertheless, like many art therapists, they quickly realise that such jobs are hard to get. Therefore, art therapists, like other professionals, find themselves entering the world of independent practice as self-employed practitioners (Hossain *et al.* 2011). As a result, the number of therapists working autonomously has started to rise significantly. In many cases this does not always happen by choice, but from necessity and financial pressure.

Responding to this state of affairs, I suggested we run a series of workshops with a focus on employment and, more specifically, interview skills, sessional work and private practice. This was positively received by most region 11 BAAT members. At that time, I had just completed further postgraduate studies on interviewing and recruitment and had an active personal interest in employment matters. I felt I could put my academic knowledge and professional experience into practice, and with the involvement of Sarah Ayache, James D. West, Anthea Hendry and Chris Wood we organised and delivered three workshops in the summers of 2012 and 2013, looking at each of the above topics. These training days were open to all newly qualified art therapists from across the region, but also to all BAAT members from the area. The Art Therapy Northern Programme in Sheffield offered us their premises. This meant we could provide three successful training days with minimum costs.

These workshops built on earlier employment training, and they have evolved and triggered new initiatives within the region and within the Art Therapy Northern Programme. These developments have received unanimous positive feedback and acknowledgement of the need for more support in relation to issues concerning employment and independent practice particularly in relation to this financial climate.

Region 11 BAAT members organised a meeting in Leeds to discuss issues related to private practice and also invited the Private Practice Special Interest Group (PPSIG) to facilitate two of their regular meetings in the north, one in Sheffield and one in Manchester. It is my understanding that this will be repeated again in the future in other regions as the PPSIG has embraced the idea of hosting meetings around the country and not only in London.

The Art Therapy Northern Programme in Sheffield also understands the value of these employment initiatives. Together with staff of the Art Therapy Northern Programme I have the desire to support trainees and develop the employment initiatives to become a more comprehensive part of career preparation for trainees and other members of the profession. This was the starting point for the 'employment workshops', as we have named them, that are offered by the Art Therapy Northern Programme in Sheffield. During these workshops, what we hope to offer is a space for newly qualified practitioners to think, discuss and raise questions on employment and independent practice. In addition, we want to draw attention to how to keep 'safe', both from a legal and personal perspective.

Private Practice upon Qualification

It has been some years since the first workshop and we now run two training days per year. During these sessions the idea of private practice is introduced and discussed. From the outset, we clearly explain that further learning may be needed if they decide to engage in private practice work at some point in the future. Newly qualified art therapists are generally advised not to engage in private work straight after qualification and not to do so until they have gained enough art therapy experience. Many art therapists support this view and believe that private practice is appropriate only after some years of post-qualification art therapy experience. Even though the experience of a clinical placement is invaluable, practitioners recognise that private practice has added complexities: it requires high levels of therapeutic and professional competence in the areas of therapeutic responsibility, accountability, autonomy and safety. BAAT also adopts a similar stance and suggests that art therapists need to have at least two years' full-time or four years' part-time post-qualified art therapy experience before they can register on the BAAT list of private practitioners (BAAT 2014). This is an attempt to ensure quality service to the public, by making sure that registered practitioners are ready for this type of private practice work. Nevertheless, BAAT also recognises that many art therapists, as mature students with prior professional qualifications, may have the skills and knowledge to practise privately from the onset of their art therapy career and therefore takes into consideration each application individually. On the other hand, the Health and Care Professions Council (HCPC) enables art therapists to become private practitioners on their successful completion of an accredited art therapy course. Some art therapists would argue that as most art therapy trainees are generally mature students, often in age and definitely in mind, who have a wealth of social care and life experience prior to engaging with their art therapy degrees, they are sufficiently qualified. At a time of registration these practitioners may already have a strong ethical and professional approach which may very well enable them to practise successfully without the support of an organisational context.

It is complicated: the HCPC, for example, acknowledges that health and social care practitioners (including arts therapists) are competent at the point of registration, but professional organisations (for the 16 professions regulated by the HCPC) vary in their advice to registrants about private practice because the different professions practise in differing contexts with different needs. The HCPC tends to work in conjunction with the advice of professional associations, and if a practitioner does not follow the advice of the professional body, the professional concerned is open to additional scrutiny as they may be seen to be working beyond their competence. Nevertheless, some art therapists suggest that since newly qualified practitioners are *technically* allowed to work privately upon registration, then the training courses should provide enough training opportunities around this topic to better equip new practitioners to practise more independently, in a similar way to other therapeutic courses such as counselling and psychotherapy. This is an interesting and undoubtedly an ongoing discussion.

Setting the Tone...

The dilemma of whether or not private practice should be introduced to trainees during their studies is explored during each workshop and is often discussed amongst art therapy practitioners already in private practice. In my experience, not many trainees express the desire to practise privately. Most commonly, trainees state that they would feel safer and would prefer to work within an organisation, even on a sessional basis, rather than engage in private work. Nevertheless, they still ask for some support in understanding the similarities and differences between independent work under the umbrella of an organisation and private practice.

During the workshops, I have made a conscious decision to cover a variety of topics such as interview preparation and job hunting, as well as private practice. Even though private practice is discussed, I encourage people to attend further training and join the PPSIG, as a single day's workshop is not enough for thinking of the complexities of this type of work. Similarly, I encourage practitioners to think about their own circumstances and competences and assess their own level of readiness for such practice and for the clinical accountability which comes with it.

Most art therapists only decide to engage in private practice many years later, others wish to work privately but never develop the confidence to do so, and some are simply not interested in private work. Nevertheless, the Art Therapy Northern Programme considers that it is important for contemporary practitioners to have some introductory knowledge around all types of art therapy practice, so that practitioners can make an informed decision on the route they wish to take. Therefore, alongside reflection and discussion, the workshops offer some practical guidance and advice based on the experience and knowledge of workshop leaders and colleagues, research concerning white-collar employment, and knowledge about BAAT.

Experience in Learning

I generally believe that the more clinical experience a therapist has prior to becoming a private practitioner the better. Nevertheless, this experience alone does not provide sufficient learning for all practitioners and other elements may also need to be in place to complement one's knowledge and skills.

David Kolb (1984) indicates that a person's learning goes through some important stages. He identifies four learning stages:

1. that of the immediate or concrete experience

2. the reflective observation

3. abstract conceptualisation

4. active experimentation.

These four stages define learning as an active experiential event, in which the person who is engaging with the activity has time to reflect, think and try out new actions and thoughts. Even though one can start anywhere within the learning circle, a single stage is not sufficient for learning, and there is the requirement for using all stages together, to complement the educational experience.

If I were to apply this learning cycle to art therapists who practise privately, I would argue that experience alone is not enough to make an art therapist a competent private practitioner. Time for reflection, discussion, thinking and activity are also required to mature and develop one's learning. This is perhaps why the BAAT PPSIG has such an important role in people's learning. The SIG provides space for discussion, thinking and reflection, and members are welcomed to share their experiences and raise questions. Equally, this is perhaps one of the reasons why art therapy trainees find the employment workshops such as those held at the Art Therapy Northern Programme and within the different regional groups of BAAT beneficial and helpful. Even though Chris Wood and I actively talk about our experience as practitioners, we are also able to offer a thinking space to the trainees where they can reflect upon their experience and the complexities of art therapy practice, whether this is under contractual employment, or sessional or private work. Despite the fact that trainees may not have the clinical experience of working as qualified practitioners, during the workshops they can internalise and reflect on the examples given as well as make suggestions and practise some of their employment skills. As Kolb's learning cycle (1984) suggests, if knowledge and active thinking are already in place, then when the experience comes, it will, it is hoped, complement and solidify one's learning.

Trainees are invited and encouraged to participate in an active discussion about their employment plans, as well as share any potential fears about their future career. The completion of the MA in Art Therapy, for many, gives rise to numerous anxieties. Sharing such anxieties in a problem-solving and containing manner can only be helpful.

The Employment Workshops in Practice

A good starting point when thinking of any post-qualifying activity is to introduce the importance of registration and the role of the HCPC. This is obviously not the first time that the role of the HCPC is discussed with the trainees, but many have practical questions in relation to their registration, the timescales and the forms, as well as the HCPC standards. Therapists wishing to practise under the protected title of 'art therapist' need to be registered with the HCPC upon the successful completion of their studies. This registration introduces professional duties and responsibilities, which all registrants need to adhere to in order to maintain their registration and professional status. Often, questions relating to volunteering arise at this point, as we talk about the first two years after qualification, the renewal of registration and issues to consider if one has not managed to gain employment within this time period.

The importance of HCPC registration for art therapists is enormous as our profession is well monitored and therefore has a well-defined code of conduct. Our registration offers professional trust and credibility to services and the public. This registration offers us the 'licence' to practise and it is up to the HCPC to withdraw this 'permission' in cases of malpractice. A brief but clear message is given to all trainees regarding the responsibilities and duties which come with the registration; even though they refer to the members' professional life, they also have an impact on one's social and personal life too. Therefore, activity which may be unrelated to one's work may influence someone's registration. Drawing attention to the use of social media and networking sites is welcomed at this point, especially after the introduction of HCPC standard 2.7 which states that practitioners need to apply the same standard of reputable behaviour at all times in all areas of their life.

Both HCPC registration and BAAT membership, even though the second is not mandatory, offer quality assurance for the public, suggesting that registered art therapists work always within an ethical, therapeutic, professional and up-to-date framework. BAAT membership not only offers advice and support to practitioners, but also a wealth of networking opportunities and informal communication as well as publicity and marketing opportunities. More specifically, BAAT members not only benefit from their memberships, but also from the support of the PPSIG. This group functions as a formal and informal forum for those art therapists who are involved in private practice and it is currently coordinated by James D. West. The group coordinator brings the group's formal business to the BAAT council, but practitioners can also freely exchange email communication and find answers to any questions through a well-established Google group. BAAT also functions as a 'safety net' when misunderstandings occur and an amicable solution needs to be found between an art therapist and a client. Even though BAAT's involvement may not be direct, the association is known to support practitioners during times of struggle. Therefore, the importance of BAAT membership and SIG registration is highlighted during the workshop. Personally, I would not encourage any private work without BAAT registration, as it is vital to have a strong professional support network, and a well-defined working framework, in this somewhat isolated role of the private practitioner.

In order to practise either independently or privately, practitioners need to be registered as sole traders with HM Revenue and Customs (HMRC), so they are in a position to file their own tax return. This may seem like a complicated process, but the reality is that it is not. There are many helpful tips and information on the HMRC website explaining the process. Additionally, HMRC officers are very helpful and happy to offer advice and support if a practitioner has any questions in relation to their tax return.

After registering with HMRC as self-employed, one of the most important things is to be organised and to have an accurate record of expenditures and income. Good record keeping will certainly make the self-assessment and tax return process easier. Some practitioners may wish to consider registering as a limited company as this reduces the liability and makes the therapy practice safer for the therapist's assets.

Nevertheless, some advice may be useful as the company needs to be registered with Companies House and pay corporation tax to start trading. In my experience art therapists start their private practice as sole traders and maybe, but not necessarily, become a limited company after some years of trading and most often when private practice is the main source of income. I am also aware of a few newly qualified art therapists who have thought hard about their art therapy practice and have consequently set up social enterprises. This enables them to access social and government funds and ensure some financial security once the funding and grant applications are in place (see Andrea Heath and Catherine Stevens in Chapter 3).

The purchase of professional indemnity and public liability insurance is necessary for any form of trading, whether one is a sole trader or a limited company, whether in session work or private practice. In many cases, both requirements can be combined in one insurance policy, but practitioners will need to double check each policy to make sure it has an adequate level of cover. There are different limits of indemnity, commonly for up to £6,000,000, and different insurance prices are offered by a variety of providers. Art therapists may find lower charges if they purchase their policy online or over the phone and therefore it is advisable to research and shop around to find the best deal. Additionally, we also advise trainees that it may be worth visiting the BAAT website, as it often offers suggestions and recommendations on insurers who are familiar with the art therapy practice, its requirements and its complexities.

An insurance policy is a legal necessity for trading but also provides a protective mechanism for private practitioners in case they find themselves in difficult situations and misunderstandings with their clients. During the workshops there is usually a general sense of anxiety in the room when this topic is discussed. The possibility of being sued often generates fear and uncertainty even for practitioners with many years of working experience. The realisation of being a 'sole trader' and its real-life implications, such as being a practitioner with an enormous amount of sole clinical responsibility and with no support and protection from an organisational infrastructure, is often a deterrent to private work.

Similarly, data protection and confidentiality are also areas which may raise doubt and apprehension to new art therapy practitioners. We encourage art therapists who engage in private practice, but also in any independent work, to register with the Information Commissioner's Office (ICO), an agency responsible for ensuring data protection of client material. This is a legal requirement if practitioners use their own computers for work, for example to write client reports, exchange emails containing case material, or to communicate with existing or potential clients. Not everyone is aware of this organisation, but as ensuring compliance with data protection is every practitioner's duty, it is not a surprise when I notice most trainees making a little note in their notebook to remember to register.

One of the most important points in independent and private work is to be self-aware in order to be safe. To safeguard wellbeing it is necessary to emphasise the importance of working within the limits of known personal competencies, as well as acknowledging the importance of good support networks and clinical supervision (see Kate Rothwell on managing a private practice in Chapter 9, Colleen Steiner Westling on risk in Chapter 10 and James D. West on self-care in Chapter 12). Practitioners need to only take on clients they feel comfortable to work with and to discuss with their supervisor if they have any doubts prior to agreeing to engage with new clients in therapy.

Supervision is most definitely one of the best ways to increase reflective thinking and enhance someone's practice. It is an educational forum where dilemmas and therapeutic actions can be discussed and it offers one of the main strategies for self-care and self-preservation. Art therapists in private practice are encouraged to seek experienced supervisors who are aware of the complexities and difficulties of private work. Art therapy trainees are very familiar with the concept of supervision and its clinical importance, but during our workshops this is revisited and discussed further due to the additional clinical risk that accompanies both independent and private work (see David Edwards on supervision in Chapter 11).

On a more practical topic, art therapists who are thinking of entering the field of private practice need to think of an appropriate venue for conducting their sessions. Having a suitable confidential space which is appropriate for art making is one important task and is sometimes a challenge for private practitioners. Issues such as risk assessment and boundaries are highlighted when a practitioner considers the venue where therapy will take place. Some therapists choose to use their own home premises, whereas others hire rooms within various establishments. Practitioners who use their homes for private work will need to think carefully about how to maintain their personal boundaries and their family's personal space when conducting therapy. Equally, consideration should be given to any safety and accessibility measures which need to be in place to accommodate their clients' requirements. Hiring a venue to conduct the art therapy sessions is in some ways simpler. A hired space can offer a neutral environment and create a safe space between work and family life. Inevitably, it enables practitioners to maintain their own professional boundaries more easily. Nevertheless, hiring a room requires a payment, and this is often one of the reasons art therapists choose to work from home. Room charges can influence the cost of each session, and consequently the therapy fees need to be adjusted to accommodate this expense. The more a practitioner has to pay for a therapy room, the higher the fee will need to be for the session to allow some financial gain. Equally, room charges can also influence the cancellation and missed sessions policy. If the therapist hires a therapy space, then in most cases the client will still need to pay for this, even in the event of a cancellation. Charges for missed sessions are often an item of discussion, but practitioners have different views on this and what they consider to be ethical as well as symbolically and therapeutically appropriate. Practitioners often wonder if there is a right approach for this, and if they should charge for every cancelled session or only for sessions with less than 24 hours' cancellation notice. Ultimately there is no right or wrong answer when it comes to such issues. Nevertheless, we invite trainees to think of their own circumstances and practical arrangements, on an individual and personal level, but to make this clear in their contract with the client and to be appropriately flexible, bearing in mind that what may be appropriate for one practitioner may not be the right thing for somebody else. Similarly, what seems to be appropriate for one client may not be appropriate for another. Therefore, we invite trainees to think carefully, assess the clinical complexity and take decisions that feel both comfortable and feasible to them and their supervisor.

On a slightly different financial theme, many trainees often wonder about what rate each art therapy session should be charged at in independent or private practice. We have had many, quite lengthy discussions on this topic over time. Some art therapy trainees often explain that they would not like to charge too much, so they can keep their prices competitive. Some others also say that they would not want to set a low fee, so they are not perceived as 'cheap', as this may suggest that their intervention is not of value. Once again, what feels right varies from one trainee to the next and it is often influenced by their own personal financial circumstances and their ideas about the therapeutic relationship. I usually encourage trainees to read the BAAT documents for a more precise figure and engage in discussions with other local art therapies to check what is the 'going rate'. Nevertheless, I can fully appreciate that trainees may need a bit of time to think through this topic. I suppose setting a fee and getting paid for offering therapy is one of the first transactions after qualification. Art therapists often describe feeling nervous about receiving money directly from their clients, as this may create strong dynamics of power and imbalance between the therapist and the client. Many explain that being paid by an organisation rather than the person who is in need of the therapeutic support feels better to them. To make this transaction easier, any financial references could be clearly outlined in the art therapy contract. The contract (often referred to in 'softer' terms as an agreement) should be thoroughly discussed between therapists and clients from the start of an intervention and within the assessment period. If both parties are happy with the content, then they can both sign this and keep it for future reference.

Creating a therapy contract is a fundamental process in private practice. It outlines the parameters of the sessions and informs clients of what to expect. It provides a formal agreement between the art therapists and the clients and in many ways creates a business-like relationship between the two. Art therapists are those who offer a service and are considered to be holding the 'power' within the therapeutic relationship. Nevertheless, they are paid for their services and can be 'sacked' if the client decides that the intervention does not progress as it should do. In a sense the therapist has a dual role in private practice, that of the employer and the employee simultaneously. This is definitely something that provokes a lot of thinking and discussion amongst trainees as the therapeutic relationship seems more complicated than organisationally situated therapist–client relationships.

Observations

I hope that this discussion has helped provide a good starting point and some necessary knowledge for art therapists who may wish to engage in private work. In most cases newly qualified practitioners would prefer to be in permanent positions within supportive organisations rather than in private practice, as they recognise the need for ongoing support during the early years of their careers. They tend not to choose private practice initially but to create forms of independent work by offering sessions. In my experience there has only been one trainee who was keen to engage in art therapy in private practice straight away on qualification, but she was also a qualified counsellor already working privately.

It is understandable that most newly qualified art therapists are hesitant in approaching private practice. The majority of art therapy trainees are self-aware individuals who know their strengths and are able to make sensible decisions. This demonstrates maturity and healthy decision making, and I think that this can help create some trust in our profession and the confidence that we are able to evaluate clinical complexity and engage in appropriate therapeutic work.

References

BAAT (2014) *Code of Ethics and Principles of Professional Practice for Art Therapists.* Accessed on 15 May 2017 at www.baat.org/Assets/Docs/General/BAAT%20CODE%20OF%20ETHICS%202014. pdf.

Campbell, D. and Meikle, J. (2011) '£20bn NHS cuts are hitting patients, Guardian investigation reveals.' *The Guardian*, 17 October. Accessed on 8 May 2016 at www.theguardian.com/ society/2011/oct/17/nhs-cuts-impact-on-patients-revealed.

Glover, C. (2016) 'Compulsory redundancies at Calderdale Royal's art psychotherapy unit cancelled.' *The Examiner*, 7 March. Accessed on 4 April 2016 at www.examiner.co.uk/news/west-yorkshire-news/compulsory-redundancies-calderdale-royals-art-11000105.

Hossain, N., Byrne, B., Campbell, A., Harrison, E., McKinley, B. and Shah, P. (2011) *The Impact of the Global Economic Downturn on Communities and Poverty in the UK.* York: Joseph Rowntree Foundation. Accessed on 29 April 2016 at www.jrf.org.uk/sites/default/files/jrf/migrated/ files/experiences-of-economic-downturn-full.pdf.

Kolb, D. (1984) *Experiential Learning Experience as a Source of Learning and Development.* Upper Saddle River, NJ: Prentice Hall.

NICE (2009–10) *Schizophrenia: The NICE Guidelines on Core Interventions in the Treatment and Management of Schizophrenia in Adults in Primary and Secondary Care.* March 2009 substantial update, republished with minor updates in 2010 (CG82). London: NICE.

NICE (2013) *Psychosis and Schizophrenia in Children and Young People: Recognition and Management* (CG155). London: NICE.

NICE (2014) *Psychosis and Schizophrenia in Adults: Prevention and Management* (CG178). London: NICE.

8

NEGOTIATING THE DYNAMICS OF WORKING WITH TRAINEE ART PSYCHOTHERAPISTS IN THE UK

—— DAVE ROGERS ——

I came to write my thoughts on working with trainees many years ago. The impetus at the time was to bring some ragged ideas and experiences into some coherent shape. We are always mindful of our responsibility to reflect on our work with clients, and when finding myself taking on trainees I began to wonder what, if anything, the differences are between working with trainees and with other clients. Trainees may well have a range of needs and distresses based upon their experience of growing up and becoming adults. In addition to these, art therapy training will inevitably create extra strains as well as opportunities for self-development towards becoming a competent art therapist. The process of being in training to help others address emotional issues and yet at the same time finding their own issues being raised in the training process can be very daunting. The role of the trainee taking on personal therapy has been recognised more formally since 1994 when the requirement in the UK for the trainee art therapist to enter into personal therapy became mandatory. Many choose verbal psychotherapy, yet a growing number enter into their own personal art therapy process. The need for these complex dynamics to be held in personal therapy, to enable these emotions to be processed, has become now firmly established. As one colleague in supervision with me commented, 'Thank goodness trainees now have their own therapy!'

The intention of this chapter is to raise awareness of some of the complex tensions and boundaries that arise for the art therapist resulting from their attachments to training organisations, work placements, personal therapists and their own art work. If art therapists providing personal therapy for trainees are aware of their own attachments, this can help them to remain more objective and provide greater validity and efficacy in their professional practice. Creative dynamics, tensions and boundaries are, in fact, constant in any creative process and are being held by both parties: the therapist and the client (in this case the trainee).

The Requirement by Training Organisations for Personal Therapy for Art Therapy Trainees

In 1991 the annual general meeting of the British Association of Art Therapists (BAAT) saw the membership vote in favour of the requirement for students to enter into their own personal therapy for the duration of their training. This would be adopted by all art therapy training courses by the year 1994. This applies an educational requirement to what is usually an individual personal choice. In terms of the student's successful academic progress the attendance of personal therapy must be maintained; it is therefore natural that the progress through therapy may become associated with other academic standards in the student's mind. In this context understandable questions will be raised, such as: Is therapy being assessed? What are your [the therapist's] links with the training organisations? If I appear unstable will you tell the college? These questions have a base in reality, and therefore the trainee enters therapy potentially carrying the illusion that their personal therapy performance is being assessed on behalf of the training bodies.

What Does This Mean for the Art Therapist?

In the role as therapist we are called upon to provide a balance to these questions by defining their therapy as 'your own personal therapy'. So, is there really any difference when working with trainees of art therapy and working with trainees in verbal psychotherapy? We can assume the trainee has chosen art therapy for a good reason for example, it might seem natural to have art therapy whilst training as an art therapist, or it might be a curiosity about another form of therapy, or a fundamental interest in art and healing. The difference from verbal therapy is the inclusion of the image, which adds the well-known triangle of therapist, image and client (trainee) into the equation.

We are observing and responding to the trainee's mark making, and at the same time having awareness of our own creative work. We, the therapists, have personal creative attachments built upon over many years, which are as important as the years of experience of being an art therapist. As art therapists we have an awareness of our own creative conflicts and tensions. We are flowing between our experience of creative work and what we observe in the client's resistance, demands and intersubjectivity with the creative process of therapy. We are creative individuals with a bond towards our own work. Daniel Vargas Gomez describes this bond, which can seem to be uncontrollable at times:

> However, although the technique itself may be random or have unintentional elements, it is still true that the painter never loses intimacy, or better, a 'bond', with the painting. This word 'bond' obviously expresses the closeness that exists between the creator and the creation, and it would be absurd to think that any such bond can lack all conscious intention. The art work cannot be completely detached from the artist: the artist can never be an outsider to his or her own work, for the painting, or any other art work, as an artistic creation, within a sense will always be nothing more than an extension of the creator. The artist can never free him/herself from the responsibility as a creator. (Gomez 2015, p.7)

So, my attachment and 'bond' to the way in which I (the therapist) create art work is always in the mix when being aware of the range of attachments of the trainee and their approaches to their own creativity.

The dynamics for the therapist are also embellished by the increasing possibility of overlap in the therapist's professional working life and the life of the trainee. For example:

- The therapist may offer student placements in their workplace.

- The therapist may work sessionally for the training institution.

- The therapist may supervise practitioners who work with fellow trainees.

- The therapist may work with more than one trainee from the same college. (Most art therapists avoid working with trainees from the same course year.)

Art Psychotherapy Is a Small World!

Some of these challenges are referred to from a university trainer's point of view in Dudley, Gilroy and Skaife (2000), which raises useful insights into the subtleties of working across educational and therapeutic dynamics. The authors helpfully touch on the relationships formed by trainees, and the need to contain the resulting splits within the training and therapy. They emphasise the importance of staff meetings and other support mechanisms for therapy teaching teams in protecting the efficacy of the training and therapy processes. In contrast, working in isolation as an art therapist in private practice does not lend itself to having easy access to work-based meetings.

We are working at a distance from organisational structures. Therefore it is essential for us to have networks including therapists, art creators, course providers and trainers. Often the networking with art creators is the area that becomes neglected as the profession has attached itself more closely to the psychotherapeutic and analytic communities and trainings.

Figure 8.1 shows how the major aspects of both the therapist's and the trainee's art therapy world can impact on each other within an intense learning process. This is purposely a simple diagram which belies the complexity of some challenging dynamics.

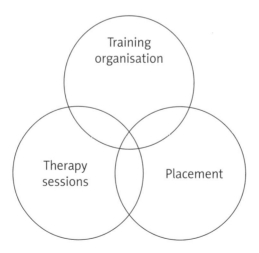

Figure 8.1 Convergent dynamics

Theoretical Framework: Attachment Theory

In some cases, the attachments that the trainee forms with the training institution, the work placement and their personal therapist may demonstrate a range of adaptable behaviours which are triggered by the significant relationships experienced in the present with personal tutors, supervision groups, placement supervisors and others. The therapist will also have experienced these attachments. Table 8.1 can be used for the trainee's model, but can also mirror the therapist's model. This is based upon the research findings of infant observation and the reaction to the Strange Situation (Ainsworth and Wittig 1969). By developing the ideas of Bowlby, Ainsworth incorporated an even wider range of potential attachments, which can also be considered within the context of providing therapy for art therapy trainees. Table 8.1 indicates the therapist's/trainee's potential experience of their training organisation, workplace or therapist using attachment theory.

Table 8.1 The trainees potential experience of the organisation/therapist

Caregivers	Secure attachment	Avoidant attachment	Resistant attachment	Disorganised attachment
Training organisation, workplace or therapist	Predictable, responsive, available, helpful, reliable	Predictably unresponsive, interfering, discouraging	Unpredictable, unresponsive, withdrawn, inept	Ambivalent, unreliable, unavailable, experienced as frightening

As training commences the trainee will initially experience a change of role, which comes with being a student: entry into a new vocation, feelings of being deskilled, commencing therapy, and beginning academic studies that might push the adult into varying degrees of regression. The student will bring this internal material to therapy in the form of anxieties, fears, confusion, ambivalence or anger, which may be split into projections, and may contain persecutory or paranoid material.

We can understand that these complexities strongly exist within attachment material and behaviours expressed by the trainee in therapy, and that the trainee's attachment response may be seen to be being played out in therapy sessions. For example, the training institution works on an assessment model, which assesses ability and flags up what is absent: students are marked and graded and always carry the fear of the threat of failure. As a parental type the institution may be experienced as an avoidant parent, preoccupied with itself, focusing on results and research and unhelpful beyond setting assignments and goals – it is then up to the student to secure results and gain the approval of the training course. The trainee may wonder whether the therapist is there to be 'the good parent' and 'save' them, to aid 'success' in their studies, or 'the good enough parent' who raises the realities of the depressive position.

The trainee may perceive the profession as a parent body which offers membership and protection, validation and belonging – but only if the trainee succeeds in their training. The therapist will hold some of the positive aspirations and negative connotations in the projections carried by the trainee and acted out in therapy: the art therapist may attract envy and hostility or represent a role to aspire to, particularly when the trainee begins the clinical placement.

No doubt some of the trainee's projections will idealise the therapist and, in terms of attachment theory and psychoanalytic technique, the therapist will foster the role of secure and available parent, developing a positive transference based within the parameters of a secure base through consistency, reliability, resilience to disillusionment, responsiveness, non-possessive warmth, unconditional positive regard and firm boundaries. Although we risk playing into the idealising projections, the intention of the therapist is always to remain positive, open and available, whilst maintaining neutrality within the dilemmas, conflicts and academic challenges expressed by the trainee.

In this context the importance of awareness in the therapist of their own attachments to the training organisations, clinical work placements, their own supervisor and their art work is paramount, as they can inevitably intrude upon the objectivity of the support they provide for their client. We know how important it is to hold these complex dynamics as therapists and to be aware of potential confusion of these processes in order to remain focused on the work and sustain clarity within ourselves. However, the reality is that things happen!

Some complexities in private practice
Example 1
The background to this example is that I had been asked to supervise a work-based trainee art therapist who was on the same training course and in the same year as a trainee for whom I was already providing

personal therapy. In my mind, I had felt that supervising a trainee from the same year at my place of work could be entirely 'separate' to having another trainee receiving personal art therapy as a client in my own therapy room. There was physical distance, that is true; and the roles of supervising a trainee art therapist at their work and being a therapist to a trainee are also very different, yet the unconscious processes can, and do, cross boundaries.

Although I thought I had guarded against this situation arising, I had one particular experience when, during a personal therapy session, the trainee told me that he 'had a secret'. His disclosure of this 'secret' revealed that he had met another trainee art therapist from the same course who said that she knew me well. They had an interesting conversation on the way to college about who I was and perhaps a great deal more.

It became apparent that taking on both 'situations' was a mistake, yet in some ways might have been a valuable one. The mistake was to imagine that the two contexts could be separated; yet they inevitably spilled into the therapy. Thinking that I could be both a workplace supervisor and a personal therapist to two individuals on the same course in the same year was more complex than I thought: an unwitting challenge, which became conscious in the art therapy sessions. I worked hard on how my imperfection as an art therapist might be resolved. In fact, the apparent 'mess-up' helped to raise the trainee's awareness of the potency and power of secrets, particularly with parental figures, and to withhold or reveal them, with impact, to the parental 'other'.

This reminded me how powerfully the training organisation forcefully impacts upon the trainee's need for attachment to the course, and in addition how the attachment to the therapist and the work-based supervising therapist is in a powerful loop. The fact that my trainee felt moved to tell me the 'secret' ('I couldn't hold on to it any longer') might, it is hoped, show the challenges of working within these overlaps. It meant that my relationship with the other trainee art therapist I supervised at her workplace had to be re-managed. Even more important for me was that during this period of my perceived 'mistake', I had not had a supervision session for some six weeks due to holidays and other practical events. This made it abundantly clear to me that the supervision I was receiving formed an essential part of my own role as a therapist, ensuring I remain clear about decision making and awareness of unconscious collusion with the trainee and training institution.

I took heart from Nathan Field's (1992) introduction to his article 'The way of imperfection' where he cautions against an obsession with the correctness of therapeutic techniques that may prove to be counterproductive and stifling. He comments that 'a striving for perfection only re-enacts the compulsion for perfectionism which is suffered by a patient' (p.139). This is helpful as it is human to err, even as an art therapist! The work with the client then became a process of recovery from what I felt was a 'mistake' of mine, yet I interpreted it as an opportunity to analyse where I and the trainees were in the dynamics of the sessions. This is not a clarion call to make mistakes for the sake of it, just to indicate what a rich environment we exist in, and the strengths and insights we need to ensure good professional practice. After the session I had the distinct image of a bus with various passengers in my mind. The questions in this image for me were: 'Who was being carried, where to and who was the driver?'

The attachment issues in this example are those of my trainee art therapist towards his training organisation and his attachment to me as therapist, and the work-based supervisee's attachment to my workplace and her allocated clients. The mélange of other childhood attachments and partnership attachments are also in the mix. My attachment to my own art therapy supervision had briefly had an interruption (my holidays and a bout of illness), which could well mean I took my 'eye off the ball' in my professional practice, finding myself in a more complex situation than I would have wished for. These discomforts are containable by experienced therapists, but we must always ensure that we approach them with absolute clarity and awareness. Clive Carswell (2007) describes the importance of this beautifully when discussing his role of counselling students:

> In addition to the capacity to tolerate and work with anxiety, we need to be able to tolerate and work with despair. A belief in the nature of despair as a transitory experience is essential, not just for success but also for survival itself. Where early experiences of despair have not been contained sufficiently by primary caregivers, the capacity to internalise tolerance of this bleak state has not been possible and this creates a basic fault within the individual. (p.17)

He extends this with the concept of the instillation of hope with which any of us who are engaged in helping trainees to survive and succeed will be only too familiar.

Carswell, however, emphasises that students and trainees need to be made aware of the fact that success without struggle is an illusion. My sense of this is that due to my own fear of failing a trainee, I might become caught up in counter-transference of becoming the over-helpful, impinging parent.

Example 2

The impact of training was clearly illustrated to me by images made during personal art therapy by a trainee art therapist in her first year. The range of confusion and anxiety about being in a demanding training at a particular time in her life is clear to see in Figure 8.2.

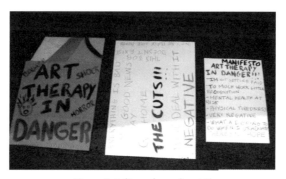

Figure 8.2 (See colour plate 13)

Not only did the stresses in her personal world press upon her, but also her internal struggle with the course content and client work was also having a powerful effect. The fears expressed for the art therapy profession were her projection of fears for herself. I need also to point out here that she was an international student whose country was thousands of miles away. Her loss of personal contact with her family and friends upset her deeply and the change of culture to that of the UK was very distressing for her at times. Much of what she felt was unfair was due to the accumulation of demands upon her life, yet she realised that she had made the decision to train in this country after carefully researching courses at home and abroad. There were also many feelings of despair coming from other trainees on her course, fearing that gaining work as art therapists was likely to be very hard to achieve. She felt this to be a very harsh situation as she'd sacrificed so much to attend the course in the UK.

At the time I had some powerful transference experiences through her image of this creature (see Figure 8.3). Within the creature there is a sense of attack upon others: by the world, the training course and myself.

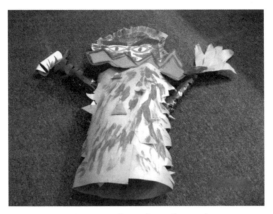

Figure 8.3 (See colour plate 14)

I felt the cardboard creature to be a representation of myself. It was helpful for me to understand that I could be imagined as an alarming assessor and a representative of the training organisation. My client may not have felt this consciously yet it held for me my own sense of transference to the experience of my own training. I was often fearful of being judged when I was being trained. So there was for me a possible confluence of paranoid feelings between my client's training, my own training and the potential collusion in the therapy room.

Example 3

I had provided personal art therapy for another trainee art therapist for quite a long time when he began asking questions and creating images that implied he had ambiguous feelings towards me as the therapist. He wanted to know who else I was giving art therapy to and what kind of people they were and tried teasing out information from me. Perhaps he was hoping I would compare him with my other clients and indicate that he was 'special'. He also wanted to know how busy I was so that he could know more about my status as 'his' art therapist. The trainee created an image of the therapist as a powerful figure who could be both rewarding and persecutory. I experienced it as a projective process, one which could be explored and understood – the projection is connected with judgement, competition and comparison, and is expressed by the trainee's questions and images.

The themes of judge, father, king and God as projections onto me, the therapist, were used to access the internal transference relationship within the trainee's internal world. These projections were also used to locate 'the therapist' in relation to the college by asking where I trained and what links existed between me and the training course. Questions sought to assuage the suspicion or the fear that I was part of this web of analysis, assessment and judgemental decision making.

As a therapist these projections are not unusual outside of the training situation with clients. Yet knowing this, it is particularly valuable to hold these projections and work with these fears and illusions to help the trainee find their own insights in the context of becoming a therapist.

Example 4

I have worked with a number of trainees who struggle with the demands of their training. Doubts, questioning, resubmitting work and potentially failing the course can make the therapist a target for anger, due in part to the therapist's evident 'success' as a therapist. Questions and insinuations also abounded as the trainee art therapist challenged me with goading challenges, such as: Whose side are you on? Do you think the college is right? Don't you think that I would make a good therapist? Will I ever make it? My art is crap anyway.

With these trainees it was vital that I could hold a balanced position, despite my own issues around authority and potential failure. The counter-transference relationship does struggle to take sides, thinking of the welfare of the trainee and whether the training institution is being unfair, hypercritical or harsh in their judgements. I felt drawn into being an adjudicator, to have an opinion and at times a fantasy of checking in with the college. But no, the need to hold the client through this won through, and I found faith in the training organisation's capacity to make academic decisions about its trainee's level of knowledge and skills in becoming a practitioner in the field of art therapy.

At times we struggle to overcome over-verbalisation, including that of metaphors, and find it difficult to interrupt the flow of words.

To suggest introducing materials and art work may feel clumsy and too intrusive to the thought process. In this case it became useful to have the confidence to say, 'There is time to make an image/marks.' By doing so we can overcome the enchantment of words by having the art work as an alternative core to the therapy.

Holding the Dynamics: The Therapist's Attachments and Counter-Transference Dynamics

Holding a theoretical framework is important for the therapist on a personal and professional level; the times when we are tempted to react to our counter-transferences (images and the trainee's personal material) are opportunities to learn and evaluate our own attachment responses to a profession which we belong to and which sets the standards and expectations with which we work. The therapist's own training experience would have placed her/him in a similarly regressed relationship with the training institution, which may evoke within us a counter-transference, which can affect our ability to provide a secure base.

Primarily as art therapists we are working with the chaos and caution of creativity. In comparison to verbal therapy we have a creative background in the visual and plastic arts. The image or object holds a strong attachment for the trainee as well as raising responses within myself as therapist. We are trained to consider the process of art making in sessions as material for understanding the concerns of our trainee/client.

> What the notion of art's role in therapy has done, however, is to create professional identity problems for students and colleagues because it blurs the differentiation between art therapy and other psychotherapies. It does a real disservice to downplay the importance of aesthetic sensibility as fundamental to the role and function of an art therapist. (Robbins 1987, p.15)

Of course, other fantasies might arise for the trainee as to the kind of art that is 'art therapy' art. In most of my experience I have found trainees very keen to use materials and to find the unique nature of art therapy to be confirmed within their own work. This helps to clarify for me the difference between my art created as an art student, art/images made during my art psychotherapy training, and my current art practice. My feelings of engagement and attachment to the art and creative work in the sessions go so deep at times that I feel envy at the trainee's ability to use the materials, my relief that they are actually using materials (I am an art therapist after all) and excitement about the depth of emotional and personal development for the trainee that is contained in both the process and product of art work in the sessions. My attachment to this process is one which has often raised my own experiences of grappling with art materials, which is often in parallel with those of the trainee.

Private Practice Extensions?

As a private practitioner it is important to be aware of what I call 'extensions' to the clinical work. How do I respond, for example, to requests that are made outside of the therapeutic hour? I have been asked if I can agree to provide my therapy notes to a solicitor to support my client in an upcoming legal case. I've also been asked to support another client's application for independent living support. More recently I've been asked by another client for a reference for a job. These have challenged my firm principles of keeping the dynamics of my client/therapist relationships firmly within the therapy setting. Yet, my background of community and social work as a helper also pulls me towards the wider community. I've brought these dilemmas into this chapter as a prudent reminder that we have to deal with, understand and sometimes interpret these extensions into the private setting. These requests are not always as straightforward as we might imagine.

Conclusion

Sometimes the splits and projections that develop can be seen when the student complains about the unfairness of the training or clinical work placement compared with how good the supportive 'all-knowing' therapist seems to be. These comments can appear to be pulling us off-centre in the transference relationship; clients may attempt to seduce us into a collusive exclusivity which we, the therapists, find helpful to view from the attachment model and considering our own internal attachment positions. These may be related to wanting to be a secure base for another, wishing to be seduced and appreciated by our clients, or even a reaction against the training institution which we continue to carry in our own internal model since our own training experience.

As counter-transference issues, these require analysis and deconstruction within our own supervision.

For the private practitioner our social and ethical responsibility is considerable in providing therapy in a confidential setting to trainee therapists. It is the trainee's right to expect the focus to be upon their personal therapy and it is our aim to provide 'best practice' to enable our trainee clients to engage with the complexities of art therapy training whilst also engaging in their own confidential process of personal art therapy. It is important to consider that we are also in the position of forming art therapy colleagues and experience both present and future overlaps of interest that require sensitive handling within the therapy as well as in the 'real world' where practitioners, students on placement and colleagues at AGMs or regional meetings can, and do, meet in the shared spaces of a small profession.

I have found that working with trainees requires awareness of the complexities as well as a high level of skill and experience. It is vital to engage in good supervision focused upon the dynamics and attachments presented by both trainee and therapist within the spectre of the training institution, the student placement and personal therapy. This is essential insurance against potential conflicts of attention as we find the bear traps of the unconscious are there to confound us in our professional practice. When overlaps occur, or boundaries become merged, we need professional competence and guidance to handle the richness of potential 'mistake-making', and enable the growth of the trainee in a tough and intriguing psychological environment.

The guidance I can offer to private practitioners when working with trainees is as follows:

- Ensure that good supervision is available on a regular basis with an experienced art psychotherapist who is also engaged in private practice.

- Join or develop a network of other art therapists working in private practice who are also working with trainees.

- Be confident about the value that you bring to the trainee's experience in therapy.

- Consider the benefits for the trainee of starting their therapy before their course has begun. This gives them a more solid basis to understanding therapy in relation to their training.

- Be open to surprises and challenges in the creative work, both that developed in the therapy sessions and that (very often unseen) made by the trainees during their time on their courses.

- Be aware of the attachment challenges to your own training. In addition, be aware of the transference to your training institutions for both you and the trainee.

- Understand the potential to be pulled toward roles such as tutor, assessor, artist, parent, colluder, the envious one and so on, by realising that these are helpful as well as potentially challenging dynamics.

- Ensure that you have worked privately with a considerable number of clients before taking on art therapy trainees.

- Explain clearly to the trainee at the beginning of the therapy why it is considered vital for trainee art therapists to have their own personal therapy, what the role of the therapist is in this relationship and the limits of any information given to the training institution. In this way, the trainee's fears and paranoia regarding the confidentiality of their therapy and reporting back to their training institution can be allayed and they will feel more liberated in their own therapy.

- 'Extensions' to clinical work outside of the therapeutic hour need to be carefully thought through. Consider all implications and consequences before taking any further action.

References

Ainsworth, M. and Wittig, B. (1969) 'Attachment and Exploratory Behaviour of One-Year-Olds in a Strange Situation.' In B.M. Foss (ed.) *Determinants of Infant Behaviour*, Volume 4. London: Methuen.

Carswell, C. (2007) 'On struggle, study and success.' *Therapy Today 18*, 10, 17–19.

Dudley, J., Gilroy, A. and Skaife, S. (2000) 'Teachers, Students, Clients, Therapists, Researchers: Changing Gear in Experiential Art Therapy Groups.' In A. Gilroy and G. McNeilly (eds) *The Changing Face of Art Therapy*. London: Jessica Kingsley Publishers.

Field, N. (1992) 'The way of imperfection.' *British Journal of Psychotherapy 9*, 2, 139–147.

Gomez, D. (2015) 'Art as an encounter.' *Philosophy Now 108*, 6–8.

Robbins, A. (1987) *The Artist as Therapist*. New York: Human Sciences Press.

Part IV

GOVERNANCE AND SUPERVISION

9

MANAGING AND NOT MANAGING

The Limits of a Small Private Practice

—— KATE ROTHWELL ——

In this chapter I will be sharing aspects of my clinical experience and learning from running a small private art therapy practice for the past 15 years where I provide supervision to therapist practitioners, and therapy to trainee art therapists and adult, adolescent and child clients. What I hope to offer other practitioners considering going into private practice is an insight into what support networks must be in place to manage within the parameters of a practice limited by the lack of support available in a public setting. I also hope to emphasise the importance of qualities not available in the public sector with the lack of availability of long-term therapeutic work.

With the reduction in service availability in the National Health Service (NHS) settings for children and, increasingly, adults, there is a move towards private arrangements. It is forecast that there will be a severe decline in infant and child clinical services available through Child and Adolescent Mental Health Services (CAMHS) and post-adoption and fostering services over the next five years. This will inevitably cause a shift towards private services for those able to afford treatment. Another deciding factor for clients who choose to go into private practice is to avoid a state-recorded health record, and some people are wealthy enough to always exercise their preference for private treatment.

To illustrate the issues I will share two case examples from my practice with clients who have conditions that may not meet the criteria for public services and evidence the importance of acquiring essential information to determine whether or not to take a case where complex behaviour is implied. I discuss what influence this can have on the management of a small art therapy practice, the importance of knowing what support networks are available to the client and the therapist, and what must be considered in any decisions made in taking on a new referral.

The first example is with an adult patient whose seemingly overt aggressive forensic history implied unsuitability in a remote private practice, but the critical deciding factor was a strong, communicative and supportive network. The second example is of a child client whose resistance to therapy contraindicated an ability to work within the therapeutic frame applied. From the outset both cases suggested an unsuccessful outcome. The success of the therapeutic endeavour is seated within the commitment of the available support network, the commitment of the client to use art making as therapy, the client's and therapist's capacity for relational attunement, and the commitment of the therapist to work with the challenges presented to understand the underlying complexities.

In every case, whether challenging behaviour remains dormant or enacted, expressive or unexpressed, the clinical practice and therapeutic frame remain constant. The deciding factor is whether, with a strong support network, any challenging behaviour can be contained, but in all cases adherence to Health and Care Professions Council (HCPC) Standards of Proficiency is required and conduct of the therapeutic practice is structurally the same in private practice as it would be in public practice. What typifies both cases described is the central use of the image-making process as the agent of change and the importance of art making to inform communication within the therapeutic relationship.

Starting a Private Practice

There are many aspects integral to starting a private practice that are essentially different to starting up a service in a public setting, not least registering as a private business, ensuring sufficient and suitable professional indemnity is in place, and acquiring data protection licensing and DBS (Disclosure and Barring Service) certification. Most vital is clinical supervision, required by the HCPC to ensure accountability. Supervision provides a necessary structure in the absence of a back-up team, ordinarily available in a public setting, when the therapist is the sole practitioner in a private practice and responsible for all aspects of the service. This can be more exposing for the practitioner without the protection of a team and therefore forces the issue of a careful and highly considered assessment to ascertain the compatibility of the practice and the therapist's skills with client need.

Discussing cases in supervision prior to the assessment will also enable a thoughtful process to consider the suitability of the client for the practice. This is vital for the protection of the therapist and for the client. It may be necessary to discuss the case with teachers and other professionals known to the client to gain a perspective of the case in order to make an informed decision as to whether to accept the referral.

There may be many expectations held by the client, or the parents/carer if the client is a child, ranging from financial implications, the therapist's skills and availability, the duration of treatment and an often dubious awareness of the art therapy approach. For this reason it is essential that an initial meeting is held to outline the terms and conditions of the contract and inform the client and carers of the importance of time and duration boundaries. This also gives the client an opportunity to ask questions and ascertain if the approach is what they hoped for and if they think they can work with the therapist. Time scale should be discussed, as should the commitment expected to allay any misunderstandings from the outset.

Reviews should be put in place to assess progress and provide opportunities to discuss changes evident in the client, whether this is observed to be improvements or deteriorations. Private practitioners may need to make use of other colleagues to work within the structure. Parents may also be considered co-workers within the frame through regular reviews, updates and informal contact. Although this model is not part of my experience in the public sector, it is not unusual for me to bring parents in to the session to discuss how the work can be bridged into home life and how they can support the client between sessions.

The network available to the client needs to be discussed in the initial meeting. This may include the immediate family and other relatives or friends, or organisations connected to the client, whether schools, teachers or other professionals, and the client should be made aware of the therapist's network by providing information on the supervisor, the HCPC and the professional body by providing the therapist's registration details, accessible online. Once an agreement has been met the therapist may inform the client's general practitioner (GP) by letter of the client's contract to enter into a private arrangement with the therapist. The letter should be kept on file with the proviso that the client's consent will be sought first before contacting a GP, but if there is an issue of safety this may be overridden. At the very least therapists must seek GPs' details. Equally the GP, understood to hold clinical responsibility, may be informed when the contract has ended and the client has been discharged from the practice. This is necessary to observe professional accountability and upholds HCPC standards that recognise that private practitioners are personally responsible for the practice and must be able to justify their decisions. Informing the GP ensures there is knowledge held at a primary level of care of the client entering into private practice, which could be a useful source of information either relayed or received if more support is required or the client needs to be referred back into public health systems. However, this is not always the case, and from my experience I have had occasion to call for police assistance and found them to be the more caring and better informed option.

The Setting

There are many important considerations and challenges to be taken into account that are integral to managing a small art therapy private practice given its location in the community. The practice discussed here is a purpose-built studio dedicated solely to art therapy, securely accommodated within a domestic garden surrounded by residential properties and accessed by a separate path leading up to the studio from a driveway. The studio space is devoted to art making. HCPC Standard 14.18 states that, 'Practitioners must be able to use a range of art and art-making materials and techniques competently and be able to help a service user to work with these.'

With this in mind there is a large table, with a smaller table underneath, on which sits a choice of spray paint, felt tips, paper towels and hand wipes. There is a well-stocked book shelf, two stacked chairs and two chairs by the table, a settee, a cupboard supplied with various assorted sizes and colours of paper and card, toys, dry materials including chalks, pencils, wax and oil pastels, and a shelving unit holding paints, pallets, brushes, inks, Modroc, clay, glue, rulers, scissors, small knives, clay tools, erasers, watercolour paints and masking tape. A child-size wicker chair with soft toys sits by a large cardboard box of odds and ends; a light box is available. All this is surrounded by portfolios from past and current work. Each client is given their own folder to safely contain their work between sessions. There is decking external to the cabin on which stands a plastic table and chairs for outdoor work. The studio is well lit with natural light from two main windows and electric light supplied by three ceiling dimmer lights, a desk lamp and a standing lamp. There are five double electricity points, a radio, hair dryer, fan and heater to regulate the temperature. There are two small clocks, one positioned for the therapist who sits on the settee and the other beside the therapist on a small table for the client. Further to HCPC Regulation 15.3, 'to be able to work safely, including being able to select appropriate hazard control and risk management, in a safe manner and in accordance with health and safety legislation', the client has use of plastic aprons to protect their clothes, synthetic gloves if unable to touch wet materials and face masks if using spray paints, and there is a first aid kit on site. Although there is no running water, a supply is kept in a large container and warm water is brought in prior to the session. Practitioners would be wise to ensure they have regular training in personal protection, CPR (cardiopulmonary resuscitation) and first aid in the event of an incident. Public liability insurance also covers the potential for accidents in the setting, and so the therapist must ensure they have adequate and appropriate insurance.

The studio has a lockable door to ensure physical security. The position of the studio affords privacy if the client wants to leave the door open during the session. The practice is a standalone room, purpose built for art therapy, which provides a unique situation different from walking into a building and through to a room possibly used for other interventions. This space is accessible and flexible. Clients can take ownership of the space and adapt it to their needs. Here they have the chance to shed away everyday life and find new ways of being. Furniture can be moved and the space changed to accommodate the activity at the time within the spatial boundaries, restricted only by the walls and floor. Though a clinical space, it is not clinical in appearance as objects are on view, there is evidence of others' use of the space in the form of marks on the tables, walls and matting, smells from art materials linger and materials get put back in different places. There are found objects brought into the studio and left whilst work is in progress, including a stepladder and multiple boxes. Children visiting the studio remark that it's like a Wendy house, adults look round and suggest how they would make use of the space. It is a retreat, a sanctuary and a safe space. It exists as a place separate from anywhere else without reference to any other place and can become whatever the client's imagination wants it to be in the time they are there.

Here the emphasis is on art making. Clients are invited to use art materials, and the provision of the space invites creativity. It is a working studio where people are using their creative side through the promotion of art making. This may be the start of a new experience for clients or the opportunity to focus solely on art making as a central means of communicating. Here art therapy is not complementary, or an adjunct to other therapies – it is the central priority.

Professional Competency

To ensure safety for both client and therapist in a private practice it is vital therapists work in their area of competency and remain aware of their level of competency. HCPC Standards of Proficiency (HCPC 2013) expect that practitioners work in the area they are capable of working in, and state:

> Your scope of practice is the area or areas of your profession in which you have the knowledge, skills and experience to practise lawfully, safely and effectively, in a way that meets our standards and does not pose any danger to the public or to yourself.

This standard makes common sense and is essential given the current lack of private practice training within the art therapy training in organisations. Furthermore professional reputation is key to private practice and links to HCPC Standard 3.1: 'Understand the need to maintain high standards of personal and professional conduct.'

These specific standards provide guidance of best and safe practice and ultimately advise practitioners to know their limits, including the range of skills, knowledge and capacity in the context of which cases to take and which to decline. Practitioners must also, under HCPC Standard 4.3, 'Be able to initiate resolution of problems and be able to exercise personal initiative,' and 13.10, 'Understand the therapeutic relationship, including its limitations.' The parameters of the practice are limited by the therapist's expertise and the practice space. This must be acknowledged to work lawfully and can be explored in supervision when a referral is made to consider realistically if what is being sought by the client can be offered by the therapist.

Referrals

Referrals to this practice are generally through word of mouth, via professional network structures or private practice listings. On receipt of a referral an initial meeting is offered to the client, and the parents/carer if the client is a child or adolescent, to discuss the issues that have brought them to seek private therapy and indeed art therapy. The next stage is to meet other family, friends or professionals to build more of a picture of the issues causing concern and what hopes are held for the therapy. Most referrals have specifically sought art therapy believing the approach will enhance the client's capacity to engage through non-verbal processes. Occasionally art therapy has been chosen because the client is interested in art, but more often there is a perception that non-verbal processes may improve communication. Usually the client has had some involvement with public services but found systems sorely lacking or the service provision has broken down causing them to seek a private arrangement.

In the two cases discussed Peter was referred by his sister, Joe by his parents. The client's family or carers were encouraged to describe the presenting behaviour they considered to be the problem. The initial meeting purely outlined the therapist's approach, the terms and conditions and the structure. This enables the client and therapist to decide if they want to continue on to assessment and if they think they can make the commitment. For some clients this may mean travelling long distances, and carers or family having to wait for the duration of the session and giving up their time on a regular basis for what may be several years at considerable financial expense. This is a serious undertaking, the success of which is debatable and uncertain from the outset, and it may be some time before changes are apparent. This will be further discussed in the case studies of Peter and Joe.

The cases detail different approaches to private art therapy and some of the very different processes that unfold in the course of therapy. In Peter's case, therapy has been ongoing for seven years. For Joe, a ten-week period was initially offered to support his transition into a new class at school but therapy has now continued for over a year.

Peter

Peter (who asked for his real name to be used) began therapy on 1 May 2009. He and his sister chose to find an art therapist in their locality because of the paucity of therapeutic opportunities in the community with relevant organisations, complicated by his high level of functioning and the demands he made on others given his acquired brain injury. Peter had an interest in art as an innate form of personal expression but also had a long forensic psychiatric history. It was for this reason the couple sought a therapist with specialist forensic experience.

In the initial meeting I was given the full history of Peter's life pre- and post-brain injury. It was explained to me by Peter that he had very specific needs for therapy and that his behaviour could be a challenge due to his disability. Both Peter and his sister made the effort to go into great detail to furnish me with all the facts I would need to decide if I could take on this work. They also appeared to want to observe my reaction to his story given the level of past expressed aggression. Peter had received individual therapy in a secure setting for many years and had a clear understanding of therapeutic boundaries. He also had a strong supportive and communicative network of family members involved in his care who were invested in his receiving ongoing therapy.

Although Peter's past history did not indicate it would be safe practice to be seen in a small private service, I agreed to assess him, feeling I had been helped to make an informed decision by his sister.

I agreed to an extended assessment to accommodate his disability and extreme short-term memory problems. In his assessment Peter was highly anxious, and at times elated and verbose. I was placed in a position of observer with little opportunity to interact other than support his requests for art materials. Peter was heavily defended against feelings of anxiety and would speak about anything that came into his mind at the time. Gradually as he became more trusting and comfortable in my presence, Peter spoke with more authenticity and opened up about his past. He was able to provide me with an extraordinary picture of the emotional impact of loss on his life, including the death of his mother when Peter was three years old and the death of his father at 16 years old, and how his father's family raised him and his brother. Peter spoke about his offences and shared times when he still felt like hurting people and what prevented him from doing so.

All the while Peter contained symbolic aggression, confusion and chaos in his art making. Though I was fully aware of the risks, I felt this would not prevent me from doing the work as I was assured by his intention to keep us both safe, and by the presence of his family who, for the first few years, brought him to sessions until it was deemed he could manage to drive himself and could be trusted to respect the time frame of the session. As Peter's independence and self-awareness deepened through therapy, his need to express his aggression through the work changed. He became more able to hear the therapist and share his thoughts. His defences softened as his attachment to the therapy grew. All the while his sister maintained regular communication on challenging issues that arose outside of the sessions and on his progression. I was supported to pre-empt what he might be bringing into session and learnt how to accommodate his unusual presentation so he could make the most effective use of what I was able to offer in therapy. Peter made positive use of the therapeutic structure, and although aggression was implied from the outset of therapy, he held to the boundaries that would keep us both safe.

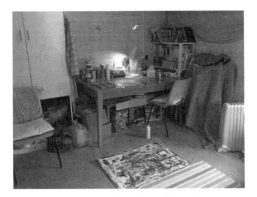

Figure 9.1 (See colour plate 15)

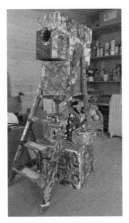

Figure 9.2 (See colour plate 16)

Joe

Joe (pseudonym), eight years old, began therapy in April 2015. Joe's parents informed me that their son began to show problems at school in Year 2. Previously there had been no concerns in class, although the parents had concerns since reception about Joe's sensory difficulties and behaviour at home. He was diagnosed with attention deficit hyperactivity disorder (ADHD), sensory processing disorder and a visual squint. He was found to have problems with auditory processing and some hypermobility. He had an educational psychologist assessment and a physiotherapy assessment, which didn't detect dyslexia or dyspraxia. Joe trialled three different ADHD medications over a six-month period, and his symptoms were considered to be under control. During the various assessments concerns were raised about autism. Initially Joe's parents could not identify with the possible diagnosis, but in the year since it was first suggested it became more obvious in Joe, especially since the medication calmed the ADHD down. Joe was referred for an NHS assessment, and a private diagnosis to speed up his access to local services was being considered.

Joe's anxiety was reported to have steadily increased in the previous year and by November he showed signs of clinical depression and was unable to leave his room. He had two weeks of school refusal and chewed his fingers so badly they were sore and bleeding. Joe was seen by CAMHS from June 2014 and in the autumn received a course of cognitive behavioural therapy (CBT) for his specific phobias. It was reported to have worked really well and his phobias improved.

With interventions from CAMHS and the charity ADD-Vance, the situation improved in December and January, and by the February half-term the parents saw significant improvements in Joe's mental health and subsequent behaviour at home. He had a successful school holiday and felt positive about his return to school. However, within four days of returning, Joe was threatening to kill himself. The situation continued to worsen and Joe became so anxious and violent at home that CAMHS referred the family to social services in order to protect his sister. Joe was refusing school and his hours were reduced in an attempt to lower his anxiety levels and his violent behaviour at home. The parents wanted private therapy to focus on identifying triggers in the school day that caused his anxiety, as he was unable to say what these were, but his family believed that he was masking his fears.

Joe had an assessment by a developmental paediatrician and was diagnosed with autism spectrum disorder, attention deficit disorder, sleep disorder and anxiety disorder, for which independent psychotherapy was recommended to address his anxiety, emotional regulation and chronic motor and vocal tics.

In the meeting with Joe and his parents he sat firmly embedded between mother and father. A small, pale, tired-looking child, he disappeared between them but also made his presence felt by demanding their attention. In conversation the parents explained that Joe struggled to get himself to sleep and often woke in the early morning after having nightmares and climbed in beside his mother, forcing his father out of the marital bed and into the spare room. Both parents looked exasperated and said it had been an extremely trying year, leaving them exhausted. Joe presented as younger than his years and behaved as if wanting to be babied.

Whilst we spoke Joe momentarily looked around the room before deciding to get up and look at the art materials. The parents became anxious that he didn't touch anything he shouldn't, but I felt some promise that what he saw sparked his curiosity. I suggested another meeting including his sister to see how the family interacted. The next time we met, the whole family arrived together and the children entered the studio with excitement. As both children expressed an interest in the art materials they were invited to use them. Again the parents spoke of the demands they faced at home trying to manage Joe, and their fears that he would one day go too far. Everyone was on tenterhooks and had hopes that the therapy would provide the support so desperately needed. Joe's experience at school was discussed, including how teachers had not adapted their practice to support him. The parents, support networks were discussed candidly later in a Skype meeting when the children were not present.

An assessment was agreed and his father brought Joe. As Joe had a robust support network both from his parents and his new teacher, it seemed there was enough commitment to support the work. After several sessions where Joe resisted engaging with art materials or allowing his father to leave him, it was decided to invite the parents to another meeting with the therapist and the supervisor, who originally passed on the referral, to discuss how to support the parents further in an attempt to move the work forward.

As an improvement in Joe's emotional world was evident after the summer holiday, I decided to tackle the issue of father and computer in session to see if it would be possible to enable Joe to separate from his comforters. Joe was again resistant and regressed but allowed his father to sit outside the studio. Joe was quiet and anxious in my company; his solution was to hide under a blanket for a few sessions until he decided he was too hot and chose to join me at the table to make art. It took over a year for Joe to arrive at a point when we could play together and for him to come into the session on his own and without his computer.

Below, Joe's parents describe their perspective of his progress in art therapy.

Parental Perspective

We were determined to persevere with the therapy despite these difficulties, as we saw no other way out of our desperate situation if it failed. It took several months of this really difficult behaviour before Joe began to relax slightly about attending. He has now been attending for 15 months and he happily gets ready and goes to the sessions and is very happy when he returns home. He no longer self-harms, is sleeping and eating better, can leave the house and enjoy life in his own way and is generally happy!

Joe attends an independent school, which has been very open and happy to engage in working with Joe's therapist. When Joe entered the new school year five months after starting the therapy, his new teacher and the therapist discussed the situation and how best to proceed. During the first term when Joe was settling into the new school year, his teacher and therapist continued to work together to undo the damage caused by his previous teacher. As we approach the end of this school year, Joe is unrecognisable from the child he was 12 months ago. His difficulties remain, but with the support of his current teacher and the continued support of his therapist, Joe is happy, and able to play a full role in school life, including sport matches, drama activities and social activities.

For us as parents the open and honest relationship between Joe's school and therapist has been key in his recovery. Both parties have been focused solely on Joe's best interests with no agenda or consideration of resources, as would be the key in the state/NHS sectors. We hope this relationship will continue to support Joe as he moves forward into the next school year and eventually into senior school.

Discussion

Private practice has no time restrictions. With parental commitment to the therapy, Joe has been supported to work at his own pace with no conditions set by targets, budget, waiting lists, capacity or resources that put pressure on a public service. The opportunity for access to a facilitating environment appears to have enabled Joe to take ownership of the space to develop self-agency to practise his potency over the situation.

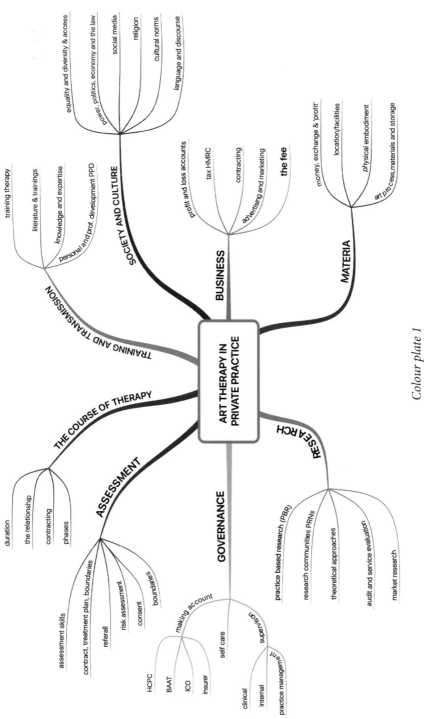

Colour plate 1

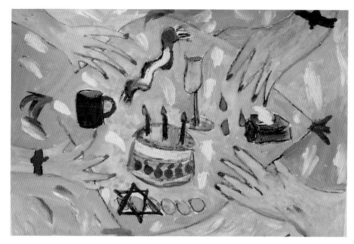

Colour plate 2

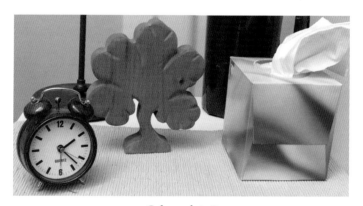

Colour plate 3

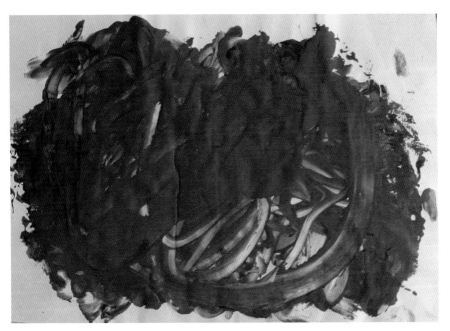

Colour plate 4

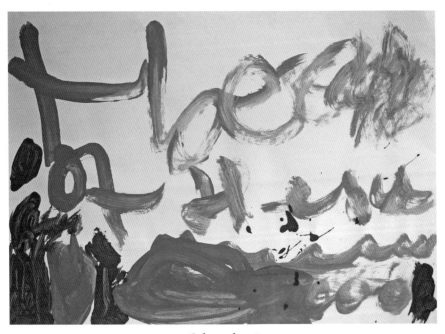

Colour plate 5

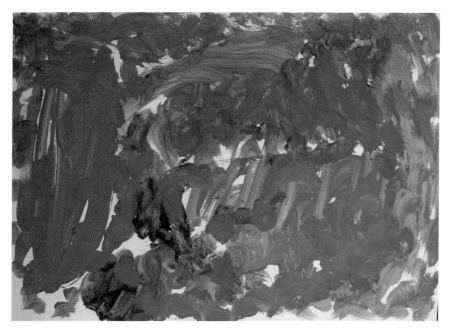

Colour plate 6

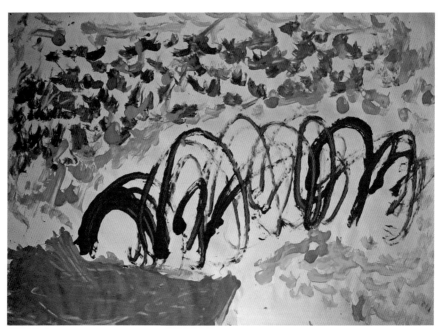

Colour plate 7

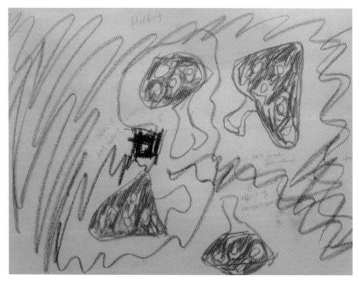

Colour plate 8

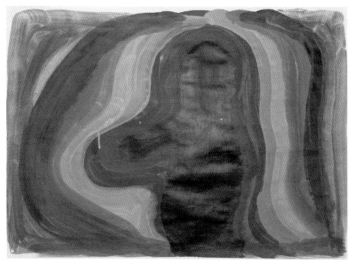

Colour plate 9

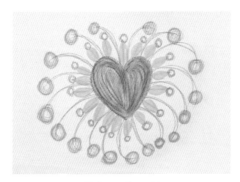

Colour plate 10

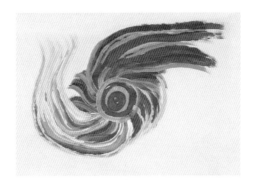

Colour plate 11

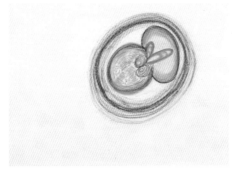

Colour plate 12

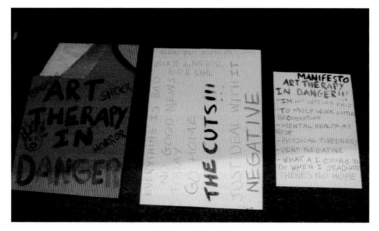

Colour plate 13

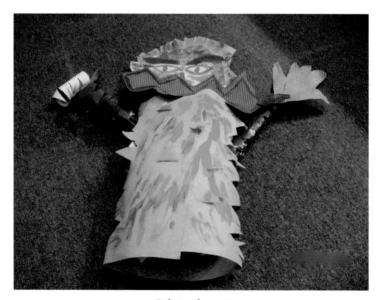

Colour plate 14

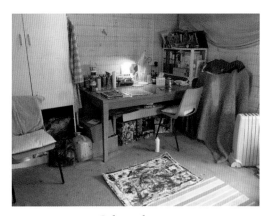

Colour plate 15

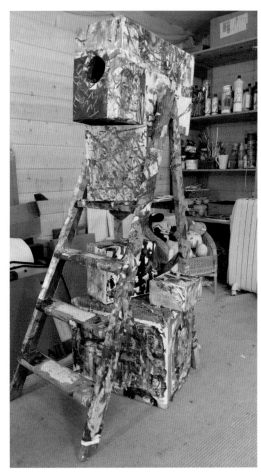

Colour plate 16

For Peter the cohesive integration and complete transparency of his support network made therapy safe and enabled consistency, preventing any need for use of aggression whilst knowing it was implied through symbolic semiotic processes, which could be communicated in non-harmful ways. This made it possible to work with Peter despite the vulnerability of the practice.

The objective of therapy in both cases was to find ways of adhering to a social environment and structure in a more harmonious way. Using the process of therapy to support both Joe and Peter to reduce aggressive defences provides the potential for emplotment (Calabrese 2008). The potential for therapeutic emplotment in practice works through a process of role modelling a more socially acceptable way of being. For Joe, knowing more about his circumstances at the initial phases of the work made it possible to support him to perceive his place in his family differently, moving from a position where he is expected to be on the defensive to one of adherence to societal norms, thereby enabling him to behave differently through a process of emplotment. Emplotment involves 'making a configuration in time, creating a whole out of a succession of events' (Mattingly 1994, p.812). This term was originally coined by Frye (1957) to explain four archetypal plot structures within the constructs of romance, tragedy, comedy and satire (Mattingly 1994). Historical plot structures can be viewed through narratives as an 'emplotment'; this offers an explanation of the 'plot' (White 1987). Therefore, 'It is the plot which makes individual events understandable as part of a coherent whole, one which leads compellingly towards a particular ending' (White 1987, quoted in Mattingly 1994, p.812).

It was Ricoeur, a hermeneutic philosopher, who positioned these ideas within structural plots of life through the concept of time and human temporality: that is, 'the state of existing or having some relationship with time' (Ricoeur 1981). Mattingly uses the constructs of emplotment to consider the use of stories created in time as essential to a sense of the meaningfulness of life when the story is unknown, to create a sense of purpose and coherency. In other words it supports a beginning, middle and ending as a meaningful whole when there is little predictability or few aspects of the plot that can be controlled. Emplotment allows for unpredictability: 'It is time marked by an effort at transformation' (Mattingly 1994, p.819).

'The therapist's clinical task is to create a therapeutic plot which compels a patient to see therapy as integral to healing' (Mattingly 1994, p.814). I see this as essential in private practice where there is little known at the start of the therapeutic relationship, where the client comes with an untold story that needs space, place and time to reveal itself through the process of therapy. There can be no pre-planned treatment script, yet the availability of the constructs of therapy needs to become known by the client through the therapist's guidance, rather than dictated through pre-placed pathways that exist in a public setting. With the inclusion of the image in art therapy, the unpredictability increases the unknowingness of the plot as a third object in the relationship yet to be created.

For the new client in private practice there is even more unknowing-ness. If the desire is there to inhabit the space and see the therapist as an ally in the potential transformation, the ingredients for emplotment can become active. The client can move from a passive to active position in his or her own 'plot'; therefore the stage is set and the actors present. The narrative element enables art therapists to gain much from considering how narrative frames the picture and events usefully and therapeutically, empowering the client as an agent. Unlike public services, where referrals often come with unsubstantiated narratives and histories created around clients in the NHS, in private practice there is the opportunity of creating narratives between therapist and client that can unfold collaboratively.

This applies to attachment theory where information on the client and their family's attachment histories need to be made known as a vital component of the assessment phase in preparation for the emplotment of the course of therapy.

Conclusion

Ultimately the lesson learnt is that the more the therapist in private practice knows about the client's familial and social structure the better. Time, duration and commitment are important ingredients in an art therapy private practice to ensure a realistic structure can be consistently relied upon, as is the therapist's awareness of their level of competency in accordance with HCPC Standards of Proficiency.

The skills gleaned by the therapist through experience are sought by the client, as is transparency about the client's support network in communications around their progression or deterioration in and outside the therapy. Having a strong support network for therapy is vital to managing complex behaviour in a small and vulnerably situated private practice.

References

Calabrese, J.D. (2008) 'Clinical paradigm clashes: Ethnocentric and political barriers to Native American efforts at self-healing.' *Ethos 3*, 3, 334–353.

Frye, N. (1957) *Anatomy of Criticism*. Princeton, NJ: Princeton University Press.

HCPC (2013) *Standards of Proficiency: Arts Therapists*. London: HCPC.

Mattingly, C. (1994) 'The concept of therapeutic "emplotment".' *Social Science and Medicine 38*, 6, 811–822.

Ricoeur, P. (1981) 'Narrative Time.' In W.T.J. Mitchell (ed.) *On Narrative*. Chicago, IL: University of Chicago.

White, H. (1981) 'The Value of Narrativity in the Representation of Reality.' In W.T.J. Mitchell (ed.) *On Narrative*. Chicago, IL: University of Chicago.

White, H. (1987) *The Content of the Form*. Baltimore, MD: Johns Hopkins University Press.

10

KNOCK KNOCK, WHO'S THERE?

Assessment of Risk in Private Practice

—— COLLEEN STEINER WESTLING ——

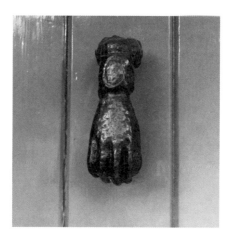

Introduction

When considering risk within the context of setting up a private practice, different images of potential negative outcomes may come to mind. In common with all these are situations that may be outside one's intention or control. How and what each therapist feels when considering the risk of working in private practice will be unique to their life experiences, which can influence risk perception, risk aversion and risk tolerance. There are the known practical risks as well as the unknown potential risks when moving from an organisational-based practice to a solo private practice. We can consider that, within an organisation, risk may be more planned for and held by the organisation, whereas in private practice, risk is held by the therapist and their supervisor. This paradigm shift may not sit comfortably with everyone.

In this chapter, we will explore the concept of risk including how we define risk; the neurological sense of fear and why it's important for risk assessment; how prolonged stress can challenge risk perception; how risk assessment can be regarded as an ongoing process; risks that private art therapists share with other modalities; and risks that may be specific to art therapists.

What Is Risk and What Do We Need to Be Aware Of?

The Oxford English Dictionary (2017) defines risk as 'exposure to possibilities of loss, injury or other adverse or unwelcome circumstances; a chance or situation involving such a possibility'. While this definition is clear, it falls short of calling to mind or body the feeling of risk, which requires an acknowledgement of fear.

Living the life of a human contains so many potential hazards that we are biologically wired for at both conscious and unconscious levels. When we consider the concept of risk with known and unknown hazards, we may feel overwhelmed and so believe that everything is a potential risk. To help us think about the topic, Reeves (2015) breaks down the risks therapists need to juggle into five contexts: 'Situational, Relational, Contextual, Professional and Personal' (p.13). We may consider these facets of our work, with the realisation that 'We are in a constant process of being at risk in different ways and at different times' (p.3). Contemplating whether we can ever control risk, or just mitigate it, brings to consciousness what we may need to be aware of and how we may codify or learn from developed awareness. We can also wonder if a codified risk assessment will truly aid risk mitigation and management, and how ongoing assessments of risk may be gauged as a client progresses and possibly changes. This makes assessing and reassessing risk with updated awareness on the contextual conditions important to our practices as a whole.

What Happens when We Are in Danger and How We Actually Respond to Risk

We have new scientific evidence from neuroscientific advances in mind/body theories and, with this in mind, we will look at the neurological process of emotional response to risk and how this may impact practical responses to risk assessment in a private art therapy practice. In order to bring more focus and understanding of why risk and fear are necessary partners towards safety, we will start from the inside and work outward.

Fear can be seen as a useful element in risk assessment as long as one stays with the feeling without avoidance or projection. Keeping the potential of a negative outcome in mind is a lot of work for the self to do, balancing neurological hemispheres of the mind from the catastrophic 'what if' sensing of the imagining mind to the ordered 'then that' sense-making of the logical mind. With attention and non-avoidance in considering risk mindfully, information can then rise to upper cortical brain regions for planning and strategising. During an experience of fear many neurological and physiological responses occur in both the brain and body. Over the past few decades, scientific advances in psychoneuroimmunology have greatly aided our understanding of how human beings process both external and internal stimuli, both emotionally and intellectually. Contributing greatly to these understandings have been the works of Joseph LeDoux, both A. Damasio and H. Damasio, Stephen Porges and Bessel van der Kolk. And, though there have been advances since Douglas MacLean first put forth his triune brain theory (MacLean 1990), it remains a useful way of viewing the brain from an evolutionary perspective.

According to the triune brain theory, the brain consists of three hierarchical levels. The first and oldest level is the brain stem region, called the reptilian brain, as it is this survival-response region of the brain that human beings share with reptiles. Next and central to the human brain is the limbic area, or the mammalian brain as it is often called, because it is the brain region capable of complex emotional processing shared with some mammals. Finally, in evolutionary terms, the youngest part of the brain, sitting on top of the first two levels, is the neocortex, the thinking brain, which resembles the grey squiggly object often illustrated as 'the brain'.

This way of ordering the brain's regions provides a generalised view for how stimuli are processed, noting that the emotional limbic region is stuck in between the lower survival networks and the higher regions of rational thought. To further elaborate, as the lower brain region relates to survival and is close to the emotional limbic structures, including the hippocampus, it also relates to memory. Risk perception, assessing and taking choices towards risk mitigation requires all three levels to be integrated and cross-referenced. Receiving information via the sympathetic nervous system (SNS), registering changes in sensations coming up from the body, and acting as the first order of feeling, the lower brain region induces primary emotions toward survival and assists in awareness of them in other people. Significantly acting as the brain's 'security guard', this region looks out for risks to the system as a whole, stimulating survival instincts and escaping danger. Additionally, the lower brain region reacts to information coming from higher brain regions in the form of thoughts, as in thinking of past experiences and projecting forward to imagine the future.

When risk perception accelerates beyond normal tolerance levels to create a feeling of intense fear, a neurological shortcut occurs to get the body to react with fight or flight. This is when the lower brain region is strongly triggered (by thoughts in the mind or sensations in the body), letting the whole system instantaneously know it is under threat by first creating a rapid (startle) response in the higher structures of the brain to wake it up to danger. Then, depending on the health and robustness of the neurological condition as a whole, either one of two paths will be taken: a long route or a short route of response. The order by which the long route occurs is as follows: first, sensory information is taken in and assessed in the thalamus, a structure acting as a 'relay station', which sends a message on to appropriate sensory areas of the brain (auditory cortex, visual cortex, etc.). There the information is evaluated and given meaning (Sounds like what? Looks like what?, etc.). This can be seen as the neurological process of evaluating whether what is before us is a risk or likely to become a hazard. The shorter route to processing fear, however, occurs when an overload of sensory information bypasses the thalamus and cortical pre-sorting and goes directly to the amygdalae for fast action, often coupled with strong emotions, as in panic. While this shortcut is very useful for survival, by quickly activating a response to danger, it can also affect our ability to think clearly. For instance, imagine seeing from the corner of your eye a mouse skitter across your kitchen floor. Instantly responding, you quickly jump onto a chair, dropping your mug of tea and plate of biscuits in the process, which shatter on the floor; after a moment, more closely observing the grey fuzzy ball and realising it is a collection of dust, you immediately release the fear, step back down and face the mess you've created out of panic. This illustrates how out of quick instinctual reactions to run away from fear, we can sometimes act on incorrect assumptions.

How Prolonged Stress Can Challenge Risk Perception

Generally, we are well equipped to tolerate and learn from periods of stress and are usually able to recoup physically and mentally once the stressful event or period of time is over. However, on the other end of the spectrum, both chronic stress (long-term fear) and sudden overwhelming trauma can set off an emergency response to the holistic brain/body system, greatly affecting the response to risk. During fight or flight responses, the overwhelmed lower brain region sets off a hormone response in the whole body to set it into action. To be specific, the system called the HPA axis (hypothalamus-pituitary-adrenal) is activated by the hypothalamus, a mid-brain structure, to release CRH (corticotrophin-releasing hormone), which signals the deep-brain pituitary gland to secrete ACTH (adrenocorticotrophic hormone), which goes on to stimulate the adrenal glands (sitting above the kidneys) to flood the whole body with the stress hormone cortisol (plus other hormones), generating the 'fight or flight' reaction. This fast-acting system for saving us from danger phylogenetically goes back to our pre-ancestral makeup as a leftover response from times when we needed quick reactions to an imminent threat like fighting an enemy or running away from a large-toothed tiger. And while this survival response serves us well when we have to deal with only occasional life-threatening experiences, chronic activation caused by consistent stressful stimulation can create imbalances to the body's systems as a whole. Additionally, chronic stress has been shown in some cases to negatively affect memory and dull concentration, both essential abilities in risk assessment. HPA axis activity often leaves a person exhausted and with the potential of being stuck in an infinite loop of ruminative negative thinking leading toward emotional and physical burnout and/or breakdown. Thankfully, the body's nervous systems (SNS and PNS) work in tandem to restore a state of balance (homeostasis). Essential to this is the PNS (parasympathetic nervous system), which when activated through rest, mind/body practices, deep breathing and so on has been shown to reduce stress in the whole system. As practitioners we face many potential risks and we are encouraged to remain open and aware of them in our work. It is therefore essential for private art therapists to practise self-care in managing stress. In order to face the difficulties and stresses of our clients' lives in practice, we must manage our own stress, otherwise we risk further compounding it in our work (for further information, see James D. West on self-care in Chapter 12).

Turning attention now away from biology and towards the outer world, but still with a view to risk, we will further explore what may inform our risk awareness.

Risk Assessment as Ongoing to the Therapeutic Process

The past few decades have seen a significant growth in research, litigation and debate, all leading to a transformation of current societal views on risk. In the UK and beyond, we have seen a rise in social and legal awareness influencing public policies, significantly influenced by the NHS and Community Care Act 1990, the Criminal Justice Act 1991, the Human Rights Act 1993, the Data Protection Act 1998 (and 2003), the Children Act 2004, the Mental Capacity Act 2007, the Equality Act 2010, the Mental Health Act 2014 and the Care Act 2014 (see www.legislation.gov.uk).

Writing from the perspective of social care work, Nigel Parton (2001) cites the findings of Parton (1996) and Kemshall *et al.* (1997) to highlight how considerations of risk have become firmly ingrained in the way organisations deliver, proceed and relate to service users and their affiliate agencies (p.61). With societal attitudes now characterised as 'blame culture' (p.69), notions of risk are kept at the front of the mind, acting professionally as we do to avoid 'hazards, dangers, exposure, harm and loss' (Parton 2010, p.62). This heightened emphasis on responsibility, liability and consequences has in response led to a development of formulaic systems for identifying and predicting potential risks to the greater public as a whole. Citing the work of Douglas (1986), Breakwell (2007) warns us however that a 'one size fits all' view of risk can be too simplistic as 'all institutions are not equal in shaping risk perception or acceptance and challenge whether risk should be assessed without consideration of issues of morality and social justice' (pp.3–4). As private therapists, we can think of ourselves as an independent institution when applying this notion to ourselves as private practitioners.

Writing about risk, Reeves (2015) states that while most therapy trainees focus on the positives they are soon 'introduced to the concepts of ethics, law, social policy, procedural demands, as well as boundaries, contracting, challenge and so on' (p.2). In the past few decades evidence gathered to create precise tools for gauging risk estimates has been developed and made available to the general public, but there remain many subjective criteria in the consideration and assessment of risks. So while art therapists working in private practice are encouraged to pay attention to notions of risk assessed for agencies and organisations, we are also uniquely positioned and encouraged into self-management and the assessment of risk for ourselves within our own solo practice. Your professional role influences what needs to be considered as a hazard even though there are universal aspects of risk that apply to all. The need for vigilance in professional judgement and accountability affects practitioners and is heightened by media reports of high-profile cases that then influence political interventions where thinking about risk can be fixated on negative outcomes (Parton 2001). A public craving to find simple solutions to problems can create concretised thinking after 'the event'. This can then lead to inflexible and limited societal mindsets, causing professional fear. Parton (2015) terms this 'wisdom hindsight' to remind us that while we are constantly making decisions about risk within a day-to-day basis, judgements about the future remain 'inherently uncertain' (p.68).

Referencing Douglas, Middens and Beck, Breakwell (2007) states that 'risk is defined in terms of two dimensions – usually simultaneously, though not necessarily. The first concerns *probabilities*. The second concerns *effects*' (pp.1–2; my emphasis). Breakwell describes probability as the likelihood of some specific negative event, as in predicting that the weather will bring rain. Considering the perspective of effect, the hazard that rain would bring is the risk held in mind. So, for instance, in an already sodden area of land, more rain might cause flooding, resulting in damages to infrastructure (Breakwell 2007). Weighing these two perspectives, probability and effect, helps form the ability to assess risk. 'The assessment of harm greatly depends upon the extent to which the outcome is acceptable (or even desirable) and this will vary between individuals and across societal institutions, according minimally to who is its victim and who is its beneficiary' (Breakwell 2007, p.2).

For effective risk assessment, holding fear in mind is essential, as without it there can be no awareness of risk. Fear of loss or harm, the foundation of risk concerns, brings forth an existential perspective of the state of 'being' between the before and after of a hazardous event.

In order to bring into focus what we can influence, mentally mapping the stages and phases of a trajectory between these two points helps prepare the practitioner to develop a well-considered risk assessment. By asking oneself what is the worst that could happen and then taking steps backward to consider at what stage the path may veer toward a negative outcome, we may be able to change the story altogether. As we do not hold foolproof predictive powers, we must keep in mind what we can 'know' from others who have gone before us, and official practice guidelines, societal beliefs and the laws of the land in which this 'knowledge' is expressed. Holding risk thoughtfully in mind requires an ability to consider how the 'big picture' may connect to potential occurrences, actions and choices closer to the here and now.

While we have thus far focused on risk, the assessment period of therapy also holds many aspects to consider when beginning with a private client. The process of meeting a new client creates an opportunity to keep an open humanistic focus on what they share, while also honing therapeutic looking, listening and sensing skills to assess what may be beneficial to reflect upon. In this way, assessment of the client is a useful forum to look out for potential risks in practice but can also expand beyond, from acute consideration towards broader frames of thinking, as during a first session, two different people from different life experiences meet for the first time where there is 'a level of complexity in how the dynamics of past relationships might impact therapy' (Van Rijn 2015, p.17). It should be borne in mind how the client has found the therapist and if this meeting is their first experience of an assessment. If someone else has referred the client having first assessed them, there is a chance that this process has coloured the way the client reflects upon it and how the new therapist holds them in mind. In the early days of a therapeutic relationship there is a possibility that the therapist may then be rejected without understanding why, and this can also be considered a risk.

Risks that Private Art Therapists Share with Other Modalities

Art therapists in private practice share many similar concerns with other therapeutic modalities. As a broad concept, risks can come from any of the following, either singularly or in combination: through our actions or inactions, through the client's actions or inactions, through actions or inactions taken by another outside of the therapeutic relationship, as well as unforeseeable natural or social occurrences negatively impacting on the therapeutic work. The consideration of going into private practice requires a person to gauge their ability to tolerate risk and to notice if their ways of thinking maintain space for planning if things go wrong. As fear and risk awareness will be consistent companions in their work, private practitioners will therefore need resilience or at least the capacity to develop it.

Addressing the practical needs of starting a private practice, Bor and Stokes (2011) comprehensively advise planning for the following concerns: financial risks, social risks, career risks, legal risks, personal safety risks, negligence and malpractice risks, and suicidal or violent client risks. Holding all this in mind can feel stressful at times, and perhaps even occasionally overwhelming, but Reeves encourages us

> to find a careful balance: to enable sufficient space and movement in the therapeutic relationship to allow for risk (for that is where important exploration may take place), while offering sufficient containment and boundaries to help ensure the risk is not overwhelming or a threat to either the client or the therapist. (Reeves 2015, p.4)

Risks Specific to Art Therapists

In the UK, arts therapists and art psychotherapists are registered health professionals, statutorily regulated by the Health and Care Professions Council (HCPC). 'WHAT?' was created by the HCPC in collaboration with the British Association of Art Therapists (BAAT) to highlight the significance of Arts Therapists as regulated professionals'. While BAAT's code of ethics for practitioners has consistently required members 'to exercise clinical judgement as a means of practising safely and effectively' (BAAT 2014, p.1), the WHAT? campaign emphasises the benefits of using an HCPC-registered professional. As HCPC-registered professionals, art therapists are required to uphold their guidance. Later in the chapter, we will look at an example that highlights what can go wrong if a person acts out the role of an art therapist without the required training or HCPC registration. The BAAT Code of Ethics (BAAT 2014) sets out the requirements for all of its registered art therapists and addresses points for those working in private practice, including:

- **Data protection:** 'Members must register with the current Data Protection Act' with regard to confidential storage of client information, both in hard copy forms and also digitally through email, texts, computer files and so on.

- **Compliance within training limits:** 'Members must not claim or imply professional expertise or qualifications beyond their training and must ensure clarity when communicating their qualifications and avoid or correct any misinterpretation of those qualifications. Art therapists and art psychotherapists have no authority to diagnose pathology or disease or give advice or opinion that would undermine treatments or medical care clients are receiving.' Though we may take knowledge from new studies, theories and published evidence, we are required to stay within the scope of our competencies, avoiding the risk of overstepping professional boundaries or promising more than we can deliver.

- **Client details and permission:** Collection and storage of client details, including name of GP and next of kin, must be kept confidential and therapists must 'obtain the client's permission to contact those...should it be necessary to do so'. If a client does not give permission, therapists are advised to make a note of this in client records and to use safe judgement as to 'whether to accept the client for private practice on a case-by-case basis'. This highlights the subjectivity of risk when a therapist decides who they take on as a client in private practice.

- **Living will:** Private practitioners are expected to create a 'living will' with 'arrangements to inform clients, in case of the therapist's incapacity or death'. In this way risk to our clients' wellbeing may be lessened as continuity of care can be provided.

- **Professional indemnity and public liability insurances:** Signing up for and maintaining professional insurances are essential due to the potential risk of the art therapist being found liable for damage of some nature. We should also be mindful that some clients may make false allegations about their therapist, and liaising with one's professional insurance company, as well as the HCPC, can help in protecting or defending one's professional integrity if required.

- **Referrals and acceptance of clients:** When considering accepting a referral, clear explanation to potential clients of 'the boundaries of fee, methods of payment, session times, notifications of holidays, notice of cancellation, and in and out of session boundaries is required'.

- **Confidentiality:** Client details, along with their process work, must be kept confidential within subjective limits based on the therapist's professional judgement. These 'limits of confidentiality must be clearly explained' when initially contracting with a client.

- **Treatment and planning in private practice:** Aspects that influence risk may include: does the client have a time-limited course or budget for attending therapy, are they working toward a goal or known issue of difficulty, and/or will taking an open-ended process toward uncovering unconscious patterns of thought or behaviour be preferred?

- **Termination of services:** We may consider how and if our trainings and official guidelines inform us about when and how to end with a client and what risks may be presented. We may also wish to take into account what can be at risk during a sudden termination beyond the therapist's control or influence.

- **Caseload:** Therapists are required to maintain a 'balanced management of the amount of clients one takes on'. Here we are reminded not to get overloaded by taking on too many clients than we may be able to keep in mind or overly complex cases which could lead to an inability to manage risk.

In addition to the BAAT guidelines listed, it is important to have a general understanding of health and safety laws with regard to all aspects the private practice space may contain, including location, entrance, surroundings, contents of the room(s), security and confidentiality, the art-making materials and tools and any other physical risks the space may create, plus a knowledge of how to manage emergencies and who to call for help. When working with child clients we also need to know, or be able to find out, who the local child protection officer is and how and when to reach out to them.[1]

Additionally, acquiring and maintaining appropriate supervision is an HCPC standard of practice and it is imperative to working in private practice. Having another mind to help consider management of risk within the therapeutic work can also enrich the process for all parties. It is important within supervision to share the collective of verbal and non-verbal, mental, emotional and intellectual processing gained from an assessment and as the work progresses. For the full 'Core Skills and Practice Standards in Private Work' document see Appendix 1.

In the UK and worldwide, art therapy courses are taught in many different schools holding various theoretical positions. Whether art therapists come from a psychotherapeutic training, where transference and countertransference are considered in the work, or from a 'making as therapy' basis, where the process of 'creation by the client' may be considered primary to therapeutic benefit, or in various combinations, the view of how we work can influence our ideas about the risks it may bring. This calls into focus the importance of HCPC-approved trainings and the registration of the art therapist.

In the *International Journal of Art Therapy* paper 'Through the eyes of the law: What is it about art that can harm people?', Neil Springham (2008) addresses what can go wrong when art therapy is practised without such training. Springham describes a court case where he was asked to be an expert witness, presenting evidence and the vetting of an art therapy practice. The case addressed a situation where a client was seen in an 'art therapy group' by a care worker with no training in art therapy. During a group session, the care worker conducted an intervention with a client, suggesting the client create an image of 'badness' and then speak to that image with whatever the client wanted to express. This culminated in the client violently attacking the image, resulting in him physically harming himself. Proper attention, containment and understanding of the client's complex needs of addiction and recent bereavement were deemed not to have been provided by the care worker. As a result of the intervention, the client suffered great pain and life-changing physical injury. As an expert witness to the case, Springham helped the court to conclude in the

---

1   For further information, visit www.nspcc.org.uk/preventing-abuse/child-protection-system.

client's favour. It could be concluded from this case that a properly trained therapist may have suggested considering the image more from an 'as if' perspective as opposed to an 'it is' neglectful stance. This highlights both the need for solid theoretical grounding and an understanding of the risk directive an intervention may generate. In the end, the court ruled that a failure in safeguarding had occurred and the vulnerable client was awarded compensation. For most therapists, the idea of being sued or asked to appear in court is a frightening concept. What we gain from Springham's paper, co-written post-case with the 'claimant', is an education in tort law formally being carried out. Tort law is described as: 'A body of rights, obligations, and remedies that is applied by courts in civil proceedings to provide relief for persons who have suffered harm from the wrongful acts of others' (The Free Dictionary 2013–2017).

For further in-depth legal considerations Andrew Reeves (2015) recommends reading Mitchels and Bond (2010), Jenkins (2013) and Reeves (2010). Reflecting on Springham's paper, art therapist and researcher Dr Sheridan Linnel (2012) offers her perspective in the article 'Risk discourse in art therapy: Revisiting Neil Springham's *Inscape* paper on art and risk'. Linnel's previous extensive research into how risk has been held within the art therapy domain has called for a non-questioning perspective where 'dominant ideas about risk were taken for granted and embedded in literature' (p.35). Citing her research into the findings of Foucault (1988), Rose (1996) and Fullagar (2005), Linnel states that 'risk management practices are necessary and crucial to saving lives, but they can also perpetuate risk adverse attitudes, pathologising and even isolating the people who are most in need of our help' (p.35).

Here we feel the fine line of professional judgement we face when receiving a referral. How do we 'know' what we think we know and how does it affect our choice in taking on a client? What are the risk factors that relate to various clients or client groups and is it ever possible to predict a client's behaviour if they do not explicitly tell the therapist what they plan to do? Considering the conditions of risk art therapy may create runs its own risk of concretely thinking we may have solid answers when often we do not. This perspective of 'not knowing' yet still trying to predict can certainly add to our stress. Balancing the task of mitigating risk as a whole requires a comprehensive perspective for risks that exist at the very beginning of a therapeutic relationship.

> It is not an easy balance to achieve and many factors can tip the balance unhelpfully, including poor boundaries, lack of attention to boundaries, personally held views on the part of the therapist, anxiety and fear, and procedural demands inconsistent with the ethos and philosophy of therapy. (Reeves 2015, p.5)

We are warned against thinking of risk in a one-dimensional box-ticking way and encouraged to consider how assessments can be limiting and too heavily relied on to be predictive. While we are attempting to assess risk, as therapists we need to consider what *we* may be looking out for but also need to encourage the client to 'be an active and equal participant in any dialogue about risk' (p.23). To maintain an open mind, avoiding simplistic perspectives on risk, Reeves suggests we consider 'the term risk exploration rather than risk assessment, as the former implies more a process of collaboration and the latter more a process of procedure' (p.23). However, there may still be times when referring to a formal assessment tool for gathering client information may be useful:

> This can be helpful information in that it can flag higher-risk clients. However, it is sometimes hoped that this application of 'science' will provide a high level of predictive value as to the intentions or actions of a particular individual: this is not the actual outcome. (Reeves 2015, p.24)

Generic assessment tools such as PHQ-9 (Patient Health Questionnaire) or CORE-OM (Clinical Outcome in Routine Evaluation; Evans *et al.* 2002) may be considered useful, though Reeves also warns that too many risk assessment tools may affect how casework is viewed culturally with further potential to influence what goes on to be researched (p.25). Reeves also recommends reading Cooper (2008), Roth and Fonagy (2005) and Lambert (2013) for further information on how assessment can affect risk in therapeutic work.

So, while we are encouraged to stay curious and interested in assessment tools and other documented perspectives, it is important to remain open to assessment as an ongoing process. Setting the intention to 'do no harm' by maintaining an open mind to the subjective field of risk and not allowing emotional avoidance may avoid hazards in our work. Whichever theoretical model of mind we may hold, it can be helpful to remember that one can never truly know what another is thinking and surprises are always possible. When using assessment tools or reading accounts of previous client-based studies, we risk making assumptions or closing down processes that may be beneficial. It is particularly interesting to consider also what risks art making may bring to the initial and ongoing therapeutic work. Further accounts of other art therapists' perspectives on the assessment process can be found in Gilroy, Tipple and Brown (2012).

Conclusion

Within this chapter, we explored the topic of risk from both physiological and practical perspectives. We have looked at potential real and imagined risks and the biological, neurological, psychological, social and professional responses that can occur. We addressed the structures offered by BAAT and others that help us hold a professional perspective and what can happen when things go wrong. We hope reading this has been useful in broadening thinking about how to assess and mitigate risks while working in private art therapy practice. We believe it is also important to consider that working at the edge of risk may often be a necessary balance in the work. Reflecting back on the anecdote of the fear response to the imaginary kitchen mouse, we need to be aware of how our own ongoing life experience of stress can influence our ability to stay grounded while finding the edge of risk. That which we fear may cause us to avoid addressing what may be most useful to us and our clients. We may go on beyond this chapter to further consider how taking risks may create potential positive outcomes. Taking the risk of working in private art therapy practice can be greatly enriching in terms of knowledge and experience as well as testing resilience at times. Mindfully reflecting on our senses as well as our intellect can fortify all aspects of our work, including our client's emotional wellbeing as well as our own, and can go a long way towards greater risk mitigation; best wishes, and good luck wouldn't hurt either!

References

BAAT (2014) *Code of Ethics and Principles of Professional Practice for Art Therapists.* London: BAAT. Accessed on 22 May 2017 at www.baat.org/Assets/Docs/General/BAAT%20CODE%20OF%20ETHICS%202014.pdf.

Bor, R. and Stokes, A. (2011) *Setting Up in Independent Practice: A Handbook for Counsellors, Therapists and Psychologists.* Basingstoke: Palgrave Macmillan.

Breakwell, G.M. (2007) *The Psychology of Risk.* Cambridge: Cambridge University Press.

Cooper, M. (2008) *Essential Research Findings in Counselling and Psychotherapy: The Facts are Friendly.* London: Sage.

Douglas, M. (1986) *Risk Acceptability According to the Social Sciences.* London: Routledge and Kegan Paul.

Evans, C., Connell, J., Markham, M., Margison, F. et al. (2002) 'Towards a standardised brief outcome measure: Psychometric properties and utility. The CORE-OM.' *British Journal of Psychiatry 180,* 51–60.

Foucault, M. (1988) 'Risk and the Dangerous Individual.' In *Politics, Philosophy,* Culture (ed. L. Kritzman). New York: Routledge.

Fullagar, S. (2005) 'The paradox of promoting help-seeking: Suicide, risk and the governance of youth.' *International Journal of Critical Psychology 14,* 31–51.

Gilroy, A., Tipple, R. and Brown, C. (eds) (2012) *Assessment in Art Therapy.* London: Routledge.

Jenkins, P. (2013) *Counselling, Psychotherapy and the Law.* London: Sage.

Kemshall, H., Parton, N., Walsh, M. and Waterson, J. (1997) 'Concepts of risk in relation to organisational structure and functioning with the personal social services and probation.' *Social Policy and Administration 31,* 3, 213–232.

Lambert, M. (ed.) (2013) *Bergin and Garfield's Handbook of Psychotherapy and Behaviour Change.* Chichester: Wiley.

Linnel, S. (2012) 'Risk discourse in art therapy: Revisiting Neil Springham's *Inscape* paper on art and risk.' *International Journal of Art Therapy 17,* 1, 34–39.

MacLean, P.D. (1990) *The Triune Brain in Evolution: Role in Paleocerebral Functions.* New York: Plenum.

Mitchels, B. and Bond, T. (2010) *Essential Law for Counsellors and Psychotherapists.* London: SAGE Publications Ltd.

Oxford English Dictionary (2017) *Risk.* Accessed on 22 May 2017 at www.oxforddictionaries.com/definition/english/risk.

Parton, N. (1996) 'Social Work, Risk and the Blaming System.' In N. Parton (ed.) *Social Theory, Social Change and Social Work.* London: Routledge.

Parton, N. (2010) *Risk and Professional Judgement: The Law and Social Work.* Basingstoke: Palgrave Macmillan.

Parton, N. (2001) *The Law and Social Work* (ed. L.-A. Cull and J. Roche) (1st edition). Basingstoke: Palgrave Macmillan.

Reeves, A. (2010) *Counselling Suicidal Clients.* London: Sage.

Reeves, A. (2015) *Working with Risk in Counselling and Psychotherapy.* Thousand Oaks, CA: SAGE Publications Ltd.

Rose, N. (1996) 'Governing risky individuals: The role of psychiatry in new regimes of control.' *Psychiatry, Psychology and Law 5,* 177–195.

Roth, A. and Fonagy, P. (2005) *What Works for Whom? A Critical Review of Psychotherapy Research* (2nd edition). London: The Guilford Press.

Springham, N. (2008) 'Through the eyes of the law: What is it about art that can harm people?' *International Journal of Art Therapy 13,* 2, 65–73.

The Free Dictionary (2013–2017) *Tort Law.* Accessed on 22 May 2017 at http://legal-dictionary.thefreedictionary.com/Tort+Law.

Van Rijn, B. (2015) *Assessment and Case Formulation in Counselling and Psychotherapy.* Thousand Oaks, CA: SAGE Publications Ltd.

11

BY PRIVATE ARRANGEMENT

Supervision in Private Practice

—— DAVID EDWARDS ——

Introduction

In the UK, counsellors and psychotherapists – including art therapists – are required to have their clinical practice supervised for the duration of their working life.[1] This is primarily because, as Wheeler and Richards (2007) note, 'Supervision has an impact on therapist self-awareness, skills, self-efficacy, theoretical orientation, support and outcomes for the client' (p.63). The importance currently attached to clinical supervision in art therapy has led to increasing attention being paid to the nature and quality of the supervision art therapists provide and/or receive. As Case and Dalley (1992) argue, 'Access to regular, good supervision is important for on-going working practice and extending the dialogue of understanding' (p.167). That is to say, clinical supervision provides new and experienced art therapists alike with the opportunity to gain creative, original and objective insights into the clinical work being undertaken.

The pivotal importance of supervision in developing and maintaining sound clinical practice is underscored by the British Association of Art Therapists (BAAT) in its *Code of Ethics and Principles of Professional Practice for Art Therapists* (BAAT 2014b), where the following is specified: '4. Members must monitor their own professional competence through clinical supervision in accordance with the Association's supervision guidelines and clinical supervisors should apply to be accredited by the Association' (p.3).

---

1 For the purpose of consistency, I have used the title 'art therapy' and 'art therapist' in preference to art psychotherapy and art psychotherapist. No distinction between these terms is implied; see HCPC (n.d.a).

Later in the Code of Ethics it is stated: '16.3. Members who act as supervisors are responsible for maintaining the quality of their supervision skills and must obtain consultation or supervision for their work as supervisors whenever appropriate' (p.8).

What Is 'Clinical Supervision'?

When applied to psychotherapeutic work such as that undertaken by art therapists, the term 'clinical supervision' is generally used to describe the process by which the therapist receives support and guidance in order to ensure the needs of the client are understood and responded to appropriately. In relation to this, the supervision process encompasses a number of functions concerned with developing and supporting art therapists in their therapeutic role. This includes psychological containment, addressing professional concerns, improving the service provided to the client, developing creative responses to clinical problems, increasing the therapist's self-awareness and helping them maintain and develop their professional practice.

In many situations, clinical supervision also involves monitoring the work of trainees and qualified practitioners in order to ensure their work is safe, efficacious and meets required professional or training standards. For example, Health Care Professions Council (HCPC) registered therapists are expected to practise professionally and competently in accordance with agreed standards of proficiency, conduct, performance and ethics (HCPC 2013). As such, clinical supervision – be this provided within the work place or externally – is now regarded as an essential component in both the training and continuing professional development of art therapists.

However, as the word 'supervision' is often employed in situations where one person inspects or oversees another's work from a position of authority, it is necessary to note that the term has a different meaning in relation to art therapy. The HCPC website carries the following statement on supervision in relation to this:

> When we refer to 'supervision', it refers to the process of an accountable, autonomous practitioner overseeing the work of someone who is normally an assistant practitioner, a student, or a health professional who is learning new skills. However, within art therapy, the term 'supervision' is used in a different context, to mean a process where the

art therapy process and the relationship with the client is supervised by another practitioner. Within art therapy, the term 'supervision' does not infer that the person being supervised is not autonomous, or that they are learning, but is instead viewed by the professional body as a regular part of art therapists' practice. (HCPC n.d.b)

In order to help set and raise standards within the profession, in 2002 BAAT published supervision guidelines for registered art therapists and introduced a register of approved/accredited supervisors (BAAT 2011).[2] This chapter will discuss these guidelines in relation to the 'private' supervision art therapists provide and receive, paying particular attention to the theoretical and practical issues involved in establishing and maintaining a productive supervisory relationship in the private sector.[3]

What Is 'Private Art Therapy Supervision'?

Arriving at a stable definition of 'private' in relation to art therapy practice is a complex matter and one that presents something of a challenge given the nature of the psychotherapeutic work art therapists undertake, the variety of contexts in which this work takes place and how this work is funded. In a paper written in 1988 my co-author, David McNab, and I defined 'private art therapy' as taking place 'when the client pays for art therapy directly at the point of service, or pays for art therapy through private health insurance' (McNab and Edwards 1988, p.16). This definition of 'private' deliberately excluded art

---

2 Details of the register of approved/accredited supervisors are available online at www. baat.org. This link is password-protected, and is only available to BAAT members.
3 Some definitions of terms might be helpful here for readers unfamiliar with the UK economy. The term 'private sector' refers to that part of the national economy that is not under direct government control, i.e. the 'public sector'; the term 'public sector' is used to describe that part of a nation's economy that consists of state-owned institutions and services provided by local authorities such as health, social services, etc. In this context, the private sector includes private health care and a wide variety of alternative and complementary treatments, including private art therapy. The term 'third sector' is increasingly used to distinguish the voluntary, community or not-for-profit (charity) sectors from both the public sector and the private sector. As noted above there is often some blurring of the boundaries between these different sections of the national economy, public–private partnerships in health care being but one example; see HealthcareUK (2013).

therapy provided on a sessional or freelance basis and which was paid for by statutory or voluntary bodies.

When we come to examine the meaning of 'private' in relation to the clinical supervision art therapists provide or receive, matters are yet more complicated. Useful though the forgoing definition might have been at the time in helping to distinguish art therapy paid for directly by the client (or possibly by their insurer) – that is to say, 'private art therapy' – from art therapy provided by the public or third sector, as far as the provision and consumption of clinical supervision today is concerned this definition is too restrictive.

First, were such a definition extended to private art therapy supervision today it would exclude much that is unique, valuable and complex about this important area of practice, overlapping as the term 'private' does in this context with others such as 'self-employed', 'freelance' and 'independent' practitioner. And, second, as statutory services contract as a consequence of successive government policies, whole areas of health and social care provision have been effectively privatised. As a consequence the boundary between private and public health care in the UK has become yet more blurred.

In an attempt to seek clarity in an area where boundaries often blur or overlap – not least, as noted above, between public and private – as used in this chapter 'private supervision' encompasses the following:

- the supervision of the clinical work undertaken by private practitioners

- the supervision of practitioners' work that takes place within the public or voluntary sectors but is supervised by supervisors who work privately; that is to say, supervisors who are wholly or partly self-employed.

It is not unusual nowadays for the work of an art therapist practising in a National Health Service (NHS) mental health unit or clinic (i.e. in the public sector) to be supervised by an art therapist practising in the private sector. This may be because they are working single-handedly and/or in a specialist area with limited access to an experienced art therapist able to provide appropriate clinical supervision. By way of contrast, it is also increasingly common to find suitably experienced art therapists employed by the NHS providing clinical supervision to therapists in the private or voluntary sector as a means of income generating or even as a means of funding their own external (and possibly private) supervision.

Furthermore, while this 'private' supervision might be paid for by the NHS – in part or in its entirety – it is very likely that the supervisor will have been chosen by the supervisee rather than the organisation whose clients will be the subject of discussion and which ultimately foots the bill. Such arrangements, while having the advantage of being flexible and economically advantageous for all concerned, can, however, also be problematic. It is not always sufficiently clear, for instance, who the supervisor is working for (is it the supervisee or their employer?) or where clinical accountability lies. The extent to which this private arrangement is, or can ever be, 'private' – in the generally understood sense of the word – is a matter of concern and one to which I intend to return later in this chapter.[4]

Clarifying the Task

The function (purpose) of supervision in relation to the work undertaken by art therapists and other health professionals (including members of the other arts therapies professions) is complex and multi-faceted. As a consequence, defining what the term 'supervision' actually means in practice can be problematic. Numerous definitions of the term exist in the psychotherapeutic and related literature, with each definition reflecting the diverse expectations and theoretical models underpinning the practice of supervision and the clinical work it supports. The Guidelines on Supervision published by BAAT (2014a) state: 'Supervision is required for good clinical practice, to ensure the continuing working development (CPD) of the Art Therapist, and for the protection and welfare of patients/clients.'

BAAT's supervision guidelines also seek to distinguish between two categories or types of supervision: 'clinical supervision' and 'managerial supervision'. Within these two categories, clinical supervision is understood to be primarily concerned with clinical matters such as techniques, the appropriate use of theory, transference and counter-

---

4   In everyday language when we use the word 'private' we are referring to something (a space, for example) belonging to or for the exclusive use of one particular person or group of people, or something such as a conversation dealing with matters that are not to be disclosed or revealed to others; see Oxford English Dictionary (2017).

transference issues and the delivery of a safe and ethical service to clients.

Managerial supervision, by contrast, is intended to provide a forum within which the supervisee might review areas of difficulty arising out of day-to-day operational and administrative tasks they are required to undertake, discuss future developments, set targets, monitor training needs and stress levels and explore the impact organisational dynamics have upon their work (BAAT 2014a). In seeking to distinguish between these two forms of supervision, it is also necessary to acknowledge that there may be areas of overlap, as is the case with the management of risk, for example. In private supervision the overlap between clinical and managerial supervision is most likely to occur when the therapist is relatively inexperienced, paying for clinical supervision themselves, is practising independently or is providing a clinical input into an organisation that does not provide any day-to-day operational or administrative support.

The outsourcing of clinical, and to a lesser extent managerial, supervision, through a private arrangement, is not without its particular difficulties however. While seemingly free from the power relations often evident in traditional forms of in-house, hierarchically based supervision, both supervisee and supervisor can, nevertheless, be subject to the imposition of managerial or organisational agendas. Those organisations that pay for their staff to be supervised externally may, for instance, require regular written reports on the supervisee's use of supervision. While the writing of such reports may be necessary during training, the value of such an approach to qualified and registered art therapists – or their clients – is more difficult to establish. Rather than providing a safe space in which to facilitate the professional development of the supervisee, supervision is at risk of becoming a form of surveillance focused on managing organisational anxiety, improving efficiency and reducing costs (Yegdich 1999, p.1196). Feltham (2002) is no less sceptical regarding the 'universal and lifelong necessity of supervision', arguing that 'the requirement that we must all engage in something identified as supervision denies professional self-determination' (p.26).

Where the supervisee is in private practice and paying the supervisor directly for the service they provide, there is, arguably, more equality in the supervisory relationship, and the supervisee can always, in theory at least, terminate the supervisory relationship at any point. Such equality does, however, come at a price. The risk here is that both the supervisee (for professional reasons) and the supervisor (for economic ones) may collude in turning a 'blind eye' to inappropriate behaviour, boundary violations or the exploitation of clients. While such risks unquestionably exist, they are by no means restricted to the private sector. As Rosemary Rizq (2012) observes:

> The NHS 'market for care' now permits mental health services to turn a blind eye to the emotional realities of suffering, instead constructing what has been identified as a 'virtual reality' where attention to targets, outcomes, protocols and policies is privileged over attention to the patient's psychological care. (p.7)

This is, of course, a major reason as to why clients, therapists and supervisors may prefer to meet outside the mental health services provided by the public sector and by the NHS in particular.

The Supervision Process

Broadly speaking, two main models of clinical supervision exist. On the one hand is what might best be described as a didactic or instructional model of supervision: that is to say, an approach to supervision in which the emphasis is primarily on the learning of theory and technique. The second model of supervision tends to focus more on the therapist's emotional response to the clients they are working with.[5] While noting that this is to some extent a false dichotomy, Case (2007a) suggests, 'This could be re-framed as a question of whether supervision is primarily for the protection and wellbeing of the client or for the continuing development and support of the therapist' (p.16).

It is, of course, in the interests of both therapists and their clients that supervision provides a safe, containing space; a space for thinking, feeling and playing. A space where the supervisee's anxiety might be reduced and understanding increased; that is to say, a space 'in which peripheral thoughts, feelings and fantasies in relation to the patient [or client] can be brought into awareness and examined'

---

5   These two distinctly different approaches to clinical supervision have their origins in psychoanalysis, and echo disagreements that emerged in the very earliest days of organised psychoanalytic training between the Hungarian and Viennese schools of thought. See Edwards (1997a) for a discussion of this legacy on contemporary supervision practice.

(Mollon 1989, p.120). Given the complexities of working outside the public or voluntary sector (i.e. privately), as well as the pressures (internal and external) on art therapists working within the public or voluntary sector, creating such a space can present something of a challenge.

In addition to the overlap between clinical supervision and managerial supervision noted above, there may also be a degree of overlap between clinical supervision and personal therapy. As Ekstein and Wallerstein (1972, p.251), for example, observe, both clinical supervision and personal therapy involve addressing 'affective problems, interpersonal conflicts, [and] problems in being helped'. Nevertheless, in spite of these areas of commonality, necessary and important functional differences exist between clinical supervision and personal therapy. Clinical supervision, unlike personal therapy, is primarily oriented toward helping therapists help the patients or clients they work with. The difference between the two forms of helping relationship is essentially one of purpose (Edwards 1993, p.218).

Wounded Healers

Rarely are the lives of therapists untroubled, and our personal lives – past and present – will inevitably have an impact on our work, as clinicians and as clinical supervisors. So too, it should be noted, does the austere economic climate in which we, and our clients, live and work.[6] As Adams (2014, p.14) observes, 'Our histories are what they are, and our motives for becoming therapists are rarely straightforward or simple.' We are all, to some extent, 'wounded healers', and these wounds may be revealed in supervision (Wheeler 2007).[7] An awareness

---

6 'In most of the leading economies in the world, the common mental disorders of depression, anxiety and stress are now the main cause of sickness-related absence [from work]… This is not surprising when the impact of the world recession is considered, with the massive downsizings leading to fewer people, having higher workloads, working longer hours and feeling significantly more job insecure' (HQ Asia 2016).

7 The term 'wounded healer', as attributed to psychotherapists, was first used by Carl Jung. As Zerubavel and O'Dougherty Wright (2012) observe, 'The wounded healer is an archetype that suggests that healing power emerges from the healer's own woundedness…and that the wounded healer embodies transformative qualities… It is important [therefore] to differentiate between the wounded healer and the impaired professional. The latter refers to therapists who are wounded and whose personal distress adversely impacts on their clinical work' (p.482).

of our wounds, motives and needs, along with an understanding of the experiences that give rise to these, is necessary so that we can, as far as humanly possible, put these aside when trying to meet the needs of others.

> Each of us needs to be very clear as to just why we go into this business of helping, for, unless we are, we are in danger of being no help at all… [We need to know whether] we are helping so as to make people love us because they need us, or admire us because we are powerful and have secrets, or because we want to prove that the world really is a just and fair place, or that ignorance can be overcome or virtue triumph, whether we are seeking clarity and understanding, or salvation, or the right to exist, or a happy rebirth. (Rowe 1983, pp.55–56)

For art therapists this self-understanding is usually gained through their own therapy. However, although personal therapy is a mandatory component of art therapy training in the UK, and has been for some time, its value as a learning experienced is not formally assessed. Indeed 'the only requirement is that the student's therapist informs the [training] course in writing at regular intervals that therapy is continuing' (Edwards 2014, p.118).[8] On a more positive note, however, as the personal therapy undertaken by art therapists in training will almost certainly be 'private' (although not necessarily 'private art therapy'), this does have the benefit of providing trainees with insights into the client's experience of therapy from the inside.

It is assumed that the personal therapy students undertake during their training is sufficient to help ensure they are 'aware of their own psychopathology and what personal issues may be triggered by transference and projections from the client' (Hogan and Coulter 2014, p.215). This is, of course, a 'big ask', particularly given the complexities involved when working privately and where the art therapist may be exposed to very powerful projections and transferences and unconscious processes without the containment usually provided by being a member of a team or organisation. In such circumstances it

---

8   While this is undoubtedly problematic, it also needs to be acknowledged that qualities such as the capacity for reflective thinking, and the ability to tolerate uncertainty, manage anxiety, maintain clear boundaries and reduce reliance on psychological defence mechanisms – all, it is hoped, potential outcomes of personal therapy – are addressed and assessed elsewhere during the training undertaken by art therapy students in the UK.

will be incumbent upon the supervisor to help contain and work with these dynamics.

The importance of art therapists having acquired a substantial amount of clinical experience prior to working privately, in addition – presumably – to sufficient self-understanding and psychological resilience to practise safely and competently, is acknowledged by de Heger (2007), who states:

> Experience gained through a diversity of clinical work, learning how to make a good assessment, to know who to work with and who not, to know what kind of intervention to offer – short, long term; supportive, interpretive, focussing on the art or the therapy, referral elsewhere, are but a few of the possible outcomes. It takes time to learn how to do all this comfortably and confidently, and, importantly, to build the network of contacts and general knowledge of other systems, professions and professionals that we might need to access to assist in the working with and holding of a client in private practice. (p.19)

The professional and ethical standards expected of BAAT members practising privately can be found in the Association's *Code of Ethics and Principles of Professional Practice for Art Therapists* (BAAT 2014b) and the *Core Skills and Practice Standards in Private Work* (BAAT 2017) produced by the BAAT Private Practice Special Interest Group in conjunction with the BAAT Council (see Appendix 1).

Establishing a Working Relationship

Although a broad consensus now exists within the art therapy profession regarding the importance of supervision, supervisors have different views on how supervision should be organised and structured; see, for example, Schaverien and Case (2007). The form clinical supervision takes, and the extent to which it is able to help the supervisee learn, develop and provide a safe service to clients, will be determined by a number of factors, including:

- The experience, professional background and theoretical orientation of the supervisor. While many art therapists are supervised by more experienced members of their profession, not all are.

- Whether the supervisor has received any supervision training. In recent years this has become an expectation, especially for organisations that fund external supervision.

The way supervision is organised can also play a crucial role in determining its usefulness. Supervision may, for example, be provided individually or in a group. Some supervisors require their supervisees to bring detailed notes as well as images to sessions, while others prefer a less structured, more spontaneous approach.

Another important variable likely to influence supervision concerns the personalities, and teaching and learning styles, of the individuals involved (Kitzrow 2001), along with such factors as their gender, age or race (Calish 1998).

Arguably, the most important factor in determining whether the agreed aims and anticipated outcomes of clinical supervision are met, however, is the quality of the working relationship established between the supervisor and supervisee. As Ormand (2010, p.379) observes, 'Supervision involves a relationship and so, like any relationship, it provides ample scope for the experience of anxiety, frustration, conflict and misunderstanding, as well as excitement and satisfaction.' It is therefore essential that both supervisee and supervisor are clear about their expectations. The kinds of questions I ask when first meeting supervisees include:

- What previous experience of being supervised have you had and what was most helpful and least helpful about it?

- What do you expect from me?

- How will you let me know if you are experiencing difficulties in your clinical work or in supervision?

- What might I expect your reaction to be if I offer you critical feedback?

- What key ideas or theories inform your clinical practice?

- Will you bring pictures, notes, tape recordings to supervision?

- When, where, how often and for how long would you like to meet?

- Who will be paying for your supervision? If it is your employer, as your supervisor, what will be the nature of my relationship with them?

- How would you like to start our first supervision session?

Normative, Formative and Restorative Supervision

There is a tension at the heart of clinical supervision in all settings, including private practice: a tension between supervision in the service of clinical governance, quality assurance, resource management and the protection of the public, and supervision as facilitation of professional and personal development. Supervisees need to be able to acknowledge their mistakes, vulnerabilities, doubts and uncertainties (amongst other things) and to seek help or support in understanding and addressing these. Set against this is the understandable need supervisees have to demonstrate they are behaving themselves professionally, helping their clients and meeting expectations. The challenge for both supervisee and supervisor in such circumstances is to help keep creativity alive (Edwards 2010) and avoid supervision becoming 'a defensive, procedural hybrid between support, monitoring and "covering one's back"' (Crowther 2003, p.106). Without sufficient trust these dilemmas and difficulties may be hidden from the supervisor and by implication from the supervisee themselves (Lidmila 1997).

In the 1980s Brigid Proctor (1987) developed the idea that supervision has three main purposes: namely, that it was *normative*, *formative* and/or *restorative*. While usually presented separately, in practice there is often an overlap between them. Though by no means the only model of supervision to be found in the literature, Proctor's provides a useful framework for considering supervision in and of private practice.

Normative Supervision

The normative function of clinical supervision is derived from the expertise, authority and 'gate-keeping' responsibilities assumed by supervisors. Where the supervisor is in private practice and supervising therapists who are also in private practice, these responsibilities span 'legal, professional, clinical, ethical and moral spheres' (Wheeler

2001, p.128). These apply to both clients and supervisees. For example, supervisors have a legal responsibility to maintain confidentiality in relation to both supervisees and their clients. They also have a duty of care to their supervisees, particularly in relation to their wellbeing and personal safety.[9]

These responsibilities invest supervisors with considerable power and both they and their supervisees may at times struggle with this. In addition, 'The very real inequalities of power in the supervisory relationship may be heightened by transference issues arising out of past good or bad experiences of being in similar power relationships' (Edwards 1997a, p.15).

This highlights the importance of high quality in-house and placement supervision during training as it is in these settings that most art therapists first experience clinical supervision and the interpersonal dynamics that may impact upon this positively or negatively.

When supervision is *normative*, the focus tends to be on issues such as accountability, quality assurance and the maintenance of professional standards. In other words, the focus of supervision is on whether the supervisee is conducting themselves professionally in relation to issues such as confidentiality and other potential boundary violations such as inappropriate personal disclosure, the development of proscribed dual relationships (including sexual relationships), the emotional or financial exploitation of clients and the therapist's fitness to practise. According to the HCPC website:

> When we say that a registrant is 'fit to practise' we mean that they have the skills, knowledge and character to practise their profession safely and effectively.
>
> However, fitness to practise is not just about professional performance. It also includes acts by a registrant which may affect public protection or confidence in the profession. This may include matters not directly related to professional practice. (HCPC 2016)

The mental health of the therapist may be one such matter. And yet, as noted above, the personal lives of therapists may at times be no less troubled than those of our clients. As this may impact on the work of both the therapist's and the clinical supervisor's fitness to practise, concerns may emerge in supervision. No matter how thoughtfully and

---

9   See Jenkins (2001) for a thoughtful discussion on supervisory responsibility and the law.

sensitively such matters may be handled, as sanctions may be applied if the fitness to practise of the therapist is called into question – including losing registration with the HCPC and a consequent loss of income – this raises important questions concerning whether or not the private arrangement between supervisor and supervisee can ever be truly 'private', no matter who ultimately pays the bill.

Formative Supervision

When supervision is *formative*, the focus tends to be on issues such as the development of skills, knowledge and understanding. This may be local, in terms of the skills, knowledge and understanding required to work in a particular setting such as private practice, or to practise within a particular model. The aim, broadly defined, is to enhance the therapist's knowledge and understanding. For art therapists this aspect of supervision will be primarily concerned with the supervisee's emotional and intellectual response to clients' imagery; see, for example, Case (2007b), Damarell (2007), Edwards (2010), Henzell (1997), Lett (1995), Maclagan (1997) and Schaverien (2007).

In private art therapy supervision paying attention to the culture or context in which the art therapist is practising might include addressing issues such as the management of risk or the withholding or non-payment of fees by clients along with other forms of 'acting out' behaviour.[10] It is perhaps important to note here, if only in passing, that therapists and supervisors may also have their own difficulties and conflicts regarding money and may have received little or no help addressing these during their training. As Haynes and Wiener (1996) observe, 'Of the three major taboo subjects of our era – sex, death and money – money is the least likely to be spoken, or written about' (p.14).[11]

---

10 Rycroft (1979, p.1) defines 'acting out' as 'an activity that can be interpreted as a substitute for remembering past events. The essence of the concept is the replacement of thought by action.'

11 See also Murdin (2012) for a thoughtful discussion on money matters in the consulting room.

Restorative Supervision

When supervision is *restorative*, the focus tends to be on helping the therapist manage the impact clients – including the clients' imagery – may be having upon them along with their emotional (counter-transference) responses to these: fear, irritation, fascination, boredom, distaste, erotic attraction and so on. As Kraemer (1990) observes, 'The novel idea which supervision has to get across is that therapy is not so much about trying to influence the patient as seeing in which ways the patient is influencing the therapist' (p.1).

In private practice, as elsewhere, art therapists may work with very traumatised, disturbed, distressed or distressing clients and are consequently exposed to the risk of experiencing secondary trauma or burnout (see James D. West in Chapter 12 on self-care).[12] For art therapists employed in organisations in the private or public sector, this work may also be taking place in a context that is itself 'dysfunctional and disabling' (Copeland 2005, p.125). In such situations it is vitally important that practitioners develop ways of coping that are not defensive or destructive. At its best, clinical supervision provides the containment necessary for this to happen.[13] As Segal (1992, p.122) observes, 'Experience does not have to be rejected or incorporated immediately but can be held for a while. Thoughts and thinking become possible.' Managing the supervision process, especially when aspects of the client/therapist relationship are re-enacted in the therapist/supervisor relationship, requires experience, resilience and an enhanced level of skill.

---

12 'Vicarious trauma' – also referred to in the literature as 'secondary trauma' – has been defined as 'the transformation that occurs in the inner experience of the therapist [or worker] that comes about as a result of empathic engagement with clients' trauma material' (Bell, Kulkarni and Dalton 2003, p.464). The term 'burnout' was first used by Herbert Freudenberger (1974) and is used to describe a state of emotional, mental and physical exhaustion caused by excessive and prolonged stress. It occurs when the therapist feels overwhelmed and unable to meet the emotional demands made of them and leads to a loss of creativity, motivation, effectiveness and productivity.

13 'Containment' is the term widely used in psychotherapeutic work to describe the provision of a relationship in which heightened emotional states such as acute anxiety might be experienced and responded to appropriately and thoughtfully. This sense of containment may be provided by a parent or carer, by a therapist or clinical supervisor, or by an organisation such as a therapeutic community.

Becoming a BAAT Approved/Accredited Supervisor

Becoming a clinical supervisor is not without its difficulties and challenges. Successfully making the transition from clinician to supervisor involves acquiring a range of new skills, in addition to developing different ways of thinking about therapeutic work. While some further training in supervision in advance of assuming the role of clinical supervisor may be helpful, most therapists acquire these skills on the job, basing their approach to supervision largely on their own experience of being supervised. Moreover, as Pickvance (1997) notes, 'The transition from therapist to supervisor usually goes unheralded and unmarked; there are no rites of passage as the therapist takes on the new role' (p.131).

While BAAT does not specify the competencies a clinical supervisor should have, the process of becoming approved/accredited is time consuming and not without its associated anxieties. In addition to providing personal information such as their training, year of qualification and membership details, applicants are also required to provide details of their continuing professional development, evidence of their registration with the HCPC, and professional indemnity insurance and supervision arrangements. Applicants must also provide a description of their 'personal and theoretical supervisory philosophy' and a statement on their 'understanding of equality and diversity' and how this might apply in their work (BAAT 2015). The rationale for requesting this information is, I understand, to help the applicant think through the implications of developing a supervisory practice.[14]

This raises the interesting and not unimportant question of motivation in relation to becoming a clinical supervisor. In the current economic climate art therapy paid positions are difficult to find, and for many art therapists private work offers additional employment opportunities. For experienced art therapists this includes the clinical supervision of other therapists working inside or outside the private sector. Private work offers the additional advantages of being relatively well paid and more flexible, an important factor for art therapists with child care responsibilities, for example. Assuming the role of clinical

---

14 From March 2015, the renewal cycle to be included in BAAT private practice and supervision became once every two years: www.baat.org/Membership/Private-Practice. This link is password-protected, and is only available to BAAT members.

supervisor also affords opportunities for professional development in addition to sharing experience and expertise in a collegial relationship.

Set against this are challenges such as the practicalities of working on a self-employed basis (including keeping records of professional standard, handling tax and other financial matters), the risk of professional isolation, the absence of holiday and sick pay and the high cost of various overheads: professional indemnity insurance, room hire, utility bills, and so on. A considerable amount of unpaid time also needs to be invested in further training (including supervision of supervision), networking and attracting potential supervisees. It is beyond the scope of this chapter to address the practicalities of establishing and maintaining a private supervisory practice in detail. There are, however, a number of useful books on the market that may be of interest to art therapists seeking to do so; see, for example, Syme (1994) and Weitz (2006).

Ending Supervision

As noted at the beginning of this chapter, counsellors and psychotherapists in the UK, including art therapists, are required to have their clinical practice supervised for the duration of their working life. While it is sometimes recommended that supervisees change supervisors periodically in order to avoid complacency and to reinvigorate the supervisory process, for many therapists the relationship with their clinical supervisor is a long-term one. Ending this relationship can raise difficult issues for both parties in much the same way that ending therapy does (Edwards 1997b). A sudden, unanticipated ending may leave the supervisee feeling bereft, vulnerable or needy, while the supervisor may feel envious, wounded, betrayed or rejected. The supervisor may also experience a sense of failure for not having been more helpful.

The decision to end supervision may be due to a number of internal or external factors such as the therapists changing jobs, irreconcilable conflicts within the supervisory relationship itself, pregnancy, ill health, the supervisor's retirement or the withdrawal of funding for external supervision (Power 2016).[15] Even when the ending of a supervisory relationship is planned and mutually agreed, difficult feelings may

---

15 See Chapter 11, 'Endings and New Beginnings in Supervision', in Copeland (2005) for a helpful exploration of the many and varied reasons why the supervisor, supervisee or the funding organisation might end a supervisory relationship.

emerge, including sadness and regret. Mander (2002) comments, 'It is not surprising that an ending in private supervision is often more difficult to initiate when there is a positive transference to the supervisor...where a plateau of colleagueship has been reached that is creative and nourishing' (p.149).

Nevertheless, as Murdin (2000) observes, 'Therapists in any of their roles have to be prepared to give up relationships that they have come to enjoy and that they have used for satisfaction, for income and for validation' (p.171). Difficult though this may be, as Murdin (2000) also reminds us, 'The ability to let go when the time comes is one of the primary achievements of any kind of therapy' (p.171).

For the relationship between the supervisor and supervisee to end well requires self-awareness and emotional maturity. Feelings of sadness and anger, along with those of gratitude and respect, need to be expressed, acknowledged and worked through as fully as possible (Edwards 1997b). An understanding of the ending process can help facilitate a 'healthy' ending in clinical supervision (Chambers and Cutcliffe 2001).

In concluding this chapter I find myself in agreement with Mander (2002) once more when she writes:

> The ending of supervision, as the beginning of it, needs to be a professional rite of passage in order to become meaningful as an emotional stage and transition, and to highlight the important relationship aspect of the supervisory experience. Then, the supervisor can become internalised and take his or her place in the supervisee's internal world as an internal good object, an ongoing influence and a model on which to draw. (p.150)

This, it seems to me, is as important in private practice supervision as it is in any other setting, possibly more so given the challenges involved.

References

Adams, M. (2014) *The Myth of the Untroubled Therapist*. London: Routledge.

BAAT (2011) Guidance note for BAAT Approved Private Practitioners and Supervisors, July 2011. www.baat.org/members/baat_private_practitioners_and_supervisors_July_2011.pdf.

BAAT (2014a) *State Registered Art Therapist Guidelines for Supervision*. London: BAAT.

BAAT (2014b) *Code of Ethics and Principles of Professional Practice for Art Therapists*. London: BAAT. Accessed on 22 May 2017 at www.baat.org/Assets/Docs/General/BAAT%20CODE%20 OF%20ETHICS%202014.pdf.

BAAT (2015) *BAAT Recognised Supervisor Application Form.* Accessed on 22 May 2017 at www.baat. org/Assets/Docs/Private%20Supervisor%20application%20form%202015.pdf.

BAAT (2017) *Core Skills and Practice Standards in Private Work* (revised). London: BAAT.

Bell, H., Kulkarni, S. and Dalton, L. (2003) 'Organizational prevention of vicarious trauma.' *Families in Society: The Journal of Contemporary Human Service 84,* 463–470.

Calish, A.C. (1998) 'Multicultural Perspectives in Art Therapy Supervision.' In A.R. Hiscox and A.C. Calish (eds) *Tapestry of Cultural Issues in Art Therapy.* London: Jessica Kingsley Publishers.

Case, C. (2007a) 'Review of the Literature on Art Therapy Supervision.' In J. Schaverien and C. Case (eds) *Supervision of Art Psychotherapy.* London: Routledge.

Case, C. (2007b) 'Imagery in Supervision: The Non-Verbal Narrative of Knowing.' In J. Schaverien and C. Case (eds) *Supervision of Art Psychotherapy.* London: Routledge.

Case, C. and Dalley, T. (1992) *The Handbook of Art Therapy.* London: Routledge.

Chambers, M. and Cutcliffe, J. (2001) 'The dynamics and processes of "ending" in clinical supervision.' *British Journal of Nursing 10,* 21, 1403–1411.

Copeland, S. (2005) *Counselling Supervision in Organisations.* London: Routledge.

Crowther, C. (2003) 'Supervising in Institutions.' In J. Wiener, R. Mizen and J. Duckham (eds) *Supervising and Being Supervised: A Practice in Search of a Theory.* Basingstoke: Palgrave Macmillan.

Damarell, B. (2007) 'The Supervisor's Eyes.' In J. Schaverien and C. Case (eds) *Supervision of Art Psychotherapy.* London: Routledge.

de Heger, J. (2007) 'BAAT Membership Group.' *BAAT Newsbriefing,* Winter, 19–21.

Edwards, D. (1993) 'Learning about feelings: The role of supervision in art therapy training.' *The Arts in Psychotherapy 20,* 213–222.

Edwards, D. (1997a) 'Supervision Today: The Psychoanalytic Legacy.' In G. Shipton (ed.) *Supervision of Psychotherapy and Counselling.* Buckingham: Open University Press.

Edwards, D. (1997b) 'Endings.' *Inscape 2,* 2, 49–56.

Edwards, D. (2010) 'Play and metaphor in supervision: Keeping creativity alive.' *The Arts in Psychotherapy 37,* 248–254.

Edwards, D. (2014) *Art Therapy* (2nd edition). London: Sage.

Ekstein, R. and Wallerstein, R.S. (1972) *The Teaching and Learning of Psychotherapy.* New York: International Universities Press.

Feltham, C. (2002) 'A surveillance culture?' *Counselling and Psychotherapy Journal 13,* 1, 26–27.

Freudenberger, H.J. (1974) 'Staff burn-out.' *Journal of Social Issues 30,* 1, 159–165.

Haynes, J. and Wiener, J. (1996) 'The analyst in the counting house: Money as symbol and reality in analysis.' *British Journal of Psychotherapy 13,* 1, 14–25.

HCPC (n.d.a) *Factsheet: Protecting Titles.* Accessed on 22 May 2017 at www.hpc-uk.org/assets/documents/10004E20Factsheet-Protectingtitles.pdf.

HCPC (n.d.b) *Arts Therapists.* Accessed on 22 May 2017 at www.hpc-uk.org/aboutregistration/professions/artstherapists/index.asp?printerfriendly=1.

HCPC (2013) *Standards of Proficiency: Arts Therapists.* Accessed on 22 May 2017 at www.hpc-uk.org/assets/documents/100004FBStandards_of_Proficiency_Arts_Therapists.pdf.

HCPC (2016) *What is Fitness to Practise?* Accessed on 22 May 2017 at www.hcpc-uk.org/complaints/fitnesstopractise.

HealthcareUK (2013) *Public Private Partnerships.* London: UK Trade and Investment. Accessed on 22 May 2017 at www.gov.uk/government/uploads/system/uploads/attachment_data/file/266818/07_PPP_28.11.13.pdf.

Henzell, J. (1997) 'The Image's Supervision.' In G. Shipton (ed.) *Supervision of Psychotherapy and Counselling.* Buckingham: Open University Press.

Hogan, S. and Coulter, A.M. (2014) *The Introductory Guide to Art Therapy: Experiential Teaching and Learning for Students and Practitioners.* London: Routledge.

HQ Asia (2016) *A Good Day at Work: Why Skilled Managers Focus on Well-Being at Work.* Accessed on 22 May 2017 at http://hqasia.org/insights/good-day-work-why-skilled-managers-focus-well-being-work.

Jenkins, P. (2001) 'Supervisory Responsibility and the Law.' In S. Wheeler and D. King (eds) *Supervising Counsellors: Issues of Responsibility.* London: Sage.

Kitzrow, M.A. (2001) 'Applications of psychological type in clinical supervision.' *The Clinical Supervisor 20,* 2, 133–146.

Kraemer, S. (1990) *Creating a space to supervise – opportunity or persecution?* Opening presentation at international conference at the Tavistock Clinic, 'Supervision as a Way of Learning: A Symposium for Trainers', July, London; published in *Tavistock Gazette 34*, 1992.

Lett, W.R. (1995) 'Experiential supervision through simultaneous drawing and talking.' *The Arts in Psychotherapy 22*, 4, 315–328.

Lidmila, A. (1997) 'Shame, Knowledge and Modes of Enquiry in Supervision.' In G. Shipton (ed.) *Supervision of Psychotherapy and Counselling*. Buckingham: Open University Press.

Maclagan, D. (1997) 'Fantasy, Play and the Image in Supervision.' In G. Shipton (ed.) *Supervision of Psychotherapy and Counselling*. Buckingham: Open University Press.

Mander, G. (2002) 'Timing and Ending in Supervision.' In C. Driver and E. Martin (eds) *Supervising Psychotherapy*. London: Sage.

McNab, D. and Edwards, D. (1988) 'Private art therapy.' *Inscape*, Summer, 14–19.

Mollon, P. (1989) 'Anxiety, supervision and a space for thinking: Some narcissistic perils for clinical psychologists in learning psychotherapy.' *British Journal of Medical Psychology 62*, 113–122.

Murdin, L. (2000) *How Much is Enough? Endings in Psychotherapy and Counselling*. London: Routledge.

Murdin, L. (2012) *How Money Talks*. London: Karnac.

Ormand, L. (2010) 'What makes for good supervision and whose responsibility is it anyway?' *Psychodynamic Practice 16*, 4, 377–392.

Oxford English Dictionary (2015) *Private*. Accessed on 22 May 2017 at www.oxforddictionaries.com/definition/english/private.

Pickvance, D. (1997) 'Becoming a Supervisor.' In G. Shipton (ed.) *Supervision of Psychotherapy and Counselling*. Buckingham: Open University Press.

Power, A. (2016) *Forced Endings in Psychotherapy and Psychoanalysis*. London: Routledge.

Proctor, B. (1987) 'Supervision: A Co-operative Exercise in Accountability.' In M. Marken and M. Payne (eds) *Enabling and Ensuring: Supervision in Practice*. Leicester: National Youth Bureau.

Rizq, R. (2012) 'The perversion of care: Psychological therapies in a time of IAPT.' *Psychodynamic Practice: Individuals, Groups and Organisations 18*, 1, 7–24.

Rowe, D. (1983) 'The Meaning and Intention of Helping.' In D. Pilgrim (ed.) *Psychology and Psychotherapy*. London: Routledge and Kegan Paul.

Rycroft, C. (1979) *A Critical Dictionary of Psychoanalysis*. Harmondsworth: Penguin Books.

Schaverien, J. (2007) 'Framing Enchantment: Countertransference in Analytical Art Psychotherapy Supervision.' In J. Schaverien and C. Case (eds) *Supervision of Art Psychotherapy*. London: Routledge.

Schaverien, J. and Case, C. (eds) (2007) *Supervision of Art Psychotherapy*. London: Routledge.

Segal, J. (1992) *Melanie Klein*. London: Sage.

Syme, G. (1994) *Counselling in Independent Practice*. Buckingham: Open University Press.

Weitz, P. (2006) *Setting Up and Maintaining an Effective Private Practice*. London: Karnac.

Wheeler, S. (2001) 'Supervision of Counsellors Working Independently in Private Practice.' In S. Wheeler and D. King (eds) *Supervising Counsellors: Issues of Responsibility*. London: Sage.

Wheeler, S. (2007) 'What shall we do with the wounded healer? The supervisor's dilemma.' *Psychodynamic Practice 13*, 3, 245–256.

Wheeler, S. and Richards, K. (2007) 'The impact of clinical supervision on counsellors and therapists, their practice and their clients: A systematic review of the literature.' *Counselling and Psychotherapy Research 7*, 1, 54–65.

Yegdich, T. (1999) 'Clinical supervision and managerial supervision: Some historical and conceptual considerations.' *Journal of Advanced Nursing 30*, 5, 1195–1204.

Zerubavel, N. and O'Dougherty Wright, M. (2012) 'The dilemma of the wounded healer.' *Psychotherapy 49*, 4, 482–491.

12

SELF-CARE IN ART THERAPY PRIVATE PRACTICE

—— JAMES D. WEST ——

Introduction

When the Health and Care Professions Council (HCPC) obliges its registrants to consider their 'fitness to practise' it does not draw sufficient attention to the specific benefits to clients of the therapist attending to self-care and the duty of care we owe to ourselves as practitioners (HCPC 2013, 2016). There is also a significant and growing body of literature about the psychological, physiological and relational risks to being a therapist that needs to be considered. In Part 1 of this chapter I review some of this literature and draw out the dominant threads. I then go on to consider this research, primarily as an art therapy practitioner of over 23 years' experience, and ask whether these internal and external dialogues of 'unfitness' are not in fact a precious source of information for both our clients and practitioners within the therapeutic engagement. Following on from the research regarding therapists' self-care, in Part 2 I move on to consider its application in the practice of 'ongoing joint assessment' and introduce a number of practical tools including a tripartite model of the self as process, the flower diagram and the modality chart. These are phenomenological tools to assist art therapists in private practice in the ongoing joint assessment of themselves and their clients with the aim of ensuring positive outcomes for both parties and to assist the linking of research to the realities of practice.

PART 1: THE NATURE OF AN ART PSYCHOTHERAPY PRACTICE – RISKS AND RESOURCES, AND THE WHAT, WHERE, WHO, HOW, WHEN AND WHY OF STRESS

It is becoming clearer through research into the field of therapeutic provision that being a therapist to traumatised clients can be detrimental to your health as a practitioner. Two recent studies of UK therapists showed evidence of this and one concluded:

> Whilst the majority of therapists scored within the average range for compassion satisfaction and burnout, 70% of scores indicated that therapists were at high risk of secondary traumatic stress. UK therapists working with trauma clients are at high risk of being negatively impacted by their work, obtaining scores which suggest a risk of developing secondary traumatic stress. (Sodeke-Gregson, Holttum and Billings 2013, p.1)

Another survey by the British Psychological Society and the New Savoy Partnership showed that:

> levels of depression rose from 40 per cent to 46 per cent from 2014 to 2015, while the number of respondents feeling like a failure rose from 42 per cent to almost 50 per cent. The survey, of more than a thousand people who work in mental health and psychology, also found qualitative data to suggest that targets, stress and burnout were major concerns for many. It revealed one quarter of respondents considered themselves to have a long-term, chronic condition, and 70 per cent said they were finding their jobs stressful. Reported stress at work also went up by 12 per cent over the survey period, while incidents of bullying and harassment had more than doubled. (Rhodes 2016)

Having established that, at least within the statutory sector where these studies were made, the practice of therapy has clearly identified risks to the practitioner, and knowing that for art therapists under state regulation there is the requirement for 'fitness to practise', we should now consider these phenomena within the context of private practice. How can positive outcomes be mutually achieved for both the therapist and the client? In private practice you are your own human resources department, practice manager and researcher. The task and responsibility of self-care is entirely your own! Therapists also face the dilemma that, while they may share 'that' they are upset in their work to their friends and loved ones, they often cannot say 'why', due to professional boundaries of confidentiality. Isolation is an added professional risk and so it must be actively countered. It is vital not to endure pain in isolation as there are major physical and psychological consequences that may well follow. It is imperative to find adequate containment through various means: supervision, peer supervision, continuing professional development and also, when necessary, a return to the unique containment of personal therapy. We will explore some of these stress effects below and then provide some of the recommended remedies pointed to by research.

Stress in Therapy

Stress is a factor affecting many clients and also presents significant risks to the therapist. Colleen Steiner Westling (in Chapter 10) has already looked at the physiological risks of stress and so I will only briefly recapitulate here by saying that embracing and acknowledging the potential for stress is the first and vital step in the journey of self-care and represents the possibility of mitigating some of its potentially damaging physiological, psychological and relational effects over time. In the course of this chapter I will consider 'affect' as a vital source of information arising within the setting between the therapist and client that must be seen as bio-psycho-socially informative to the therapy. I then will discuss the research that points to phenomena that may appear as 'negative affect' and 'countertransference' in the setting but can lead to a 'fuller' engagement, contributing to 'compassion satisfaction', positive outcomes and psychological protections for both the therapist and the client. 'Compassion satisfaction' can be considered as the opposite of 'compassion fatigue', representing a broad range of positive outcomes for the therapist in the provision of therapy.

In 1999 it was recorded that stress was considered as a cause of between 75 per cent and 90 per cent of visits to primary care in the United States (Elkin 1999). It is a very widespread contemporary phenomenon. The sociologist Alvin Toffler (1984) pointed to the excess of change in modern life as the main driver of stress.

If we imagine driving a car with the brakes and the accelerator fully engaged, this gives a picture of the effects upon the body if a heightened and sustained fight/flight/freeze response over time is maintained. These instinct-driven states, triggered by stress, are by definition experienced as states of incongruence when the instinctual drivers to action and inaction are counterposed in this way. A significant trigger for stress occurs in situations that induce a sense of having no control or of being endangered. Our instinctual responses, designed to be time limited, when endured over long periods, pose major health risks and potential damage to all the vital organs of the body (kidneys, liver, heart, stomach), broader systemic risks to circulation (such as stroke and dementia), disruption to the defences of the body as a whole, evidenced in the field of psychoneuroimmunology, and a consequent inhibition of the body's capacity to heal and renew itself. Joanna Findlay looks at this physiological health phenomenon from an art therapy practitioner's perspective (Findlay 2008). The stress response also takes the higher brain offline and so becomes mentally debilitating and likely to reduce the capacity of the subject to act effectively (Van der Kolk 2014).

The subject's perception of the threatening situation is key to understanding the physiological response and also to mitigating its negative effects on the mind, body and relationships over time. These phenomena apply equally to therapists as well as their clients, and I will keep returning to this mutuality of the experience of stress, suggesting the need for a holistic, systemic and ongoing assessment of the therapeutic scene. Vital therapeutic information is contained in these largely somatic messages that can in time provide hope and healing through the collaborative engagement of therapy, but only when attention is given to this bio-psycho-social feedback appearing in the modes of communication and opened up aesthetically and symbolically through the process of the art therapy session.

In recognising the triggering factors of stress through the experience of loss of control and in the perception of danger, there is a double risk apparent for therapists, who inevitably endure periods of 'not knowing' in the process of 'holding' the client and also of being vicariously traumatised as secondary witnesses to the distressing material presented to them in words, images and the raw affect of their clients' retelling. Over the years as a supervisor I have often wondered how art therapists sustain their practices and mitigate these risks when sometimes few explicit steps in self-care appear to be being taken. I am now more likely to actively pursue these questions. It has become clear that the therapist in making their own artwork pursues a vital process of self-care. Findlay provides a good review of image research and the relationship between the production of artwork and its potential for protection and healing (Findlay 2008). The research suggests there are aspects of the art process or the artful performance of the role that are inherently protective to the therapist who presides over and facilitates the therapeutic process for the client. Thankfully for therapists, this shows that there are positive reasons to pursue this career, despite the risks, as an alchemical process of transformation can be identified when the client transmutes their difficulties and challenges into strength, wisdom and resilience, vicariously providing a tragic gift and reward to the therapist. The research also points to this in the following way:

> Of particular note was that exposure to trauma stories did not significantly predict secondary traumatic stress scores as suggested by theory. However, the negative impact of working with trauma clients was balanced by the potential for a positive outcome from trauma work as a majority indicated an average potential for compassion satisfaction. (Sodeke-Gregson *et al.* 2013, p.1)

Vicarious Traumatisation, Compassion Fatigue, Burnout and Secondary Post-Traumatic Stress Disorder

These are some of the dramatic names given to the phenomena of the negative physiological, psychological and relational effects of enduring prolonged negative 'affect' as a therapist. Fortunately for prospective therapists there is also mounting evidence that the effects of being affected as a therapist can not only be 'endured' for a fee, but that a collaborative union with the client can leave both parties revitalised, well motivated and ready to face the challenges that life will always present with excitement, a sense of play, hope and flexibility. The term 'exquisite empathy' will be considered later as an expression of this phenomenon.

Van Der Kolk (2014) shows how trauma can be countered by a combination of 'top-down' treatment, which brings knowledge to the process, and 'bottom-up' treatment, where a deeply felt and contrary positive experience to the negative trauma can free patients from the effects of the traumatic past and bring them into a full and hopeful appreciation of present safety. Similarly, the art therapist Lobban (2012) found with veterans that traumas held in the mind can be drawn out and integrated through art making and group narration. Smith (2016) in a literature review of art therapy with veterans points to claims across the research literature that there is a positive 'impact of externalising the art image in order to facilitate processing of memories…and the transition from non-verbal expression to verbal processing of trauma' (p.72). The process necessarily requires a holistic understanding of treatment to return the patient to this assurance of relational safety. Van der Kolk goes on to say that the aims of trauma recovery should be to:

> reestablish ownership of your body and your mind – of your self. This means feeling free to know what you know and feel what you feel without becoming overwhelmed, enraged, ashamed, or collapsed. For most people this involves (1) finding a way to become calm and focused, (2) learning to maintain that calm in response to images, thoughts, sounds, or physical sensations that remind you of the past, (3) finding a way to be fully alive in the present and engaged with the people around you, (4) not having to keep secrets from yourself, including secrets about the ways that you have managed to survive. (Van der Kolk 2014, pp.203–204)

This statement logically applies as much to the therapist encountering trauma vicariously as it does for the traumatised client having experienced the event directly. Later on in the chapter we will consider the resources available within an art therapy session to achieve these outcomes mutually and consider further the vital modal transitions and sequences apparent in recovery from trauma.

In the research cited it is not clear whether it is an advantage or disadvantage for a therapist to have experienced trauma personally and found recovery from it, but while it is easy to see that it could positively encourage compassion and empathy, the risk of being re-traumatised is clear, potentially leading to a visceral over-identification. Sodeke-Gregson et al. (2013) state, 'A higher risk of secondary traumatic stress was predicted in therapists engaging in more individual supervision and self-care activities, as well as those who had a personal trauma history' (p.1)

There are, however, other significant examples of therapists using personal trauma as part of the journey to becoming a therapeutic agent for others, most notably in Jung's notion of wounded healer (Dunne 2015) and Victor Frankl, a survivor of Auschwitz, who also went on to develop logotherapy, providing examples that seem to contradict this generalisation. Frankl's 'The Case for a Tragic Optimism' (Frankl 2008) in fact provides a manifesto of how this objective can be achieved. The recent research of dual identities of service user and mental health professional (Richards, Holttum and Springham 2016) and more recent research by the British Association of Art Therapists (Huet and Holttum 2016) into dual experience in therapists would likewise suggest a potentially more complex and nuanced picture of the positive use of the therapist's own mental distress. The modality chart discussed in Part 2 can be used to examine the phenomenological detail of the joint engagement and to help the therapist distinguish and address what belongs to whom in therapy through a detailed empirical consideration of the physiological, psychological and relational evidence, helping to disentangle the personal associations that inevitably and usefully appear in the collaborative field of therapy.

I once received a call from a client who stated nothing of the detail of his trauma in the conversation but simply communicated an urgency through his need to book a prompt assessment the following week. I awoke that night and found myself struggling to breathe. Having made a connection with the call that I had received I was then able to put it aside and returned easily to sleep. I have experienced occasional night frights relating to my own past traumatic experience but the phenomenon and pattern of this experience did not fit the usual pattern of my own reactions. It was only when I met the client for assessment and his personal history was disclosed that I realised that I had experienced something of the major physical reactions of a terrified child that matched my client's physiological reaction at the moment of their being traumatised. It made me aware that somehow a physiological state had been communicated in our telephone conversation; presumably through voice tone and the stated urgency alone. We discussed this phenomenon and it appeared to assist us in building the therapeutic alliance. After a therapy that lasted a number of years the client was released from these somatic reactions to childhood trauma and identified other additional relational, psychological and work/life benefits, so we made an ending. The comparative analysis of the specific phenomena of somatic reactions past and present was used here to point to the importance of the therapist's and client's ownership of the process within the engagement over time and to show how attention to detail and sequence is essential both to the therapy and the self-care of the therapist.

Reflections in the Mirror Neurones – Empathy

Neurological research (cited in Rothschild 2006) also shows why therapists are at profound risk of stress within their role. We now know through developmental and neurological research that the individual prehistories of both the therapist and the client meet in the setting. Both parties are conjoined in this endeavour, consciously and unconsciously, verbally and non-verbally. The new research suggests that what is referred to as the 'therapist's countertransference' is also something that should be taken more seriously as a real relational phenomenon evolving from this deep neurological and animal connection which presents both a vital source of implicit and intuited information and a potential physiological stress risk to the therapist. Ignoring the notion of countertransference would now seem irresponsible when we consider the health risks that may well follow for the therapist and the consequent loss of relational information from the setting that would necessarily follow. Scientific study here appears to support and evidence the reality of the embodied intersubjective field of psychotherapy originally put forward by the much maligned Victorian neurologist Freud (who nonetheless expressed an ambivalent attitude to countertransference himself, seeing it as an interference to the clean objective process of analysis). The neurological research of Siegel (2011) also appears to back the 'faith' of psychodynamic therapists since Freud that one day science would evidence intuited neuroplasticity and the potential healing and civilising functions of communication occurring in therapy, taking it beyond the fixations of objectifying diagnosis and providing a scientific basis for therapeutic change.

Exquisite Empathy and Compassion Satisfaction

These terms relate to the potential positive outcomes for therapists in providing therapy and the subsequent thriving that can come from it. The research of Harrison and Westwood (2009) is groundbreaking in its discovery of 'exquisite empathy', identifying this counterintuitive phenomenon that explains why the therapist's proximity to the client's world protects the therapist and how the provision of therapy, despite its tragic engagements, can be a source of satisfaction and an opportunity for celebration and enjoyment for the therapist.

> This finding surprised us, because we went into the research thinking that empathic engagement was a risk factor rather than a protective practice. However, when clinicians maintain clarity about interpersonal boundaries, when they are able to get very close without fusing or confusing the client's story, experiences, and perspective with their own, this exquisite kind of empathic attunement is nourishing for therapist and client alike, in part because the therapists recognize it is beneficial to the clients. Thus the ability to establish a deep, intimate, therapeutic alliance based upon presence, heartfelt concern, and love is an important aspect of well-being and professional satisfaction for many of these clinicians. (Harrison and Westwood 2009, p.213)

This last document, considered as part of our reflection on the needs and strategies of therapists faced with potential vicarious traumatisation in their work, discovered nine major themes appearing in the clinicians' narratives which can provide us with an initial list of nine self-care strategies for art therapists experiencing the effects of affect in their work in private practice. They also map nicely on to Van der Kolk's (2014) aims for trauma recovery stated earlier and once again point to the mutuality of journeys for the therapist and the client within this trauma territory. These are the nine themes:

1. countering isolation (in professional, personal and spiritual realms)

2. developing mindful self-awareness

3. consciously expanding perspectives to embrace complexity

4. active optimism

5. holistic self-care

6. maintaining clear boundaries

7. exquisite empathy

8. professional satisfaction

9. creating meaning.

Significantly for the art therapist in private practice, most of these can be achieved through active engagement with the work, through networking circles and in the therapist's own art practice. The themes all suggest that it is the work itself that provides the protection rather than seeking an external remedy. This answers the question I raised earlier as to how art therapists, who in my experience are often not explicit in their self-care activities, achieve these outcomes nonetheless by throwing themselves into dedicated work and art making as facilitators/artists and through the parallel aesthetic engagements of their personal art practice. The list of strategies reveals how this self-care is easily accomplished when 1, 2, 3, 4, 5 and 9 are clearly achievable simply by engaging in the art process and the other points (6, 7, 8) relate more specifically to the meanings taken from, and the artful management of, the therapeutic engagement. HCPC (2013) standard 3.4, which requires art therapists to 'recognise…the obligation to maintain fitness to practise [which] includes engagement in their own arts-based process' (p.8), is fully justified.

If we add to the protective strategies the additional two noted below by Sodeke-Gregson *et al.* (2013), we have an 11-point model for the self-care of art therapists in private practice to support them through their most challenging work:

10. practice research and development

Practice-based research will be covered more fully in the research section of the book, but it is clear that the research and development of your private practice helps build a sense of control that will diminish stress, enhance meaning and understanding of the therapeutic engagement and also help you to build professional autonomy through your work. In private practice this could also include the development of business strategy and ethics as an integral part of the research process.

11. working within research-based guidelines advised for certain clients

Ignoring guidance was found to be indicative of a greater likelihood of compassion fatigue in therapists (Sodeke-Gregson *et al.* 2013). Providing therapy as part of a professional research community may benefit the therapist's confidence in practice but it is also advisable to be critically aware of general formulae recommended for treatment of certain conditions. In terms of specific treatment for trauma the therapies that are offered tend to be behavioural in orientation. Cognitive behavioural therapy (CBT) and eye movement desensitisation and reprocessing (EMDR) are specifically recommended by National Institute for Health and Care Excellence (NICE) guidance. Focusing on the present therapeutic moment is seen as essential, and the global monitoring of five CBT areas (Fitzgerald 2013) offers a systemic and holistic view of the interaction of situation, thoughts, emotions, physiology and behaviour in relation to the triggering situations that may send the client into a reliving of the past trauma. Susan Hogan (2016) offers a thorough and useful critical assessment of CBT art therapy. Van der Kolk (2014), however, points out that the more 'cognitive' CBT becomes, the less helpful it may be in the process of integration for trauma. Looking into the sequential interactions of these interacting fields is useful to both the therapist and client in understanding the trauma, the recovery process and the protection of the therapist from the secondary effects of strong affect. The most frightening aspect of trauma is the slippage from the 'here and now' into the 'then and there' and the consequent mis-recognitions and disorientations which are often accompanied by unmediated reactions, visceral emotions and major physiological consequences. If the therapist can hold a steady ground in the here-and-now reality, the alliance is likely to help the client to work through the trauma into the safety of the present relational moment.

These studies suggest that a closer and exquisitely empathetic engagement is a protection to the therapist, providing greater likelihood of compassion satisfaction and the prospect of a mutually helpful art therapy engagement benefiting both parties. This 'mutuality' has to be considered in private practice for it to be viable, and so I conclude that the art of self-care must necessarily be considered in art therapy training towards private practice. The art therapy trainer Michael Franklin explores the need of 'mindful self awareness' and compassion for self and other in his study of art therapy training (Franklin 2014).

Appropriate Supervision

Of the 11 self-care strategies, most can and should be supported and encouraged within clinical supervision. Two areas of research pertinent to this investigation and the further evidencing of this field of intersubjective research are Casement's (1985) notion of 'internal supervision' and Kagan's (1980) 'internal processing recall'. Both authors preceded the new neurological research developments discussed above and this suggests the need for further research. Both, however, pay attention to and support the central concept of the therapist's reflective practice, encouraging active research and enquiry in practice and emphasising the importance of the feeling data of countertransference in this process of enquiry. Casement encourages this in the form of internal supervisory dialogue, whilst Kagan encourages the use of video in recording the therapist's response to their recall of the process of the session. Both suggest a value in teasing out the internal evidence of the *effects of affects* through an exploration of the deeper unconscious intersubjective communications occurring in and after the session.

Conclusion

This section considered the evidence and real risks to therapists of stress and vicarious traumatisation in therapeutic engagement and also some of the strategies and supports that can be put in place to ameliorate the process and to try to ensure a greater likelihood of positive outcomes for both clients and art therapists by using 11 strategies of self-care. Part 2 'introverts' the research process and looks at it from the therapist's practical and theoretical perspective in order to provide a text that, in the round, is both useful and true to both research and practice. We will also consider three tools that can be used in the 'ongoing mutual assessment' of the practice field.

PART 2: PHENOMENOLOGICAL TOOLS FOR ONGOING JOINT ASSESSMENT – A TRIPARTITE MODEL OF THE SELF AS A PROCESS, THE FLOWER DIAGRAM AND THE MODALITY CHART

In Part 1 an emphasis was placed on general research into therapists' stress and their potential for vicarious traumatisation. In this section the emphasis will be now be placed on the meaning and the use of 'affect' in therapeutic practice, moving us from an external perspective of therapy to a specifically practice research-focused perspective. The case for 'ongoing joint assessment' as a protective strategy for the therapist and client, and as a means to understand the broad potential for the art therapy, has been outlined above, so I will now introduce models of the self and the relationship and a modality chart to assist art therapists in private practice in this 'ongoing joint assessment' with the aim of ensuring positive outcomes for both parties and also to foster links between research and the realities of practice. The British Association of Art Therapists' Core Skills and Practice Standards in Private Work document (Appendix 1) points to the central importance of a thorough assessment within private practice. Therapy is a joint work sustained by the ongoing attention of both parties 'in' and 'for' themselves in the 'work'.

The Tripartite Structure of Any Body's Self

The sociologist Stan Rosenthal's and the psychoanalyst Thomas Ogden's tripartite models of the self as a process are of use in this assessment.

Having acknowledged the stress risks present in the therapeutic engagement in Part 1, it is now time to consider the potential of the therapist's use of their embodied self and the art process as a rich source of information that may be neglected if therapists do not attend with care to this dynamic interaction. The field of 'affect' includes the therapist's own peripheral actions both in and outside therapy as potential sources of information, including their emotional life, their art, imagination, dreams and relationships, both conscious and unconscious.

In the 1990s I offered a regular yearly talk at Goldsmiths, University of London, preparing trainees for independent sessional work. I found Stan Rosenthal's model represented in his book *The Self as Process* (1983) very useful in considering self-care for therapists who were working independently. In addition to Rosenthal, Thomas Ogden's tripartite model of the self, expressed in *The Primitive Edge of Experience* (1992), was equally helpful. Ogden takes Klein's model of infant development (paranoid schizoid and depressive positions) and adds a third position (autistic contiguous) to create a mobile and systemic notion of the self as a process. Rosenthal's thesis likewise is that the 'self as process' is composed of three interdependent aspects: the psyche (internal self), the soma (the body) and the social (external self). When trying to convey how to look after yourself in independent and private practice, this notion of joint assessment and self-care is both advantageous and democratic as it uses the same tools used for client assessment in the therapist's own self-assessment. In private practice where the setting is more often the therapist's home (see Chapter 14), where all organisational elements of the statutory provision have been transferred to the therapist and the setting, it intensifies the need for an effective and ongoing assessment of the complex and related systems and processes. The multiplicity and minutiae of 'the process' as they appear in the setting require theoretical supports and filters to hold, understand and symbolise it. The self triangle posed by Ogden and Rosenthal provides a basic model that maps the likely relational, transferential and interactional fields of the therapy.

As I have stated, Ogden places three 'modes' as poles in the triangle which expand on Melanie Klein's two developmental stages and correspond to Rosenthal's model as follows: depressive–social, paranoid schizoid–psyche and autistic contiguous–soma (see Figure 12.1). Ogden de-pathologises what can easily become static diagnostic labels and sets them into a structural, relational and systemic relationship, divesting them of fear and providing a 'normal' map of the psyche in its planar movements between these extremes. This triangular plane can help the private practitioner in the assessment of ongoing individual intra-psychic and inter-psychic processes which may be playing out between the therapist and client, and also provides an opportunity for reflection upon the broader relational and cultural fields, transforming a simple fixed diagnosis into an examination of sets of systemic and interdependent relational potentials.

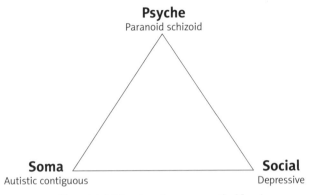

Figure 12.1 The tripartite structure of selfhood

For the private practitioner this brings the 'big players' of mental health into a more dynamic, relational and developmental perspective. It also helps us to see how 'illnesses', that may cause a collapse into one or other of the corners of the triangle and that may lead to formal diagnosis, can be seen as movements away from at least two of the other modes of experience and so reinstate a potential for them to be reinvested, reevaluated and reassessed as part of the therapeutic journey. This may be productive for the client and have value in the development of self-care strategies for the therapist because the psychological movement of either participant in this systemic relationship will necessarily 'move' the other party within the planes of its functioning.

Beyond the specific theoretical agendas and prejudices inherent in every psychological model, the underlying adherence to a tripartite structure of the self points to the fact that we generally find ourselves cast into this world as embodied, desiring, social beings and that this will lead to a recurrent interplay of these bio-psycho-social concerns. Though simplification and reduction undoubtedly abound in human concerns and also acknowledging the human tendency to seek out reductive uni-causal and mechanistic determinants, this model usefully counters this tendency and suggests there will always be at least three major levels of causality in play in any human concern. We must accustom ourselves to bio-psycho-social interplay. Weegmann and Cohen (2002) make this case well in their study of the psychodynamics of addiction, but it can undoubtedly be applied more broadly.

Ogden and Rosenthal's tripartite self has a number of correlations with other models (see Table 12.1).

Table 12.1 The tripartite self as it appears in other
models of selfhood and perception

Rosenthal	Ogden	Freud	Lacan	Peirce	Berne	Mindell
Psyche	Paranoid schizoid	I (ego)	Imaginary	Icon	Adult	Mind: verbal/ auditory
Soma	Autistic contiguous	It (id)	Real	Index	Child	Body: kinaesthetic/ proprioceptive
Social	Depressive	Over I (superego)	Symbolic	Symbol	Parent	World: world/ relationships

The important point is that these models offer the therapist a way
of considering the relational process of therapy in a deeply intersubjective way.

When I first qualified in 1994 I recall making the mistake of trying
to work out strict ownership of pathological material within the therapy.
This caused a major diversion from the work at hand and a considerable
waste of time, energy and distress to me personally. I have since learnt
to promote the primacy of the intersubjective field between therapist
and client and disavow strict notions of subjectivity and objectivity.
I take ownership of 'my stuff' but also recognise that most of what
appears in therapy is intersubjectively posed. This helped me to develop
a capacity to tolerate strangeness and bewilderment in therapy without
needing to prematurely rationalise and support my sometimes reluctant
capacity to 'wait and see', nurturing an understanding and trust that
things will usually become clearer in time as more information comes
forward if I am able to be open to it.

This tolerance of ambiguity acknowledges the profound
interrelatedness of the conscious and unconscious in the self processes
of both the therapist and the client. Clear boundaries are vital in
containing this process of curious holding and puzzling through
the material. Worrying too much about ownership and pathological
diagnostic labelling detracts from the qualitative assessment of the
phenomena that appear in the process by unnecessarily and prematurely
fixing them. A skilled supervisor may help the therapist notice and
hold this process as it occurs, enabling them to bring a fuller awareness
to it and also bring full witness and presence to the client's art and
therapy by simply 'being there'. It is essential that there is an ongoing

joint assessment of the field as part of this process, encouraging playful curiosity and wonder as opposed to objectification, reification and prescription. The notion of countertransference seen in this light is one sided and insufficient, excluding the possibility and reality of the client's thoughts and feelings about the therapist's material and unconsciousness, which are inevitably present and yet often fearfully disavowed by both therapist and client in wishful investments of power. My aim would be for a more democratic awareness rather than notions of stable pathological structures, unearthed and objectively identifiable as 'the client's illness', because this structuring appears contrary to the conception of dynamism and change that must be central to any notion of psychodynamic therapy.

In Ogden's triad each mode has its special area of concern as a defence and as a creative potential. The *depressive* defence has its negative tone but is often expressive of the discursive 'shoulds' and 'oughts' of the social law, norms and conventions (the symbolic). A depressive process tends to exclude the needs of the body and the freedom of imagination that could redeem and revitalise it. The *paranoid schizoid* defence invests in the imaginary realm but tends to deny the social contract and the body's needs, comforts and routines. The *autistic contiguous* defence finds comfort in bodily routines but neglects the social symbolic order, the freedoms and flights of play, metaphor and imagination. These defensive hazards and imaginative potentials are there for all of us, but as a tool of ongoing joint assessment the tripartite model provides a very adaptive schema for the consideration of the tone of the therapeutic relationship and in the assessment of where the therapist and client may find themselves within the process. For example, I may find myself distracted and disembodied in relation to my client's emotional embodiment and usefully explore what may explain our positions in the interpersonal transference and then consider where they may have originated in the personal prehistory of each party and then how an adaptation may subsequently be negotiated within the ongoing interaction. Langs (in Smith 1999) points to the real risk to the client in a therapist's focus on the client's illness which may say more of their desire to 'have the answers' than paying due attention to the full process and creative use of the relational intensity. Ogden's model facilitates the witnessing of complementary and compensatory dances that occur between the client and therapist, revealing the roots of the issue relationally.

You may tell me of your depression and I feel a strange sense of elation. You talk of sadness and I feel anger. You speak of your mother sweetly but suddenly I recall a figure in my past who was deceitful to me. All these require a 'why' and a 'why now', and my experience as a therapist and supervisor tells me they are rarely either solely the therapist's stuff or merely the client's transference but usually a joint and complementary work. This work can be a joy and a pleasure if it is engaged in with an open heart for self-development and compassion, but if it is taken on from a fixed place of identity and a fearful narcissism it is likely to become a battle that can be damaging to both parties. If I disavow the depression I feel when I am with you, I can lose both the possibility of looking into the present context in which it may be arising and how it may have arisen relationally and historically for you (and for me). If I cannot hold my sadness in relation to your risk of vulnerability, I cannot then support you. If visceral and embodied fear sends me into distraction, I cannot reflect on this and then help you to re-symbolise your body into the community of language; we both are then left in a sort of wilderness by this resistance to relate. Jointly the work of self-discovery shifts both parties into what can become an exciting and affirming appreciation of life's tragi-comedic turns. This joint attention to mental wellbeing presents a revelatory narrative which in its complementarities and identifications challenges the technological objectifications of the medical model and draws attention back to the formative interaction of human selfhood through the relational process.

These phenomenological tools aim to enrich and enhance the process, to 'thicken' the description and help both parties become better aware of their joint and single ownership of aspects of the process as they arise.

Counsellors will be aware of the Johari window that plots out the known and the unknown for self and other (see Figure 12.2).

	Known to self	Not known to self
Known to others	Arena	Blind spot
Not known to others	Façade	Unknown

Figure 12.2 The Johari window

If we now push this diagram into the logical form of a Venn diagram we get a picture of the complex knowledge zones, both conscious and unconscious, within the client/therapist relationship. In an artistic turn we can call it 'the flower of knowing and unknowing' (see Figure 12.3).

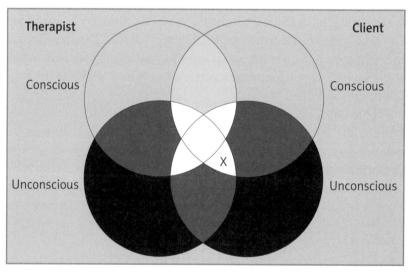

Figure 12.3 The flower of knowing and unknowing

This flower diagram draws our attention to all the fields of experience that must be logically present if the notion of conscious/unconscious process is accepted between therapist and client. It is of relevance here to our topic of both self-care and assessment to identify certain major potential recurrent blind spots within the therapeutic interaction. A prime example would be zone 'X' which relates to 'What the client knows about the therapist and yet the therapist is unaware themselves'. Whilst it is logically presented, this zone is often foreclosed in the therapy relationship by both parties. In practice, however, clients may begin to make remarks towards the end of the therapy which reveal that observations have been made about the therapist all along, but were withheld from open discussion, until now. This reveals the client's knowledge of the therapist's undeniable characteristics of which they may have been previously unaware themselves, or at least unaware that the client was aware of them. These tardy remarks reveal this withheld knowledge and simultaneously identify a sense of growing equality in what Freud called 'the dissolution of the transference', which is a welcome sign of the approach of a therapeutic ending. Therapists should not wish to be invisible to themselves or their clients through their misuse, or defensive use, of the authority they inevitably hold and that is only temporarily invested in them. In private practice, posturing is unlikely to be beneficial to the client, the therapist's business or the therapist themselves, but these investments and projections are a very real part of the process for both parties.

In the flower diagram I have purposely shaded the areas of the client's and the therapist's unconsciousness darkly to highlight both the Freudian and Jungian notion that the repressed unconscious is generally 'darker' and potentially more sinister than the wider unknown, but also to promote the idea that enlightenment comes from reflection with others and that this potential relational knowledge is key to understanding psychodynamic psychotherapy. The lightest central area represents the most mutually reflective zone, bringing together, as it does, the mutuality of the therapist's and client's reflections. Purely cognitive reflections are identified as only bringing light to light, and so the possibility of illumination through integration with the unconsciousness process is then limited or severely truncated. Cognitive behavioural therapy, as Van Der Kolk (2014) pointed out in Part 1, becomes more effective as it works in a simultaneous 'top down' and 'bottom up' process. The embodiment inherent through the physicality and sensuousness of arts therapies returns a balance to narrow cognitive processing, suggesting that the flower of knowing and unknowing can bloom in any art therapy practice as long as it is not curtailed by simplistic and reductive attempts at evidencing. The very act of drawing and painting necessarily involves symbolisation and the use of kinaesthetic, proprioceptive, visual and auditory modes. We hear the charcoal scratch across the paper, showing our marks to ourselves and others, as we feel the expression and see its potential meaning. A complex blend of constructed, recalled sensation, memory and imagination is invoked in every aesthetic and artistic act. It is in this process of drawing attention to, valuing and activating all the modes of experience that the modality chart described below can assist the art therapist to appreciate and order the huge array of phenomena presented in the field of an art therapy practice.

The Modality Chart

A quotation by the psychoanalyst Wilfred Bion offers a starting point to consider again the paradoxical and multilayered scene of therapy, its curious aesthetic data and the centrality of the fleeting and unique moments of its research project. The modality chart (Table 12.2) aims to assist the therapist to manage the density of this data, and like Bion's Grid (1989) it is an attempt to aid the therapist and client to enjoy, endure and understand the forming knowledge of the therapeutic context.

> Instead of trying to bring a brilliant, intelligent, knowledgeable light to bear on obscure problems, I suggest we bring to bear a diminution of the 'light' – a penetrating beam of darkness: a reciprocal of the searchlight… So that, if any object existed, however faint, it would show up clearly. Thus a very faint light would become visible in maximum conditions of darkness. (Bion 1990, p.20)

Table 12.2 The modality chart

	Proprioceptive	Visual	Auditory tonal	Auditory digital	Kinaesthetic	Relationship	Dream	Context
Greater/ lesser								
Internal/ external								
Links								
Time								
Positive/ negative								
Recalled/ constructed								
Conscious/ unconscious								
Midpoint								

In this paradoxical statement Bion uses the metaphor of light in an inverse fashion to the metaphor of light explored in the flower diagram above, but it nonetheless represents illumination occurring through the therapeutic relationship. Bion had earlier quoted Freud, writing in a private letter, that 'I often try to blind myself in order to examine these obscure places' (p.20), suggesting again a struggle between cognition and an alternative sensibility. The flower diagram shows the logical reality of some of these potential fields of knowing and unknowing, and I have already suggested that in order to gain the insight of the knowledge of the senses that cognitive preoccupations must be suspended or temporarily bracketed. Is Bion proposing that to be aware of feeling (the proprioceptive) requires a switching from the visual and auditory digital for us to blindly 'see' as therapists? Is this also the 'negative capability' written of by Keats, often referenced by Bion, encouraging aesthetic sensibility and bracketing the need to 'know'? Artists certainly use metaphors provisionally rather than dogmatically with a sense of fit rather than of logical consistency. The art therapy approach outlined by Rappaport in *Focusing-Oriented Art Therapy* (2009) facilitates a bridging of the gap that exists between the body's 'felt sense' and the symbolised knowledge on which it depends for content and congruence. Bion's beam of darkness represents an attempt to see things afresh, and so he asks us to be informed by the dynamic present and the body, over prior mental representations and conventions. He followed years later with a statement that is rarely quoted in its full viscerality:

> Discard your memory; discard the future tense of your desire, forget them both, both what you knew and what you want, to leave space for a new idea. A thought, an idea unclaimed, may be floating around the room searching for a home. Amongst these may be one of your own which seems to turn up from your insides, or one from outside yourself, from the patient. (Bion 1980, p.11)

He asks the therapist to attune themselves to the actual scene and setting of the embodied and relational 'now' and to submit themselves to the strangeness of its unique intensity. The loss of control and relational 'affect' are also alluded to when he states, 'In every consulting room there ought to be two rather frightened people: the patient and the psycho-analyst' (Bion 1990, p.21). In our culture this idea seems antithetical, but it may be an indication of the cultural loss of our congruent self-regulation. Our inflated scientific and technological control does not appear to correspond to an ease-fulness and grace but rather with mental dis-ease and the widely evidenced symptoms of cultural and personal stress identified earlier in this chapter.

The Evolution of the Modality Chart

The modality chart was not intended as a tool for quantitative measurement and generalisation. In fact it originally evolved through a personal engagement with a difficulty in recalling dreams. I had often found that the recollection of dreams occurred for me not as instant recall of a clichéd visual film sequence, but more often as a single element that endured into waking experience (often a simple feeling or an idea), and then from this surviving trace I could follow Ariadne's thread to a fuller recall of other sensory and symbolic content and then on again into the construction of narrative, a sequence. I continue to find the modality chart useful in this personal process and in playfully expanding the potential of all the reflective reconnections that are likely to be 'there', for myself, for clients and for supervisees. It has become a sort of phenomenological butterfly net to gather fleeting information and also to discover the patterns and silhouettes of consistently absented data from past scenes. In this sense it can support the process of Bionic darkening that facilitates the broader experience of the ephemera of therapy practice and so it can be used as a qualitative tool in the collaborative research endeavour of art therapy practice. The aim is not to tie down the facts but rather to assist the therapist and the client to make links more freely with deeper and deeper resonance into the webs of association and the threads of significance. It should not be used deterministically but can be of use in the formation of hypotheses and in reality testing.

There are other examples of similar prompts to thinking. Aristotle (1992, p.5) originally proposed his 'categories' (of substance, quality, quantity, relation, time, place, position, state, activity, passivity) in order to explore the nature of the empirical world and the *qualia*, or 'whatness', of our experience of things. In the 18th century Kant transformed these into his 'categorical' and 'a priori' ideas of the mind which he thought were necessary for us to experience the world. Van Manen (1990) proposes the use of Heidegger's 'existentials' of 'spatiality, corporeality, temporality and relationship' as the fundamental tools of phenomenological research in a similar vein. De Bono (2010) proposes his 'six thinking hats' to encourage exploration of multi-modal creativity in practical, scientific and business endeavours, relating them to six identified neurological capacities. Dilts and DeLozier (2010) developed their 'neuro-logical levels' in a similar way to draw attention to the recurrent factors apparent in learning. Gardner's (1993) 'multiple intelligences' and Silberman's (2015) 'neurotribes' and 'neurodiversity' likewise respect the different orientations and preferences of individuals and groups. The modality chart follows in this rich tradition to facilitate a deeper regard for and an orientation towards the actual presented data of art therapy practice in place of static diagnostic formulation. The aim here is to assist the therapist to stay with the rich data of therapy practice and avoid flight into the security of theoretical preconception, prejudice and projection.

The chart was further developed in my role as supervisor to therapists of other modalities (visual art psychotherapy and dance movement psychotherapy) in the contexts of both state and private practice, encouraging in me an attention to both detail and the noting of significant absences. It was also developed through a growing sense that the richest information exists in these details, asides and the almost inexpressible feelings that characterise the therapeutic scenario which are often missed or ignored by generalising research aims, theoretical prejudice and the prior impositions of outcomes and hypotheses. It can help to appreciate the unique sequences and modal switches which often have their own significance and to assist in a fuller and fairer retrospective reconstruction of the lost elements of the session, in post-therapy reflection and their return in subsequent engagements. Reflection, sense making and research are by definition after the fact so, while I would agree with Bion that the therapist should enter the session without 'memory, desire or understanding', he clearly did not suggest the therapist should remain blank in perpetuity. His Grid is a testimony to his own post-therapy elaborations and preoccupations.

Building the Modes

It is necessary that the sensory and aesthetic concerns of artists should allow for a strong aesthetic and sensory research orientation in art therapy. The modality chart first involves an engagement with our five senses, referred to as the 'modes' in psychology. Aristotle's exploration of the five senses of touch, taste, smell, sight and hearing (Aristotle 1992, p.174) is one of the first thorough analyses of our sensory equipment and provides one of the bases of our contemporary understanding of the five modes of experience. Moving to a more contemporary psychotherapy model, Arnold Mindell, a Jungian analyst and founder of process-oriented psychology (POP), writes of these modes as 'channels' and adds to the Aristotelian five senses by adding the 'world' and 'relationship' that acknowledge our attachments and the social and environmental givens. In *River's Way* (1989) he develops the idea of these channels of experience into a phenomenological 'process science'. I was fortunate to have Sheila McClelland (1996), an art therapist and a process-oriented psychologist, as my tutor in my training, who introduced me to Mindell's work.

Neuro-linguistic programming (NLP), in which I have subsequently trained, also draws on a rich North American postwar tradition that develops the idea of 'modality preferences' and 'representational systems' and pays particular attention to the visual, auditory and kinaesthetic modes. NLP, like Mindell, collapses Aristotle's 'taste' and 'smell' into 'feeling'. Table 12.3 shows how each of these modal models has contributed to the evolution of the modality chart.

Table 12.3 The modes compared with other similar models

Modality chart	Aristotle	Mindell	NLP
Proprioceptive	Touch, taste, smell	Proprioceptive	Kinaesthetic
Visual	Sight	Visual	Visual
Auditory tonal	Hearing	Auditory	Auditory tonal
Auditory digital			Auditory digital
Kinaesthetic		Kinaesthetic	Kinaesthetic
Relationship		Relationship	
Dreams			
Context		World	

The chart was developed in various practice contexts as a phenomenological and process-oriented tool to assist in the provision of therapy, as an aid to supervisorial exploration, as a playful exploration of personal experience, and for self-monitoring and self-care. Both POP and NLP are fundamentally phenomenological in their drawing on and building on the schemas that are readily accessed by any individual through 'lived experience'. Adaptations of our sensory equipment occur throughout our development, through cultural difference and in disability, and can be usefully explored to provide us with therapeutic application in developing better rapport and in supporting clients who experience deficits. Being over 50 and dyslexic provides me with ample opportunity to develop my own compensatory bridging strategies.

Mindell (1989) describes the aims of 'process orientation': to 'determine the evolving structure of processes, i.e. their channels, primary and secondary characteristics', and to develop 'the ability to work with signals in their own various channels, to amplify these signals and bring them closer to awareness'. The attention to sensory experience is inherently part of the art therapy process, and a detailed exploration of the modes can only enhance the art therapist's skills. Mindell also usefully draws attention to the importance of our noticing 'double signals', 'unoccupied channels', 'edges' and the significance of 'channel switching', 'composite channels' and 'synaesthesia'. He presents a model that is ultimately a systemic field theory that encourages a holistic engagement. The modality chart can assist the therapist in the provision of Van der Kolk's 'top down/bottom up' therapeutic approach, integrating and exploring past tragedy and the countering joys of the complex bio-psycho-social process, through the aesthetic moment shared by client and therapist in art therapy.

The chart can be used by practitioners independently of their theoretical allegiances as it aims to encourage our full attention rather than support a particular theoretical hypothesis. There was also an aim in its creation to provide a common ground to facilitate communication and respect the richness of the therapeutic experience of clients and therapists, and facilitate communication between the modalities of the arts therapies, where there is an urgent need to evolve aesthetic languages and theoretical structures from practice up rather than adapting ill-fitting theories borrowed from the meta-psychologies of other professions which often lack good fit with our own practices.

This chart has subsequently also been used and developed in my National Health Service (NHS) work, particularly in the joint supervision of both art and dance movement psychotherapy (DMP) and also with mindfulness practitioners, where it was enhanced to assist a collaborative appreciation of the complex modal phenomena provided by different 'arts modalities' and the unique benefits they each can provide for clients. We are all united in our art therapy practices by the reality of our own and our clients' whole body experience which the chart recognises. This conception of the unity of the senses in the body also counters medicine's tendency to allocate a professional for each body part and then end the conversation, disrupting both the patient's body and their experience. It is also important that art therapies are not aligned too narrowly with their allocated senses. The chart can help deconstruct these impositions. For example, 'feeling' (proprioception) often plays a greater role in visual art therapy than 'sight' (visual) in its practical therapeutic application. Artists feel as they draw and move the stylus in a synaesthesia that brings together touch, sight and gesture and symbolism. Artists often see colours as harmonic sounds just as musicians may see the colour of musical harmonies. There is often an assumption that art therapists use the visual; music therapists use the auditory; and dance movement therapists use the kinaesthetic exclusively. Empirically observed, this is evidently nonsense. All art therapy engagements are complex and multi-modal because the therapeutic interaction always involves the whole bodies of both the therapist and the clients. It is important for all art therapists to develop an understanding of these full modal processes both to protect our unique professional skills and better understand the power of these processes in their practical therapeutic applications.

The chart can be used in solitary mindfulness and self-care strategies to help clarify what remains 'lodged' in the therapist's body away from the therapeutic scene. It can have use in personal therapy, supervision, and explicitly or implicitly in explorations with clients within the session. My own application of this chart includes dream recall, exploring complex countertransference and complex post-traumatic stress disorder (PTSD) with clients and by myself, as a creative and playful reparative form of mindfulness, in self-hypnosis, and also in considering the use of the modalities in my own artwork, art teaching, assessment, supervisorial reflection and the consideration of appropriate referrals.

Change is the dynamic aspect in psychodynamic therapy. It can be identified through modality changes towards greater adaptability, cognitive flexibility and aesthetic enrichment. Nature is characterised by flux and change. Fixity and stasis are therefore identified as a defence or a loss of our natural adaptability and flexibility. Lack of change and adaptation in this sense is 'unnatural' and yet the practitioner's rigidity and the client's stasis are often promoted by professional affiliation and diagnostic categorisation within the state sector. As clients explore change, the chart can help the therapist identify and understand these changes and support the process. It can also help to identify and explore repeatedly recurring patterns, and 'unresourceful' strategies in the modal sequences expressed over time.

Sequence and Strategy in the Use of the Modality Chart

In NLP the notion of 'strategy' is identified by strings of sensual representation often considered concretely by us as 'reality'. The modality chart can help the client and therapist to consider these sensual sequences of behaviour and thought and then the value of adopting different strategies through congruent change, deconstructing and reconstructing maladaptive strategies that may follow from traumatic experience. Noticing and becoming aware of the unconscious steps involved in a traumatic reaction can help to change them and reengage active choice making. If every time I encounter x then y inexorably follows in my process, if I can first become curious of this process and represent it to myself or another, I can then start to change it and start changing aspects of the sequence and finally open up to fuller dynamic exploration and integration. Many clients in art therapy do not gain this sort of 'insight', but change and benefit comes from the containing art process and the therapist's 'holding' their clients through change even when it occurs at an unconscious level. Consciousness and cognition are sometimes overvalued in terms of their curative effect. The modality chart can explore these changes as they occur at many different levels, both conscious and unconscious. Art therapists are often working non-verbally, accepting 'the not knowing' and aware that the temporary switching off of the cognitive function (auditory digital mode) can also be an important part of the creative process. Yet in this way we can monitor the effects and affects of the engagement in the modes over time in both ourselves and our clients. I will now outline the modes (summarised in Table 12.4) and then their qualifiers (see Table 12.5) as they appear on the axes of the chart.

Table 12.4 The modes

1. Proprioceptive	P	Feeling interior to the body, touch, including smell and taste
2. Visual	V	Vision/spatial awareness, the image, mental images
3. Auditory tonal	At	Raw sound, music, including voice tone
4. Auditory digital	Ad	Talk and self-talk, interpretation, symbolisation, verbal concepts
5. Kinaesthetic	K	Movement, the feel of movement, actions, gestures
6. Relationship	R	The experience of relationship with people, things and places
7. Dream	D	Dreams and dreamlike phenomena, e.g. transference, unconscious, phantasy, narratives, myth, film
8. Context	C	Location, ecology, world, context, big picture or story, vision, frame, discourse, wider system, gestalt

The order of the modes is based roughly on their developmental primacy and the preferences of the practitioners who have used it. Seen developmentally, it seems preferable to have *proprioception* first and *context* last. This reflects how we arrive into the world as infants initially without clear vision, developing our sensory awareness and then a growing capacity to symbolise and finally beginning to relate more and more broadly as reflective individuals within our social spheres. The chart can also be seen as a set of interdependent looping circuits because, without *context* (earth, world, society, family, dyad and linguistic context), there can actually be no primary observing human selfhood. The chart is not presented as any sort of hierarchy or linearity and varies greatly in each individual's preferences.

The first four modes, P, V, At, Ad, are sensual and correspond to Aristotle's identified five senses. The philosopher Bertrand Russell may have considered these modes as the source of empirical 'sense data' and sensory evidence. As we have mentioned above, smell and taste are included within *proprioception* because they are experienced as internal to the body and are developmentally strongly evocative of primary feeling. The subdivision of auditory into *auditory tonal* and *auditory digital* is imported from NLP to distinguish raw sound from the auditory experience of self-talk experienced as thinking or experienced externally as 'others' voices' and auditory hallucination, depending on the contextual reading of the frame. Mindell associates the mind with the visual and auditory modes and the body with kinaesthetic and proprioceptive modes. He considers these within an interdependent and holistic union of process, 'Mind, Body, World'.

Within the behavioural approaches of NLP and CBT, sequences of behaviour can be broken down into simpler sequences of experience or 'strategies' that the client is then encouraged to reflect upon, adapt and disrupt, and can be supported in other congruent choices considered and tested through 'behavioural experiments'. It is possible to write experience in shorthand, and this plays an important part in clinical hypnosis, which was one of the forms of treatment that led to the development of NLP. Great attention is paid to individual sequences and the patterns of experience (Dilts *et al.* 1980). I will illustrate. Let us say a client arrives in a flustered state for the session, provides rationalisations for lateness, sits down and then begins to sob, turning attention inwards, and then begins to consider past images of a traumatic childhood experience…falls silent and begins to paint…finishes the painting and then says with feeling and a sigh, 'This is my world!', and then relaxes… We then go on to look at the work and the process together. The therapist of course will have their own sequence going on in parallel to the client's process and they can examine this process in supervision and then bring an enriched picture and embodied resources back to the work.

It is useful for the therapist to be aware of these sequences because these personal patterns often have sufficient stability to be indicative of a general attitude to life, making us recognisable each as characters in the world. This client's pattern or strategy could be written as follows, where the 'i' and 'e' qualify the modes here as either 'internal' or 'external':

> Arrives in a flustered state to the session (K,e), provides rationalisations for lateness (Ad,e), sits down (K,e) and then begins to sob (P,i), turning attention inwards; and then begins to consider past images of a traumatic childhood experience (V,i)… falls silent (depends what is being done in the silence?) and begins to paint (P,i, K,e, V,e)…finishes the painting and then says (Ad,e) with feeling and a sigh (P,i), 'This is my world!', and then relaxes (C,i,e)…(P,i). We then go on to look at the work and the process together (R…C).

(K,e)…(Ad,e)…(K,e)…(P,i)…(V,i)…?…(P,i, K,e, V,e)…(Ad,e)…(P,i)… (C,i,e)…(P,i)…(R…C). Pattern recognition is vital both to art and therapy, as both involve the sequencing of the symbolic and aesthetic process with understanding. The chart can help us to examine patterns and provide alternative routes that could be taken. It can assist us in a thorough assessment of the phenomena encountered rather than our getting too involved in the assertion or disavowal of theoretical constructs. If the data of a client's patterns cannot be held within the therapist constructions then it may be time for the therapist to seek alternative theoretical constructs and new theory. It could also be time for the client to seek another therapist! As therapists we all have strengths and weaknesses, and adequate rapport and flexibility is very important in therapy as it will increase a sense of empathy, being listened to, and being seen.

The last four modes (kinaesthetic, relationship, dream and context) are more complex and are built from the smaller sense-based units. They nonetheless display a sufficient unity as experiences or gestalts to be considered as modes but they are more conventionally symbolised and socially interactive. They shift the focus towards depth and complexity in therapy, often in relation to the theoretical orientation of the therapist. My dreams, my vision, my world, my story, my relationships and the actions are more complex wholes than what I see, hear, feel at any moment. These modes shift the therapy focus away from simple behavioural sequences towards more complex understanding and towards judgement, values, hopes and more abstract conceptual constructs. If we take a Rogerian position: conflicts and incongruence often arise between our required behaviour and these larger constructs, and so finding a congruent solution becomes essential to the course of therapy. A client may arrive with exam nerves but then realise, following a dream that somehow spoils the tidy rationalisation of the problem, that there is an underlying issue of self-esteem in performing practical tasks generally which evolved from a critical parental voice that still demands attention after all these years.

Each K, R, D, C can be broken down into the sensory elements P, V, At, Ad. A dream, for example, as we explored above, may be experienced as a sequence of visual, auditory and proprioceptive elements which, on elaboration, build into an aesthetic world, a narrative or an ethical claim or value. A memory of an interaction may likewise be made up of sensory sequences (e.g. I saw his red face and then heard him shouting and then I felt (V,e…A,e…P,i)) with the significance (Ad) coming later with deliberation.

Context is the most complex mode but it can nonetheless be experienced as a unity or whole. The workplace may be the context in question, but this may be linked to memories of other social settings and their associated discourses (school or family home), and even though it is the last mode in the chart it is vital in our consideration. All sequences only make sense within larger wholes, gestalts, discourse or frames. A painting may depict an elaborate set of relationships within such a scenario, setting or context (environment or culture, historical moment) and without which the smaller sensory units will not make sense. It is often the larger ecology of relationships and discourses that hold the 'game' together and so contain the keys to a conflict, and yet each mode provides opportunities for questions, reflections and sense making, enabling the client to discover a broader range of choices and ways of understanding their dilemma, independent of the therapist's particular theoretical constructs which may represent the therapist's own vain attempts to make sense and have a world view and a context for meaning making. The therapist's theoretical constructs must always be seen as secondary to the integrity of the client's world and the help that one can give another through collaborative reflection.

The Qualifiers Used in Building the Modality Chart

If we place the modalities that we have chosen on one axis and the processes by which they can be qualified on another, we have a chart of 64 potential interdependent areas of likely relevance that reveals the creative richness, intensity and complexity potential in an art therapy session. It goes some way to explaining the frequent complaint made by art therapists about the excess of information and volume of material that can be present in a single session. The chart can help therapists draw out relevant and recurrent patterns in the full range of experiences without reducing and diminishing the process and so value its complexity as part of the therapy's resources.

I am aware that NLP notions of 'sub-modalities' have played a part in my thinking around choosing these 'qualifiers'. In Eriksonian hypnotherapy, on which NLP draws, clients are encouraged to adapt their experience by changing the intensity, colour and size of recalled images and memories of traumatic events. This exemplifies a way that clients can take back playful agency of their constructions of reality and of the past. This has clear benefits to those living in a post-traumatic world, as the literature presented above suggests. The trauma remains as a reality, but the way it then plays upon the client can be externalised, transformed, deconstructed, reconstructed and re-visioned, returning active engagement and agency to the client. The abundant resources available within the arts therapies can help this process in so many different ways.

Table 12.5 The qualifiers

Greater or lesser
Is the phenomenon experienced with greater intensity over time or is it diminishing? Is the client relating more? Is their pain less? This qualifier provides a sort of scaling that can become meaningless when taken out of the context of the other related information. It provides the numerical basis of many outcome measures which can have value both within and outside the therapy.
Internal/external
Is the phenomenon experienced as internal or external to the body? For example, an idea may be experienced as an internal thought or an external truth. A visual hallucination may be experienced as external by the client but may be assumed to be internal to the client by the therapist because the immediate phenomenon is not mutually evident externally to the therapist as a reality. Jung wrote a great deal about the value of introversion (internal focus of evidence), comparing himself with Freud the extrovert (external focus of evidence). Our senses are characterised by their internality and externality. Aristotle's original examination of the senses looks into the internal and external objects of each of the senses.
Links
Identifies the linking and switches across the modes identified by Mindell. Why does the client change the channel at this particular point from proprioceptive feeling to a visual memory? Why do I stop thinking about something and start singing? This acknowledges that linking and switching usually has its own significance. The qualifiers also provide opportunities to explore phenomena that appear to fulfil more than one criterion. The notion of 'edges' (Mindell 1989) provides for significant experiences that are shifting or disavowed, both inner and outer, positive and negative, 'double signals', 'composite channels', 'synaesthesia', and expressing a conscious or unconscious intention to change. Sometimes 'when' and 'why' a channel switch occurs is of as much significance as the content.
Time
Is the phenomenon experienced as occurring in the present or in the past, or in relation to the past or in relation to the future? The notion of time also has significance in relation to hope, depression and the process generally as occurring in time or through time. Phenomenology and existentialism pay great attention to the phenomena of time orientation and our being through time, space and in our embodiment and relationships.

Positive or negative

Is the experience broadly speaking a positive or negative one? Does the client's experience of the phenomenon have a particular tone. Is it joyful? Are they sad when talking about it? Do they appear to be generally more content due to the therapy or are they clearly disturbed and unsettled by what they are encountering? In this area the therapist can assess the resources and commitment of the client to work through their difficulties which may involve encountering unpleasantness and disturbance as part of the journey. Sometimes consent needs to be explicitly gained for this reason. This field would also include positive and negative shape: figure (positive) and ground (negative).

Recalled/immediate/constructed

Is the phenomenon experienced as remembered, imagined or experienced in the present moment? This qualifier is used in NLP (Bandler and Grinder 1990) to assess whether an idea is the consequence of a creative mental construction or is recalled in memory. I cannot recollect my future but I can construct it in imagination. Depression is often hinged on a repeatedly recalled past, while a paranoid psychosis may involve a certain creativity and imaginative elaboration in its constructions. I have added a midpoint of 'immediacy' between recalled and constructed for what happens in the jointly witnessed 'now' moment of the session.

In/out of awareness (conscious/unconscious)

Is the phenomenon experienced with awareness or on the edge of awareness, or is it out of awareness? It may be evident to the therapist that the client knows something but is not yet conscious of it nor able to symbolise it. Across time Mindell may see this as the interplay of primary and secondary processes. For psychodynamic therapy of a Freudian, Jungian, Kleinian or object relations or gestalt orientation, this category is seen as essential to therapy, providing a dialectical interplay of figure and ground. It is understood that much of our experience occurs on the boundary or beyond our conscious awareness, but nonetheless that insight and congruent awareness of it can be gained over time. Breath is largely an autonomic function, so it can therefore become a good indicator of emotional affect and provide a bridge between the unconscious body process and the intentional self. It is only through regulating breathing that we can influence our sympathetic nervous system. Voice tone and speed of speech delivery may be an indication of body states beyond the content of speech. In the midst of a stress reaction, slowing speech and three deep breaths can usually help both the client and the therapist to find a more comfortable pace, more capable of reflection. The physiological in the CBT 'five areas' acknowledges this unconscious bodily realm (Fitzgerald 2013). The body often silently holds our personal story away from day-to-day awareness. In trauma the unconscious past impinges on present conscious functioning.

Midpoint

Each of the previous qualifiers (apart from 'Links') have a midpoint that can represent either an absence of information or a negation of information in the mode. Paradoxically it can also represent a healthy homeostatic balance. It is therefore worth considering if the mode is not noticeably represented in the process whether this is due to its cultural or individual repression, useful adaptation and sensory preference, or a balance that leaves it in neutral. What is the quality of its silence? The absence of information is therefore seen as informative. If the client never speaks of family: is this significant? Do the other modes point to something else being present that is as yet unstated? The modes are interdependent and mutually informative.

In concluding this section I hope I have shown how the chart can help support both the client and the therapist in exploring their 'lived experience' of therapy and that this study may lead towards a discovery of the phenomenological essences of art therapy in practice which can be verified within the intersubjective experience of the therapeutic alliance, through intersubjective peer verification, and then externally by other research formulations that value both the client's and therapist's unique insights into the process. Below is a version of the modality chart drawn with my own pictograms corresponding to the modes and qualifiers to show how it can be more conveniently conceived for portability and reference. I spent a number of weeks in my spare time throwing an eight-sided dice twice each time to explore the relevance of the 64 zones randomly and discovered on each occasion it evoked interesting and relevant therapeutic associations. Why don't you try it?

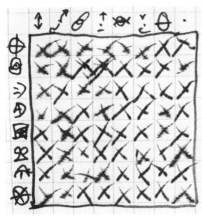 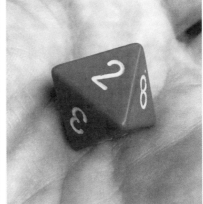

Conclusion

In the course of developing this understanding of self-care in private art therapy practice, first through an examination of the real trauma risks to therapists and then through the development of integrated models for practitioners to use, my hope is that this points towards further reflective practice research which may lead to further evidencing of the value of art therapy interventions more generally. This undoubtedly requires a conception of research that requires, as the sociologist Herbert Blumer (1989) stated in defence of his own methodological position, that we 'respect the nature of the empirical world and organize a methodological stance to reflect that respect' (p.60).

What is the nature of the empirical world we witness as therapist and client researchers in the collaborative engagement of art psychotherapy? How do we respect it and develop a methodological stance that respects its nature? I hope this chapter has gone some way to reveal something of the nature of our world with a sense of enduring wonder for its peculiarity, its breadth, and the value it both discovers and creates within the complexity and abundance that is native to it. This field *can* be researched with both an empirical and phenomenological focus to ensure an evidence-based practice that relies on practice-based research, able to balance and occasionally challenge the dominant models of research that appear sometimes to risk undermining the very practice they seek to evidence. However, it is vital not to diminish the richness, freedoms and potentiality of the art therapy process by limiting the research focus. Some of these questions will now be taken up again in the chapter on research in private art therapy practice that follows in Part V.

References

Aristotle (1992) *A New Aristotle Reader* (J.L. Ackrill ed.). Oxford: Clarendon Press.

Bandler, R. and Grinder, J. (1990) *Frogs into Princes*. London: Eden Grove Editions.

Bion, W. (1980) *Bion in New York and Sao Paulo*. Strathclyde: Clunie Press.

Bion, W. (1989) *Two Papers: The Grid and Caesura*. London: Karnac.

Bion, W. (1990) *Brazilian Lectures*. London: Karnac.

Blumer, H. (1989) *Symbolic Interactionism*. Los Angeles, CA: University of California Press.

Casement, P. (1985) *On Learning from the Patient*. London: Tavistock Publications.

De Bono, E. (2010) *Six Thinking Hats*. London: Penguin.

Dilts, R. and DeLozier, J. (2010) *NLP II*. Capitola, CA: Meta Publications.

Dilts, R., Grinder, J., Bandler, R. and DeLozier, J. (1980) *NLP I*. Cupertino, CA: Meta Publications.

Dunne, E. (2015) *Wounded Healer of the Soul*. London: Watkins Publishing.

Elkin, A. (1999) *Stress Management for Dummies*. New York: Wiley Publishing, Inc.

Findlay, J.C. (2008) 'Immunity at Risk and Art Therapy.' In N. Hass-Cohen and R. Carr (eds) *Art Therapy and Clinical Neuroscience*. London: Jessica Kingsley Publishers.

Fitzgerald, S. (2013) *The CBT Workbook*. London: Hodder & Stoughton.

Frankl, V. (2008) 'The Case for a Tragic Optimism.' In *Man's Search for Meaning*. London: Rider.

Franklin, M.A. (2014) 'Mindful Considerations for Training Art Therapists: Inner Friendship – Outer Professionalism.' In L. Rappaport (ed.) *Mindfulness and the Arts Therapies: Theory and Practice*. London: Jessica Kingsley Publishers.

Gardner, H. (1993) *Multiple Intelligences*. New York: Basic Books.

Harrison, R.L. and Westwood, M.J. (2009) 'Preventing vicarious traumatisation of mental health therapists: Identifying protective practices.' *Psychotherapy Theory, Research, Practice, Training 46*, 2, 203–219.

HCPC (2013) *Standards of Proficiency: Arts Therapists*. London: HCPC.

HCPC (2016) *Standards of Conduct, Performance and Ethics*. London: HCPC.

Hogan, S. (2016) *Art Therapy Theories*. London: Jessica Kingsley Publishers.

Huet, V. and Holttum, S. (2016) 'Art therapists with experience of mental distress: Implications for art therapy training and practice.' *International Journal of Art Therapy 21*, 3, 95–103.

Kagan, N. (1980) 'Influencing Human Interaction – Eighteen Years with IPR.' In A.K. Hess (ed.) *Psychotherapy Supervision: Theory, Research, and Practice.* New York: Wiley.

Lobban, J. (2012) 'The invisible wound: Veterans' art therapy.' *International Journal of Art Therapy 19,* 1–16.

McClelland, S. (1996) 'The Art of Science with Clients.' In H. Payne (ed.) *Handbook of Inquiry in the Arts Therapies.* London: Jessica Kingsley Publishers.

Mindell, A. (1989) *River's Way.* London: Penguin.

Ogden, T.H. (1992) *The Primitive Edge of Experience.* London: Karnac.

Rappaport, L. (2009) *Focusing-Oriented Art Therapy.* London: Jessica Kingsley Publishers.

Rhodes, E. (2016) 'Wellbeing issues facing psychological professionals.' *The Psychologist 29,* 6, 425. Accessed on 1 July 2017 at https://thepsychologist.bps.org.uk/wellbeing-issues-facing-psychological-professionals.

Richards, J., Holttum, S. and Springham, N. (2016) 'How do "mental health professionals" who are also or have been "mental health service users" construct their identities?' *Sage Open 6,* 1, 1–14.

Rosenthal, S. (1983) *The Self as Process.* Cardiff: Institute of Human Development.

Rothschild, B. (2006) *Help for the Helper.* New York: W.W. Norton & Company, Inc.

Siegel, D. (2011) *Mindsight.* London: Oneworld Publications.

Silberman, S. (2015) *Neurotribes.* London: Allen and Unwin.

Smith, A. (2016) 'A literature review of the therapeutic mechanisms of art therapy for veterans with post-traumatic stress disorder.' *International Journal of Art Therapy 21,* 66–74.

Smith, D.L. (1999) *Approaching Psychoanalysis.* London: Karnac.

Sodeke-Gregson, E.A., Holttum, S. and Billings, J. (2013) 'Compassion satisfaction, burnout, and secondary traumatic stress in UK therapists who work with adult trauma clients.' *European Journal of Psychotraumatology 4,* 1–10.

Toffler, E. (1984) *Future Shock.* New York: Bantam Books.

Van der Kolk, B. (2014) *The Body Keeps the Score.* New York: Viking Penguin.

Van Manen, M. (1990) *Researching Lived Experience.* New York: New York Press.

Weegmann, M. and Cohen, R. (2002) *The Psychodynamics of Addiction.* London: Whurr Publishers.

Part V

RESEARCH

13

RESEARCH, EPISTEMOLOGY AND THE FEE IN ART THERAPY PRIVATE PRACTICE

—— JAMES D. WEST ——

This chapter is written in two parts. Part 1, The Scene of Research for Private Practitioners, considers how the exchange of the fee in private practice changes the nature of accountability. I will consider the implications this has for the epistemology of research in this setting. Part 2, Means, Methods and Methodologies in Researching Art Therapy in Private Practice, considers some of the forms of research that have particular relevance for a collaborative practice-based research (PBR) in this context.

PART 1: THE SCENE OF RESEARCH FOR PRIVATE PRACTITIONERS

Introduction: Questions and Definitions

The field of research is vast and full of controversy and so I will seek to address a number of key issues for practitioners regarding the research of private art therapy practice specifically. The key questions I will aim to address are, first, 'What characterises research in a private art therapy practice?' and then, 'What kind of research is possible, appropriate and ethical within this field of inquiry?' My aim is to represent the possibility for practice-based research to art therapy private practitioners, encouraging them to work collaboratively with art therapists in the statutory sector, learning from the wealth and diversity of our different practices, in the interests of all our clients. I believe it is important that we recognise the increasing diversity of practice and respect the different epistemologies (theories of knowledge) that evolve from these varied contexts. This will help us to make new and creative theoretical syntheses for innovative research and present a critical voice to the dominant research traditions whenever necessary.

What Is Research?

The Organisation for Economic Co-operation and Development (OECD 2015) in its Frascati Manual defines research as follows, linking it to practical research and development (r&d). It states that research is the:

> creative and systematic work undertaken in order to increase the stock of knowledge – including knowledge of humankind, culture and society – and to devise new applications of available knowledge...
> A set of common features identifies r&d activities that aim to achieve either specific or general objectives, even if these are carried out by different performers. For an activity to be an r&d activity, it must satisfy five core criteria. (p.28)

According to the Frascati Manual the criteria the activity needs to be fulfilled are that it should be novel, creative, uncertain, systematic, transferable and/or reproducible. I have purposely chosen a definition that is a global standard to avoid the current narrow and hierarchical research standards of the National Health Service (NHS) identified and explored by the art therapist Gilroy (2013). The OECD definition for our purposes here usefully twins the term 'research' with 'development' and acknowledges the place of the pursuit of knowledge in the broader context of social benefit through innovation.

The broadest and the easiest way to envisage research generally within a private practice is offered by the business thinker Roam (2009), who backs up his pragmatic approach with recent neuroscience research. He characterises visual thinking and research through four visual words in the following sequence: *look, see, imagine* and *show*. It is delightful in its simplicity! We *look* and gather data; we *see*, categorise and make sense of it; we then use *imagination* to compare it with what we already know for fit or invent new hypotheses and theoretical ways of 'seeing' the data; and finally we share our knowledge by *showing* it. The process can endlessly loop, yet the order of the sequence is vital because, as fearful human animals, we often *see* before we *look*. This simple visual process metaphor has surprising fit with the vast array of complex research methods and methodologies that are fiercely defended as 'gold standards' by various interest groups within society, the political establishment and academia, each often calling out the other's methods and methodology as invalid. It is very clear that research is not an objective and neutral field with truth apples falling easily from its trees! In order to avoid these expansive controversies and polemics I will try to remain within the pragmatic territory that defines private art therapy practice. A private practice can retain a relative autonomy of these debates due to the local, material arrangements that defines it as the *self*-employment of a *sole* trader and therefore an *independent* practice. It is also worth noting that progress in science owes a great deal over the centuries to the endeavours of private individuals and that reasoned dissent and a level of irreverence is a necessary companion to the process of research and development.

Why Do Research in Private Practice?

In the early days of formal art therapy research Helen Payne (1996) stated that through 'the practitioner engaging in researching their own practice they become connoisseurs of it' (p.33). This remains good advice and a clear motivation for research that is in the interests of both clients and practitioners. However, it is also the case that as paid professionals we should consider the expertise that is expected and transacted by the fee. The fee presupposes an exchange of goods, and so therapists have a responsibility to consider what 'goods' they are offering in return for the fee. Research also provides us with a place to assess the nature of the transaction and an assurance of professional competence for the client, encouraging us to listen to their feedback regarding the process. It asks us to reflect and show efficacy, efficiency and outcomes, and consider how the client and therapist can have some assurance that the therapy helps them learn something, solve something, gain something, change something and consider reflectively what that 'something' may be. In Chapter 12, I pointed for the research that suggests r&d can also be a protective factor to the health and wellbeing of the therapist in their work. Through an involvement in research, however tangential, the therapist can also become better able to understand the research literature they may use to inform 'best practice' and understand their clients' needs. Private practitioners must therefore be active in research.

So what then would this active research look like? In an art therapy private practice, where the therapist is both practice manager and practitioner, collaboratively involved in research with the client, it is easy to lose sight of the significance of the densely packed abundance of process data. In this context as in other fields of research, *data* exists, and so *information* can be drawn from it which can help to build *knowledge* with the aim of *informing* the stake holders and wider groups of professional colleagues and the public. So, how best to research, manage and communicate this in ways that are ethical and congruent to the therapeutic aims of a private practice that exists primarily as a transaction of 'goods' between the therapist and the client?

Is Therapy Research?

If therapy is not seen as an active collaborative research inquiry, then how can it actually be conceived? If it is not defined as research in itself then there is a danger of it becoming a merely technical exercise of identified and prescriptive service provision, likely to leave the client dissatisfied and the therapist deskilled. I will represent therapy as an endogenous research project to counter the assumption that research can only occur in the academy or the hospital clinic and be performed only by external 'researchers' who are often not practitioners

(McLeod 1999). Clients who seek private art therapy are generally not seeking a technical intervention or a prescribed solution to their dilemmas; in my experience as a therapist, they can often feel worn down by their own experience of the accountancy-driven agendas of the workplace, and so are averse to submitting to the same quantifying methods driving 'their' therapy. They should nonetheless expect a professionally provided space and an engagement with art materials and an art process held within a therapeutic relationship that collaboratively, experientially and experimentally researches the dilemmas they bring. All art therapists have a basic MA research qualification and so they are ready to begin this practice research.

The English word 'research' comes from the old French *rechercher*, meaning to seek out or search closely (and this is rooted in the Latin *cicare* – to wander – and *circus* – a circle). The etymology suggests that what is essential to the activity of research is a cycling and reflective review of our experience, either individually or collectively, as a way of establishing what we think we know, but also in order to discover new knowledge through a process of ongoing inquiry. Research seen in this way is likely to disturb norms and pre-judgements, as it requires a receptivity for new information and knowledge in both the client and the therapist. It cannot exist to satisfy vested ideological positions, whether they are scientific, political or academic, and so it is vital to explore our research practice *reflectively* and *reflexively*, considering our investments, motivation and intentionality and our ethical stance within the practice of inquiry. In the context of private practice the investments are clear, simple and overt in the way that in the statutory sector investments and intentions in research are often hidden and formed within highly complex group and organisational dynamics (professional, managerial, political and industrial interests, academic investments, large-scale and long-term planning and finance). In the simple small-scale local economy of a private practice, the therapist can return to the unique needs of the paying client and their particular story. Small is indeed beautiful (Schumacher 2014). The state sector will always tend to lose this micro-narrative within the larger wheels of organisational, professional and financial accounting stories. The art therapy profession's involvement, acceptance and support of private practice can offer a useful 'outside' to these larger discursive practices that many of us in dual employment find both refreshing and illuminating. An art therapy private practitioner in the UK nonetheless has a primary professional responsibility to account to the client as employer but is also required to fulfil practice standards outlined by the profession in the Health and Care Professions Council (HCPC 2013, 2016) documents that regulate us as state-regulated professionals.

Data Loss

All researchers must be cautious of data loss. Ben Goldacre (2013) makes a critique of current state health guidance that is often based on the research funded by the pharmaceutical industry, and questions its convenient loss of inconvenient data that invalidates the scientific research procedure it rhetorically promotes. As private practitioners it may be useful for us to consider in like mind what data we may wish to lose on the way to supervision, or may struggle to submit even to ourselves. However, it is often this problematic data with uncomfortable fit with our current perspective that is crucial to practice research, because research and practice both require the challenge of new data that can form fresh theoretical and ethical perspectives that a critical incident (for example) may suggest. It is vital that we explore these moments of challenge and discomfort that occur in practice non-judgementally, as these very 'problems' of practice are often the source of research questions for practice research and personal professional development (PPD). We will return to critical incidents and research in the second part of this chapter, where I will look at methods and methodologies specifically.

The EBP Agenda for Research

Art therapy in the UK developed within the statutory provision (Waller 2013) and evidence-based practice (EBP), and the National Institute for Health and Care Excellence (NICE) continues to stand by a hierarchy of research evidence that effectively excludes the practice-based research that could be undertaken by individuals within their practices and which practitioners must consider as evidence within the process of reflective practice required of them by the HCPC. As Gilroy (2013) points out, 'in this orthodox EBP framework experimental studies are graded at lower levels, expert opinion is the lowest level and qualitative research is excluded altogether' (p.15).

This has resulted in a situation where art therapists will often hear it glibly declared by non-practitioners that there is 'no evidence for art therapy' and many uncritically accept this, bind their wounds and carry on, buoyed up alone by personal faith in the process. This statement could, however, be turned around and restated more fairly as a question, 'Why is the data of art therapy excluded by the methodological assumptions of mainstream research practices?', resulting in a situation where most process data from art therapy practice is currently lost to research. The question of 'what science is' that stands behind these debates is not at all settled and is hotly disputed between the various sciences and within many academic disciplines including psychology, sociology and the history of science. Whilst no one can doubt the technical achievements of science and technology since the Renaissance, for good and for ill, the debate now needs to be rebalanced to take account of the 'lived experience', actions and practices of clients, therapists and researchers (Dewey 1981; Dilthey 1976). Cartwright (2007) presents a thorough assessment of scientific reasoning and methods pointing to the 'vanity of rigour' that the current hierarchy of evidence presents and its exclusion of numerous scientific methods evident within the history of science. She also challenges the widely accepted assumptions that place randomised controlled trials (RCTs) as a 'clincher' at the pinnacle of the research hierarchy to produce the 'best evidence' for every context, and points to the major problems of application that such evidence presents to practical application in the community. Natural science methods clearly have their place as a method amongst other valid methods, but the current hierarchy is creating a distortion of evidence and research activities that all practitioner researchers should question with more rigour.

Sadly, much of the current research discourse that surrounds art therapy in the state sector actively supports clinical data loss, whilst the very rich data of art therapy practice is placed beyond the scope of research through the hierarchy of accepted evidences – and yet, paradoxically, for practitioners it still provides the uncertain but creative heart of our practice. The uncertain nature of the signification of the image, countertransference feelings and the multiple and perplexing behaviours that characterise much of the data and process of our practice need an adequately reconceptualised research forum that helps us to hold and handle this data, so that it can be better used in the interests of the clients we serve. The conceptual nets in use will determine the efficacy of this practice research project and must be adequate for the task. It makes no sense panning for gold with a gauge designed solely for large stones! Cost and impracticality put most of the 'accepted' research 'gold standard' models of research out of the hands of private practitioners, which raises the question of what remains *doable* in terms of practice based research.

The current research hierarchy of the EBP orthodoxy inevitably favours pharmaceutical interventions that can more readily control variables and deterministically follow chemical mechanisms. Whilst this positivistic methodology has legitimately evolved as an agenda from the Cochrane Reviews, where doctors and independent researchers were asked to systematically review and rigorously test their medical treatments, it has been extended well beyond its epidemiological remit into fields the of public life, where it has questionable methodological validity. This has led to recommendations that indicate a failure of research rather than a failure of practice.[1] In these recessionary times such guidance is then translated into policy to justify anti-social policy actions with devastating effects in the community.

Art therapy is a social, symbolic, relational and aesthetic intervention. It is not a chemical intervention and neither is it a treatment for disease. It produces highly complex and often unique data evident within each engagement. This is not to say that there are no stable patterns or consistent benefits from which to make inferences (Uttley *et al.* 2015) but rather that simple mechanistic research methods are clearly ill fitted to the research task. To ask the practitioner to reduce the art therapy process into a medical metaphor of dosage means it will no longer reflect the open, creative and adaptable therapeutic process at the heart of practice and so then inevitably rules out its efficacy as an intervention when seen in these terms. An art therapy private practice can and does proceed in a reasoned way and can evaluate its evidence within an appropriate practice research forum. To deny there is 'evidence' within art therapy downgrades the general capacity for verification that is central to most human endeavours, whether they are

---

1   NICE Clinical Guideline 115 on alcohol-use disorders (2011) finds evidence to support the pharmaceutical treatment of addiction, the use of acupuncture and cognitive therapy, but largely excludes the social and relational treatments that have been at the heart of rehabilitation in the UK. This appears to suggest a failure of research rather than a failure of the treatment. Questions concerning the aetiology of addiction, the transmission of addiction through inter-generational attachment patterns, behaviour, deprivation and trauma, which are evident to practitioners, are also diminished in their significance, and genetic transmission is offered as a causal factor in explaining aetiology.

the daily tasks of living, the origination of scientific ideas, or business innovation and creativity within the arts. There is a need for a softer notion of provisional and ongoing inquiry and of socially emergent themes, with a better understanding of the ongoing interaction of tacit and explicit knowledges in practice over time. I will draw attention to some research developments and traditions which represent a newly burgeoning and creative research field.

Natural Science and Human Science Research

There is a debate that can be traced from the American pragmatists and the social psychologist G.H. Mead (2015) (who posed the question of whether human selfhood can be considered outside its social symbolic context), then on to the sociologists Blumer (1989) and Habermas (1984). The communication theorist Craig (1995) here similarly represents the problem of applying natural science methods to human science problems. He makes a distinction between different epistemologies appropriate to different worlds of human action and shows the need to build a new normative theory:

> …conceptions of scientific theory continue to dominate discussions of communication theory… Scientific theory is concerned with what is, not what ought to be; the goal of scientific theory is to discover general explanations of phenomena that increase our ability to understand, predict, and control events. Normative theory, in contrast, is centrally concerned with what ought to be; it seeks to articulate normative ideals by which to guide the conduct and criticism of practice… Practical action depends on an interpretive understanding of situations and requires deliberation about purposes and moral standards (normative reflection) as well as means (technical rationality). The term praxis has come into use as a way of emphasising this fuller conception of practice as reflectively informed, morally accountable human action. (p.249)

John Searle (1977) made a similar point regarding this dilemma as it appears in philosophy and the study of language:

> One of the oldest metaphysical distinctions is that between fact and value. Underlying the belief in this distinction is the perception that values somehow derive from persons and cannot lie in the world, at least not in the world of stones, rivers, trees, and brute facts. (p.175)

He then goes on to rigorously counter this argument.

I hope to show the relevance of the case that Craig and Searle make for language and practical action for art therapists whose practical concerns are currently limited by our adherence to limiting methodological frames.

The epistemological shift that private practice encourages can motivate us to explore more appropriate means to research our field with new conceptions of research, theory and practice that meet the needs of practitioners and their clients with greater congruence and respect the centrality of the art process that is central to an art therapy intervention. Craig (1999) usefully outlines seven traditions drawn on by communication theory that provide relevant fields for art therapy research as a field of communicative and practical actions (rhetorical, semiotic, phenomenological, cybernetic, socio-psychological, sociocultural and the critical tradition). Some of these research traditions will be considered further in Part 2 of this chapter.

There often appears to be a wish in art therapy that a magical investment in 'scientific proof' will legitimise our profession; and yet, paradoxically, the healing that art therapy brings is through an embodied, relational and communicative process that contrasts with the focuses of allopathic medical research. There are already neurological experiments and outcome measures showing positive wellbeing outcomes for art therapy, but there is now also a growing need, in my view, to reconsider the essence of what art therapy is as a relational, social, communicative and embodying aesthetic process.

Habermas (1984), Heidegger (2011) and Husserl (1970) all point to a need to reconsider our Western thought forms, practices and epistemology, and the psychological, social and material consequences of the worlds we create with them. None deny certain beneficial effects of our advanced technological and instrumental reasoning, but all urgently demand we consider our idealisation of a particular mode of thinking that is applied to all dimensions of our existence. This critique still rings true in this century and has been followed by other voices, most recently by Unger (2004) and his critique of 'necessitarian' culture and politics. Habermas made a historical study of Western epistemology and concludes that politically and socially we should re-evaluate the current application of technical and instrumental reasoning following the apotheosis of the scientific discourse. He naturally questions who benefits socially and economically from this epistemology when it is presented as the sole truth. Whose interests does it serve? He raises important ethical, social and political questions. The irony for me, after 23 years of practice, is that it is now in private practice that art therapists often feel they can hold onto 'their values' and a way of practising that reflects those values, increasingly exiled by the instrumentalism evident in the statutory provision.

The Implications of Context on the Epistemology of Research

Typically the scenario of private practice is characterised by a collapse of all the departments found in the statutory treatment context, often into the single space of the therapist's home. All the professional roles of the hospital context (apart from medical treatment) can be found within the relationship of the client and the therapist in the context of private practice. For many therapists this is an unbearable and frightening prospect, whilst for others it offers the possibility and prospect of relative autonomy and a holistic practice where the fragmented roles and specialisms of the hospital are reintegrated into two basic roles: that of the therapist and the client. The therapist takes on the roles of management, assessment, human resources, accounts, advertising and public relations and, most importantly for our discussion here, research and development. It also raises the question of where the responsibility for research lies when the client is paying a fee, and it could be argued that the client, in paying the fee, is funding the clinic and is therefore funding practice research within therapy. It is in this adapted framework of inquiry that research into art therapy private practice must be made and we must recognise the symbolic and material significance of this shift of power and resources, as it fundamentally reframes the epistemology, research agenda, methodology and method. The therapist in the statutory context is providing data and research evidence in their being accountable to an external source because therapy is funded by the tax payer, and so research in this context is fulfilling all manner of agendas, as it is caught in the broader contested politics of the state-funded health service often referred to as 'our NHS'. The client in private practice funds the therapy, and so the therapist is primarily internally accountable for research within the therapeutic frame to the client/funder. The client can legitimately talk of 'my therapy' with a similar sense of ownership. Therapists in this context must accustom themselves to the 'reality' of this shift of dynamic, role, meaning and accountability.

Agency and Patience

The client has considerable power and agency in this context, though they may often not initially realise it; realising this power often becomes a significant part of the therapeutic journey. Clients in private practice have no obligation to be 'patient', and frequently aren't. Their agency and control in the process is emphatic and symbolised by the fee. There is also a clear collaborative research agenda built into the therapeutic contract. Even if the presenting problem or symptom is not resolved by the therapeutic engagement, the client often leaves with a sense of having obtained a greater self-knowledge and agency that is usually considered part of a fair exchange of goods. Art therapy in the state sector can sometimes ignore the importance of the relationship, the exchange between therapist and client, and the value this may have in their recovery. Frances Walton points to this potentially beneficial effect of private provision in Chapter 2.

If we follow the medical metaphor and seek to identify the 'active ingredient' in the dosage of art therapy as we would if we were a pharmaceutical treatment, we face immediately numerous ethical and human science dilemmas in locating this activity to which Craig, above, has pointed. Aristotle devised the categories of 'action' and 'passion' to examine the nature of things in the world empirically. The term 'patient' retains an echo of this original conception and implies that in medical treatment the doctor or medication are the 'agent' in treatment. This metaphor cannot work if art therapy in fact depends on enhancing the agency of the 'patient', which most therapists would consider is a primary aim of therapy and its effectiveness. We hope the client leaves more able and with greater choice than when they arrived. This is one reason why most therapists have adopted the term 'client', because it promotes the 'patient's' activity and agency in the interaction where the term 'patient' denies it. If the active ingredient in therapy follows from a combination of the client's will, the therapeutic relationship, the setting and the art process, the researcher is faced with levels of complexity and flux that make a mechanistic medical metaphor unworkable. A change of our discourse is therefore necessary for the identification of the therapeutic effect of art therapy to be recognised (*looked* for), identified (*seen*), understood (*imagined* in significance) and researched (*shown*).

The phenomenon of the patient as employer in private practice provides an opportunity to reflect on the research aims and research epistemology that evolve from this particular context, and contrasts with the state provision in ways that produce useful insights into practice more generally. Private practice places an emphasis upon the unique needs of the client who is at once the patient and employer and who often appears without a specific diagnostic label, making notions of 'quotas' and the 'clustering' of patients, used in the state sector, largely irrelevant. This provides us with an opportunity to pause and question our theoretical and research orientations more generally, and asks us to consider what sorts of evidence and research methodologies are useful and appropriate within the private practice context. These recessionary times have made the critical engagement of art therapy with EBP, encouraged by Gilroy (2013), even more crucial, when the shortage of funding appears to encourage discourses of reductive inductive empiricism within the state provision. In private practice the accountancy and managerial agendas are re-absorbed into the client/therapist relationship and so also the agenda for research towards the practical aims of the client who funds it. Private practice can provide clear interest and motivation to both the practitioner and client because both are positively, literally and materially contracted into an invested engagement within the therapeutic process. Research in this context must therefore be orientated towards this reality and provide art therapists and clients the opportunity to build a new agenda for it within therapy.

Counting, Accounting and Audit

The collapse of the organisational departments in the statutory provision into the single forum of a domestic private practice means that it is possible to have a more holistic attitude to data collection and also a more holistic research agenda that does not emphatically divide audit and research in ways that are customary in large organisations. All the data that appears within private practice is potentially data for practice research. For example, an invoice that is primarily a quantitative means to account to Her Majesty's Revenue and Customs (HMRC) is also a record of attendance and therefore a quantitative and potentially a qualitative measure of client satisfaction, if the reasons for ongoing attendance (numerically identified) are combined with verbal reports in a review. The data of private practice is polysemic and encourages a mixed-methods approach by private practitioners in assessing their practice. Though this discourages us from taking positions on quantitative and qualitative research methods, the art therapist as both artist and therapist in private practice has good reason to promote 'quality' over 'quantity' in their aesthetic orientation and also because the client is seeking a 'quality' of relationship and of service. Art therapy in private practice can be a bastion of quality in the face of the widespread dehumanisation of our organisational culture, and from this place it can re-establish the heart of practice for re-export.

Gilroy (2013) gives a thorough assessment of audit and research, and Huet and Springham (2013) in their *Audit Pack* (available to British Association of Art Therapists (BAAT) members on the BAAT website) present audit within the framework of state provision and the organisational accountability to the tax payer. The epistemological shift that occurs when the client funds therapy in private practice has its inevitable transformative effect on audit. As well as reuniting audit and research, it also removes the layers of administration and management to which the art therapist has been traditionally accountable in the statutory context. The agendas of 'efficiency' and 'efficacy' that currently drive both audit and research in the state sector must be renegotiated by therapist and client into a more holistic and potentially more intuitive and qualitative assessment of progress. These agendas of efficiency and efficacy are still present, but interwoven in complex ways within the therapeutic and transferential agendas of the therapy and the practice. What does it mean to account to yourself, as manager, and to your client, as funder, alone? This requires a shift in research culture and what Bateson (2000) referred to in his study of addiction recovery as an 'epistemological shift'. The documents mentioned above regarding audit remain very relevant, but need translation to a more endogenous research focus within private practice. Gilroy (2013) lists 'relevance, equity, accessibility, acceptability, effectiveness and efficiency' (p.70) as criteria for auditing a successful service provision; these criteria are clearly relevant in a private therapy provision but with the proviso of a major shift occurring in the 'to whom' of accountability that transforms the agendas of both audit and research. The research agenda that can follow from audit must likewise be tailored to this field, and the sourcing of data is likely to be more pragmatic and pluralistic, drawing upon the multiple agencies of the practitioner (manager/owner/therapist/researcher) and client (funder/client/service user/customer/patient/researcher) within the process.

Audit, Outcomes and the Fee

As the seasoned art therapist Joan Woddis, now approaching 90 years, is frequently heard saying, 'Everything that happens in the therapy is about the therapy.' It is an important but simple motto that recognises the holistic and systemic nature of data management that exists between the client and the therapist, and the conflation of all the practical, managerial, financial and research agendas that combine meaningfully in therapy. Everything in private therapy is symbolically loaded, and so audit and research must be considered in terms of their symbolic potential in relation to the therapeutic aims of the therapy. The symbolism of the exchange of fee, the therapist's livelihood and professional research must be reconsidered in this light as, and when, they become a focus within the therapy on the journey. As editor, I requested all the authors in this book consider and draw out the symbolic interplay of this particular dimension of the exchange of the fee in private art therapy practice as a defining feature which vanishes in the state provision.

The current major movement in art therapy research is in the *measurement of outcomes*, largely due to the accountability of the therapist to external bodies, particularly management and accounts, within state-funded health and educational provisions. In private practice, accountability is to the client alone, and so this suggests that accounts are to be made to the client in an endogenous circuit of exchange. This necessarily returns therapy to the study of its own products: the image, dreams, stories, and the relationship with the client. In all contexts an account of the meaning and efficiency and efficacy of therapy is rightly made to the person that funds it. In private practice this shifts the whole agenda of therapy research back to the therapy itself and away from external bodies. The benefit of this epistemological shift is that it re-centres the accountability for the research agenda back towards practice specifically and the client's progress rather than the generalised and burgeoning management/research/accounting culture. This refocusing of the research agenda encourages the therapist to re-evaluate the forgotten research agenda native to therapy as a vital process, and asks us to reconstruct the memory of practice itself as a valuable and primary research. In art therapy it refocuses us on the collaborative internal process of the research into the image, dreams and the relationship that are the process and product of art therapy. This internal research dovetails with the current movement towards qualitative research, reflective practice and reflexive research. My aim in Part 2 of this chapter is to show some of the resources that are available for that research. It is not that art therapists should ignore EBP and the epistemology promoted within the state provision, or indeed any relevant evidence that has been gleaned from other more controlled environments, but rather to allow for the scene of private practice to experience its own research virtues and its particular research needs. These evolve between the therapist and the patient/employer, respecting the particularity of this setting and the specific epistemology it encourages for research.

Re-Coupling the Carriages of the Research/Practice Train in Art Therapy Private Practice

All private practitioners are owners of small private businesses that exist for the benefit of the client and the therapist. R&d is a key part of any business strategy and service development. Without reflection and research into a business it is unlikely to succeed and so will necessarily fail in the provision of its service in the community. The success of a business and the provision of a service to the client are inherently linked within the microeconomy of a private practice. How this essential practice research occurs is not limited to any particular method or methodology, and for many art therapists it appears to be an almost entirely intuitive activity, but it nonetheless must be undertaken in the practice within ethical limits that are congruent to the aims of the therapy and not disruptive of it.

Market Research

The need to understand the local market for your business enterprise is also very real and a necessary concern for the private therapist that must also be researched. Private practitioners must be very aware of the context of their business, in a way that contrasts with the legitimate general natural science research aims of medicine and the hospital context. Most private practitioners do this research intuitively, but there is no reason why this cannot be undertaken in the way that larger businesses assess their market. It is vital to consider where your practice sits and 'do the research' in relation to the needs and number of clients that are likely to use your service (the demographics). Wishing and good will alone are not sufficient! There needs to be 'reality testing' and a consideration of yearly outcomes and viability in parallel to the 'reality testing' processes inherent to the psychotherapeutic engagement. It seems easier for art therapists to accept this market research challenge ethically if they consider it in terms of the service provision for their clients. Whichever way it is done, market research is a real need for a private practice, as there is no point in offering a service that no one wants or can use, no matter how intrinsic its value as a practice.

Summary of Part 1

If we accept therapy itself as a field of inquiry abundant in data we can then go about making sense and forming meanings through a process of reflection and interpretation, made collaboratively with clients and intersubjectively validated in order to find local solutions to local problems. In this way a particular and specific knowledge base can be formed. This process is inherently beneficial to the client as it respects their agency within the process of therapy and is appropriately constructed to fit their lives. A desire for the client to research themselves is usually a motivation to seek therapy and should be actively sought by the therapist as part of the initial assessment for therapy. The therapist is likewise transformed by this collaborative research project which counters positivistic notions of 'pure objectivity' that aim to remove subjectivity from research. It is also in this way that the therapist builds greater self-knowledge and experience to benefit future clients and themselves. If the therapist refuses this reflexive, intersubjective and collaborative research role in therapy, it is their clients and themselves that will then suffer this impoverishment, and in private practice this may be literal. A positivistic notion of therapy research is likely to be detrimental to the progress of the client and the therapist in their mutual development. The knowledge formed in this context is not owned by the therapist, abstracted or general but is specific and local; it is the product of a professional relationship that models collaborative inquiry and experimentation. An aim then must be to move from this local *praxis* to research, re-coupling the practice/research train, producing *endogenous* practice-based research and evidence, and then moving outwards towards *exogenous* research and back, being careful to maintain the essential link of research and practice in order to produce relevant, applicable research and guidance to the profession and continue to build the general stock of art therapy evidence for posterity.

PART 2: MEANS, METHODS AND METHODOLOGIES IN RESEARCHING ART THERAPY IN PRIVATE PRACTICE

I considered the scene of an art therapy private practice with regard to research and epistemology, context and accountability in Part 1. I will now consider the 'how' of research in a private art therapy practice context, bearing these points in mind, and re-evaluating the potential for 'practice-based research' with examples of research methods and methodologies that appear to be compatible with this aim.

This overview will be structured in relation to the course of therapy. Helpfully, the art therapist researcher Gilroy (2013) points out how the three major traditions of qualitative research reflect the process of research: 'If **phenomenology** seeks to *describe* and **heuristics** seeks to *discover* through personal introspection then **hermeneutics** seeks to *interpret...*' (p.104; both italic and bold are my emphasis).

This shows the fundamental place of the qualitative research methodologies within the phases of the research process. Usefully it also corresponds with our visual metaphor of *looking, seeing* (observation), *imagining* (introspection) and *showing* (interpretation) adapted from Roam (2009) in Part 1. In structuring this tour of research through the course of therapy we can sidestep some of the more divisive debates over method and methodology which detract from the general aim of illumination in all research and focus on methods and methodologies which appear to have good fit with the art therapy private practice context. I will also use this opportunity to point to some of the research methods and methodologies that have been used within the chapters of this book.

The phases of research and of therapy can be considered under the following process headings: (1) Before, (2) The beginning, (3) The middle, (4) The ending and (5) After. Just as research questions frame the research, it is noticeable that seeing each phase of the therapeutic journey as research suggests that particular research methods and methodologies are better suited to each phase. Having already been critical of the notion of a hierarchy of research methodologies, I will try to be even handed in assessing how different research methodologies follow from different questions in the phases of the research and therapy process. In this sense, I do not recognise a 'gold standard' of research. Method in human and natural science should be determined by its appropriate contextual and practical application. Table 13.1 shows how each method and methodology can be placed roughly within the phased process of the course of therapy.

Table 13.1 The course of therapy in terms of research

	1. Before	2. Beginning	3. Middle	4. Ending	5. After
Visual thinking	Looking	Seeing	Imagining		Showing
Qualitative research methodologies	Phenomenology/ description		Heuristics/ discovery		Hermeneutics/ interpretation
Visual research methodology:					The show & curatorial research
Panofsky (1983)	Ekphrasis	Iconography	Iconology		
Rose (2016)	Site of production	Site of the image itself	Site of circulation		Site of audiencing
Research methods	Surveys of clients and therapists; archival research; infant observation in training	Biographical research; baseline measures for outcomes; participant observation; in-therapy interview and reviews; visual research; semiotic analysis; researching transference and counter-transference and evidence of unconscious processes; visual response and creative writing	Discourse analysis; visual research; narrative research – re-authoring; action and social action research; grounded theory in practice	Assessing outcomes achieved; ongoing social action; audio image recording	Outcome measures data analysis; post-therapy interviews; customer satisfaction survey; analysis of transcript and recordings and visual documents in formal research; curatorial research
Systemic inquiry	Commissioning	Co-design	Co-reflection	Co-action	Co-curating
In or out of therapy	Outside	Inside	Inside	Inside	Outside

Questions: An Introduction to Part 2

Before I begin an assessment of methods and methodology I would like to reset the frame of our considerations with an art historical vignette to foreground the arts-based and social research orientation of an art history inquiry.

Different questions suggest different methods of discovery. The types of questions we ask privilege certain methods and methodologies (Yin 1994). If we consider the basic questions we can use – *who/ what* questions, *how much/how many* questions, *where* questions, *when* questions, *how* questions and, last but not least, *why* questions – these questions can provide us with some basic tools of inquiry and a starting point for further reflections on the type of research to employ in exploring our chosen territory.

A Van Gogh Vignette

A recent book (Murphy 2016) and television programme about the discovery of new evidence to settle certain longstanding questions about the life of Van Gogh (*who* and *how* he was) concluded, after a number of circling iterations, with new evidence, new questions and new answers. Along the way a supplementary question became central: 'How much ear did he remove?' A drawing by the physician Dr Rey, who treated Vincent for the self-inflicted injury, was discovered in the course of archival research (the drawing is redrawn in Figure 13.1). It showed definitively that he had removed most of his ear. This evidence contradicted longstanding stories built around accounts gathered close to the time of the incident. This single piece of art-based evidence (a drawing) changed the 'best hypothesis' narratives that had been constructed by experts around his actions. The amount of ear removed was seen as an indication of his level of distress and it was then framed in social and symbolic terms, reconsidering all the other evidence that surrounded this grotesque donation to an adolescent girl, who was a friend and who he knew from Paris, and not a prostitute as had also been supposed. This new evidence changed the meaning of the strange gift and consequently our view of him. The new information, of his gifting his whole ear rather than the lobe, was all set in the context of other known actions and events that led to new 'emergent' conclusions about his character and motivation.

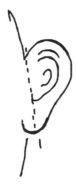

Figure 13.1 Redrawn by the author 'after' Dr Felix Rey, 'after' Van Gogh

It is apparent that these questions – 'who/what?', 'how much?', 'where?', 'when?', 'how?' and 'why?' – were evident in this research and were answered by various methods including archival search, interviews with surviving family members of the young woman in question, and various types of logical thinking. Key words in the previous paragraph point to some areas in research pertinent to art therapy as a symbolically and socially interactive therapeutic intervention (e.g. discovery, questions, answers, supplementary question, treated, the injury, contradicted, assumed, data, accounts, time, incident, evidence, 'best hypothesis', constructed, experts, indication, level of distress, social and symbolic terms, changed the meaning, our view of him, discovered, supposed, new information, context of known actions and events, new 'emergent' conclusions, character and motivation).

The physician's drawing, which became the key information ('a difference that makes a difference' in Bateson's (2000, p.315) definition of information), was made for the American author Irving Stone in 1930 as part of his own research for a biography of the artist. He had sought the doctor out and had kept the drawing in his records. *Who* were the players in this drama? *How* much of the ear was removed? *Where* did it happen? *When* did it happen? *How* did he do it? And finally, a new 'best hypothesis': the *Why*? The researcher *looked* at the data and through numerous interpretive hermeneutic cycles *saw* its significance, sought more evidence and *imagined* the meaning of the evidence set within the actions of the participants of the drama and finally pieced it together, *showing* what it all meant as research and its value in our transformed understanding of what had happened. A new tragic narrative was *formulated* on the basis of new evidence providing a 'better' settling of the data and, it is hoped, a truer, fairer and more accurate understanding of the man.

This process of inquiry illustrates a small-scale amateur art historical research that echoes the research of art therapy practice and promotes the retelling, reimagining and the settling of matters of a personal history. Unlike art historians, art therapists have access to the voice of the artist/client and are co-witnesses of the art made, adding to a sense of collaborative research and sense-making as a therapeutic engagement in the present. The example shows how the mind/bodies of the players, within social and historical contexts, make a story and how our contemporary concerns are represented in the research process and its subsequent understandings and findings. This art historical research also typically uses the three logics of *deduction* (reasoning), *induction* (likelihood) and *abduction* (guesswork or 'best hypothesis formulation') which provide another important set of tools to complement the basic questions available to the practitioner/researcher at no additional cost. For art historians, the search for retrospective diagnosis and pseudo-psychiatric labelling has now moved towards a more contemporary interest in shared meaning and motivation; and this reveals the forming discourses of our current research agendas. There is also a recognition that all our representative actions, whether as artistic or scientific researchers, are set within a 'circuit of culture'.[2] There is no outside to this social fact which demands of us always to maintain a reflexive and reflective stance as researchers.

※ ※ ※

The rest of this chapter goes on to use the course of therapy as a structure to explore research methods and methodologies but, as will become clear, a number of them occur in cyclical rather than linear processes within research and in the course of therapy, and so resist my simplification. This said, it seems that this limitation is outweighed by the benefits of setting them in a structure that draws attention to their virtues. The following table of contents outlines the structure of the research strategy and the course of therapy through time.

---

2   The sociologist Stuart Hall reflects on du Gay's 'circuit of culture' which places the cultural fields of representation, regulation, consumption, production and identity into a dynamically interdependent relationship (Hall 2013).

1. Researching Beforehand: The Market, the Context, Demographic Research, Surveys and the Choice of Therapist
2. Researching the Beginning and the Background: Assessment, Initial Formulation and the Treatment Plan
   2.1 Assessment and the Treatment Plan in Private Practice
   2.2 Setting Outcomes, Measures and Baselines at the Start?
   2.3 Supervision as a Forum of Practice Research
   2.4 First Appearances: A Phenomenological Approach to Art Therapy Private Practice
3. Researching the Interior of Therapy: Insiders, Constructs and Discovery
   3.1 Insider Research/Personal Knowledge, Ethnography and Heuristic Research – Discovery
      3.1.1 Insider Research
      3.1.2 Heuristic Research – Discovery
   3.2 Action Research, Social Action Research and Systemic Inquiry – Situated Experiments in Therapy
      3.2.1 Social Action Research, Emancipatory Theory and Practice
      3.2.2 Systemic Inquiry
   3.3 Case Study Research – Making a Case or Painting a Portrait?
   3.4 In-Therapy and Post-Therapy Interviews and Reviews
   3.5 Literature Review and the Critical Review of Theory in Prioritising Practice
      3.5.1 Literature Review
      3.5.2 Critical Review of Theory: Potential Data Loss Again
      3.5.3 Taking Pleasure in Reality (Testing)
   3.6 Grounded Theory
   3.7 Reflectively Practising Towards Research: Reflective Journals
      3.7.1 Research Journals
   3.8 Pictured and Storied Lives: Art and Narrative Therapy and Research
      3.8.1 Visual Re-Search in Art Therapy Private Practice
         a. Retrospective Review and Art Historical Research
         b. Art Writing and Art Speaking as Research
         c. Art Making as Research – Visual Response
      3.8.2 Knowing the Signs – Semiotics
      3.8.3 Narrative Research and Discourse Analysis
4. Researching the Ending
5. Researching After: What Is There to Show?
   5.1 The Show: Curatorial Research
   5.2 The Gallery

1. Researching Beforehand: The Market, the Context, Demographic Research, Surveys and the Choice of Therapist

Before therapy begins there are a number of areas for possible research, for both the therapist and the client, in preparing the ground and choosing therapy.

For the therapist: We have already discussed the importance of knowing your location, your market and the sort of research that can be done by the practitioner through *archival research* of data, such as local government information, local directories and so on, to gather knowledge about the local clinical context. Your clients will likely be drawn from this local demographic with all its characteristics and culture. Take an interest! Be curious! Do some *fieldwork*! Your research may vary also according to your specialism and this may include discovering local support services for clients (e.g. client on the autistic spectrum, addictions); these support networks can be important for referral form therapy. If you are working with children, awareness of local Child and Adolescent Mental Health Services (CAMHS) educational structures, social services and local safeguarding contacts may also be advisable. The British Association of Art Therapists (BAAT) special interest and regional groups may also be informative in terms of client groups and areas of practice.

For the client: There is the possibility of researching the profession of your therapist, their registrations and trainings prior to engaging in therapy, and considering what therapy may be most helpful to you through your own current understanding of your dilemmas. Do you wish to see a man or a woman? Is their sexuality a factor in your feelings and thoughts? Are the class and ethnicity of your therapist important to you? It is worth remembering that 'the assessment' in private practice is as much an assessment of the therapist by the client as it is of the client by the therapist.

A therapist also cannot be chosen and assessed if they cannot be found, and so therapists must make themselves available to be discovered in the world of the client! The codes and standards of the HCPC (HCPC 2013, 2016) and of BAAT (BAAT 2014) are available to the public and represent the professional standards and ethics expected of art therapists in the fulfilment of their role. These documents can be valuable for the clients in understanding the safeguards for them represented by these bodies and standards. The training documents of the ten art therapy training courses also reveal the curricula undertaken by art therapists and the expertise acquired within these trainings. McLeod (1999) critically evaluates professional training manuals as a form of practice research.

2. Researching the Beginning and the Background: Assessment, Initial Formulation and the Treatment Plan

2.1 Assessment and the Treatment Plan in Private Practice

Gilroy, Tipple and Brown (2012) have considered the evidence base for assessment methods in art therapy practice in a useful edited volume. For clients seeking private art therapy, 'the assessment' covers a complex process that generally includes treatment formulation, planning, fees and contracting. This process is held by the therapist, who will judge how far to actively involve the client in information gathering and planning, taking into account the level of distress and the client's capacity for involvement. The BAAT Core Skills and Practice Standards in Private Work document (see Appendix 1) was first drawn up between the BAAT Council and the Private Practice Special Interest Group (PPSIG) in 2015 and revised in 2017. It was developed, in research terms, through a *cyclical process of professional reflection, review and revision*. The standards place a significant emphasis on the importance of assessment, contracting and treatment planning in private practice. Assessment provides a starting point for the ongoing process of dynamic formulation and review and the process of 'ongoing joint assessment' recommended in Chapter 12 on self-care. The assessment is also a time to consider the client's reasonable expectations and the potential outcomes of therapy, and some of the challenges the work may present. The journey and the outcomes cannot be fully determined in advance, but can be broadly outlined with a knowledge of the presenting problems and the personal history which is taken (*biographical research*). Evidence of therapy as a researching endeavour is shown in the uncertainty of the process, which can cause a level of anxiety to both parties. The therapist is expertly trained to hold this 'not knowing' in themselves and the client, and makes an assessment of the client's psychological, relational and material resources available for the journey. At this stage the therapist may have numerous 'tacit' research questions about what may be useful areas to expand upon and explore to the benefit of the client. The British Psychological Society's document *Good Practice Guidelines on the Use of Psychological Formulation* (British Psychological Society 2011) shows the relevance of a 'dynamic formulation' that can be integrated into the art therapeutic assessment without obstructing the creative flow of the productive and free art process.

The BAAT Code of Ethics (2014) also outlines the general obligations that fall upon private therapists in the initial stages of therapy as follows:

Treatment and Planning in Private Practice

Members who work in private practice must make art therapy plans that:

(i) seek to attain and maintain the client's optimum level of functioning and quality of life;

(ii) delineates the type, frequency, and duration of art therapy;

(iii) sets goals that, wherever possible, are formulated with the client's understanding and permission and reflect the client's current needs and strengths; and

(iv) allows for review, modification and revision. (p.11)

2.2 Setting Outcomes, Measures and Baselines at the Start?

Often clients will wish to know the outcome of therapy at the start. Whilst it is hard to evaluate the ending at the beginning of a process, desired outcomes can be considered periodically both formally, using standard measures, or informally, depending on both the client's and therapist's preferences and aims. Many therapists use formal measures that have been developed in statutory clinical contexts. In the BAAT survey of art therapy private practitioners, analysed by Anthea Hendry in Chapter 14, 56 per cent indicated that they use formal outcome measures some of the time. It is important for the therapist to understand the origin of the measures used and their intended function and appropriate use, if they are to yield useful data for research within and beyond the therapy. The BAAT library lists an extensive list of outcome measures currently used within the profession.[3]

Seen critically, the word 'outcome' used to mean something that occurred at the end of a process, yet culturally we have come to expect that an outcome, by a perverse transformation of language, be determined at the start of a process. This appears to be a discursive development where assumptions of control and entitlement parallel the contemporary consumerist discourses that pervade our relationships, actions and reflections. The negative effect of this is that we may lose sight of the value and quality of the journey. Many clients seeking private art therapy wish to rediscover a place of ontological appreciation which, as a purchase, contrasts radically with other purchases they may make. Clients are purchasing a time and space and an engaged relationship that is, by definition, attentive and available to them, but yet curiously uncertain in its meaning, which is always to be determined within the interaction. The client, as customer, asserts their specific control and desire within the field, but the engagement simultaneously raises questions about commodity, value and identity within the relational exchange. The circuit of culture, mentioned above, reappears and potentially enriches the territory and reflection in the assessment of the 'cultural' appropriateness of the measurement of outcomes and the setting of baselines for ongoing scaling at this stage.

---

3   http://baatlibrary.org.

The status of art therapy in the state provision has placed an inordinate emphasis on outcomes driven by accountancy-led agendas of 'value for money' (predominantly questions of 'how much?' and 'how many?'), sometimes to the exclusion of other, equally important questions. I have already mentioned that in private practice the client's agency and our direct accountability to them allows us to ask pressing questions about the balance of qualitative and quantitative data in research, as well as the measures we may feel are appropriate to use to research therapy. The incommensurability and indeterminacy of the art process and of ourselves as clients/artists could be reframed in this context as a valuing of transformative artistic freedom in therapeutic terms, rather than as an avoidance of accountability and efficacy – as it is sometimes framed in the statutory services. The emphasis on collaborative research and reflexivity in private practice may offer inroads to alternative and new methodologies which evolve more congruently from the context with a better fit to the values of art therapists in private practice and the therapeutic aims of our private clients. There is scope to work with both the statutory 'requirements' and these internally emergent research agendas simultaneously and in this way honour both our own, and our clients', full capacities, moving towards a more satisfying, integrated and holistic approach to both research and therapy.

Cognitive behavioural therapy (CBT) has been very successful in producing quantitative evidence from the therapeutic engagement through formal quantitative scaling of the therapeutic intervention, and, more importantly, suggesting that the therapist and client are co-researchers to the client's specific issues. We can develop this notion of collaborative practice research that seems natural and fitting to the therapeutic scenario further. Most therapists would agree that there are aspects of therapy that are open to scaling, done formally or informally. However, it must also be recognised that this may exclude other possibilities that a free-floating and free associative attention offers in therapy and which, like the image, is harder to gauge quantitatively. However, as in the phenomenon of dreaming, we can reflect on it retrospectively and interact with its message, but we cannot force it, prescribe it or direct its production. Schön (1983), in his study of reflective practice in professional and scientific fields, shows how the objectives of research are actually and practically achieved. He shows that we can reflect upon the process at the time (reflection in action) and after (reflection on action). It is necessary sometimes to respect the process as it happens and then invite reflection upon it in the playground of practical learning. Therapists should be very reluctant to give up this idea of practical research and experimentation, especially when in private practice it is our unique selling point (USP) as arts-based practitioners in the saturated market of verbal and cognitive therapies. The art process itself often finds its goal in process and often through 'error', finding its value and aim as it proceeds through the stages of material transformation. For clients and systems that emphasise control and rigid expectations, it is a gentle transformative and humane remedy that leaves a trail of material markings of the journey for later consideration, reflection and research.

The scientist Michael Polanyi (1969) represents some of the paradoxes and procedural problems in research generally that are relevant to the setting of outcomes at the start of a process. Retracing a paradox, he points to Plato's identification of the researcher's dilemma, stating that

> to search for the solution of a problem is an absurdity. For either you know what you are looking for, and there is no problem; or you do not know what you are looking for, and then you are not looking for anything and cannot expect to find anything... (Polanyi 1964, p.6)

This may explain why the client's 'presenting problem' is rarely the 'real problem', revealing therapy both as an uncertain researching process and also a heuristic process of discovery that must have one foot in mystery, uncertainty and the unknown, in order to be open to new perspectives and insight. It also indicates that, within therapeutic inquiry, a clear and inflexible research agenda and outcome, or too rigid a definition of the problem or hypothesis, may actually derail the valid process of heuristic inquiry. It highlights that a degree of courage and compassion should be identified in the client and in the therapist at the initial phase of assessment because, though the work of therapy can be evidence based, the researching journey cannot be prescribed in advance and this lack of control may produce considerable anxiety and stress in both parties.

2.3 Supervision as a Forum of Practice Research

Supervision can help to alleviate the stress and anxiety of the unknown by acknowledging that this uncertainty is a reality of the inquiring process and a necessity in practice, and so neither a failure to know, or a failure of competence. In Part 1 of this chapter we identified that a primary aim of research is to avoid the loss of 'inconvenient' data. Supervision can be very helpful in this respect to therapists and to their clients. It can help us bear the challenge of data load and the anxiety of 'not knowing' that comes forward in the research process, yet this may conflict with the client's and the therapist's prior constructions, assumptions and theoretical prejudices. Therapy then will usually lead to insight, and a shift in epistemology (knowledge claims) for both parties engaged in this unique inquiry, which will, it is hoped, be beneficial to the client on their journey and also promote personal and professional development in the therapist.

The supervisor can reassure the supervisee of the value of retaining an active research attitude by assisting them in their 'making sense' of the patterns and links that form and reform kaleidoscopically in the data of therapy and within the parallel supervisorial relationship. This psychodynamic approach to supervision contrasts with models of supervision that stress adherence to a model. The supervisor of a private practice can also help to unravel the complex layers of investment that involve clients' wishes, therapeutic outcomes and transferences – sometimes rich in ethical entanglement with the therapist's business interests. In supervision, research is given additional resources by another witness and a contained forum for reflection, supporting the therapist through the learning that comes from critical incidents in practice and turning these fearful moments into opportunities for research, reflection and learning. Helpfully, as David Edwards points out in Chapter 11, the supervisor is also a private practitioner, and so parallels can easily be drawn with the private supervisorial relationship that resonate in the supervisee's own practice. This notion of interplay and resonance between various resonating frames of reference can be seen holistically in private practice and will be examined later as an example of *systemic inquiry*.

2.4 First Appearances: A Phenomenological Approach to Art Therapy in Private Practice

The philosopher Immanuel Kant (2012 [1781]) suggested that he knew nothing of 'things in themselves' directly and even declared, 'I have no knowledge of myself as I am, but only as I appear to myself' (para. 25). Later Arthur Schopenhauer (2012 [1819]) began his *magnum opus, The World as Will and Representation*, with the statement: 'The world is my idea.' More contemporaneously, in the last century, Alfred Korsybski (2010) stated that 'the map is not the territory' (p.58). It is worth rereading these statements and considering their profound implications for tidy notions of 'objectivity' in science and 'subjectivity' in art.

The three paradoxical statements represent the general problem of our human assessment of reality, and provide artists with the latitude to 'play' and scientists the possibility to 'invent'. We can represent the world to ourselves and others but somehow remain caught between our concrete lived reality and our insufficient generalised representations of it. Images, symbols, sounds, gestures, feelings, words and logic all assist us, as scientists and artists, in a necessarily always ongoing assessment of 'reality'. Freud (2006 [1906]), possibly as artist and scientist, referred to this ongoing process as 'reality testing'. Phenomenology takes this dilemma seriously and asks us to build a science based upon our experience of the apparent world and its consistent and persistent forms.

Developed by Edmund Husserl (1962) in the early 20th century, phenomenology aimed to return scientific endeavours to Kant's 'appearance' of 'things in themselves'. He requested that practitioners and researchers attempt to 'bracket' theory and knowledge, and develop an attention of the world as it 'appears' to us in our immediate consciousness. The value of this approach to art therapy practitioners seems self-evident because it revalidates our, and our clients', 'lived experience' and returns the focus of therapy to its sensual (aesthetic) appearance. Therapy can create a unique space of reflection, so rare in modern living, where 'information overload' pushes us constantly away from ourselves, to ground our reflections on our lived experience. This phenomenological approach can be found in the existential and aesthetic writings of Sartre (2003, 2004), Merleau-Ponty (1962), Heidegger (2010) and Dufrenne (1979), and has been a central concern in the writing of some art therapists, notably Skaife in the UK (2001) and Betensky (1987) in the US. It is also promoted as an appropriate methodology for art therapy research by Gilroy (2011, 2013).

The psychologist Willig (2008) outlines interpretive phenomenological analysis (IPA) as a rigorous method of psychological research that draws upon this tradition. In the social sciences, phenomenology is considered as one of the main qualitative research traditions (Cresswell 1998; Wertz *et al.* 2011).

A phenomenological hermeneutic methodology brings together the science of appearances (phenomenology) and the art of interpretation (hermeneutics). It appreciates the phenomenon of the art process and pays attention to our experience as it happens. The embodied process of aesthetic experience and its interface with the collaborative 'meaning making' of therapy are central to both art therapy and phenomenological methodology. They both ask for engagement and close committed attention in place of scientistic distancing of the subject from its intentional objects. It encourages an active and engaged inquiry through investigation of subjective partiality and yet retains an investment in thoroughness, depth and rigour. Art-based research is by definition an interpersonal and interactive research. It asks us as therapists and clients to connect with our intersubjective phenomenological experience so as to become reflectively and reflexively aware of that of which we were previously unaware – which is the essence of research.

Van Manen (1990) in *Researching Lived Experience* shows how a hermeneutic phenomenological research has relevance for all dedicated practitioners and resists some of the typical dichotomies of research discourse: subject/object, theory/practice and practice/research. He argues that there is a sense of deeply inhabiting the topic of research through practical experience. The value of phenomenological research is that it is deeply grounded and situated in the very circumstances it aims to research: namely our intersubjective, embodied, lived experience as therapists and clients. He states, 'A phenomenology of practice does not aim for technicalities and instrumentalities – rather, it serves to foster and strengthen an embodied ontology, epistemology, and axiology of thoughtful and tactful action' (Van Manen 2014, p.508).

Once again, as with Craig (in Part 1 of this chapter), ethics are seen as a reflexive and integral expectation of this sort of practice research; ethics are not seen as an 'add-on' to counter the positivistic objectification of the client. We will return again to the topic of the research ethics of practice research towards the end of this chapter.

Private practice foregrounds the need for practice research and asks us to make an ethical assessment of what is at stake in the interests of our clients and ourselves. The aim of phenomenological methodology is to use our subjective experience collaboratively, to ask questions and share about how things consistently appear to us in lived experience, and then to collaboratively draw out the essence of those experiences. As a method or stance it privileges the aesthetic orientation of art and can help us promote a sensuous quality of experience and qualitative questioning about the nature of what it is to 'be', in a dialogue about the appearance of things for the client and the therapist in therapy.

3. Researching the Interior of Therapy: Insiders, Constructs and Discovery

In this section I will consider the interior of therapy as a forum for endogenous research.

3.1 Insider Research/Personal Knowledge, Ethnography and Heuristic Research – Discovery

3.1.1 Insider Research

It should now be clear that keeping rigid distinctions between phenomena, heuristics and hermeneutic research methodologies is not strictly possible, as these processes are interdependent and always involved in a process of cyclical engagement. Hermeneutics (the art of interpretation) reveals our understanding as a circling engagement with texts, relating the parts to the whole in ongoing cyclical phases of analysis and synthesis (Dilthey 1976; Gadamer 1975).

Another challenge to the notion of 'objectivity' in research is represented by Viktor Frankl (2008), who in his discussion of his reasons for presenting an autobiography as a way of retelling the experience of Auschwitz stated poignantly:

> To attempt a methodological presentation of the subject is very difficult, as psychology requires a certain scientific detachment. But does a man who

makes his observations while he himself is a prisoner possess the necessary detachment? Such detachment is granted to the outsider, but he is too far removed to make any statements of real value. Only the man inside knows.(p.20)

This statement reveals the importance of 'insider knowledge' in making a valid historical account and as part of his therapeutic narration. His story becomes a research document that would now be probably called an auto-ethnography. When we consider the autobiographical paintings of Frida Kahlo, Freud's personal dream research (1980) or C.S. Lewis's (2013) exploration of personal grief, we discover 'native' explorations of the subject's own socially situated subjectivity that reveal a self 'objectively' in a context of others. In Chapter 12 on self-care for art therapists in private practice, I showed the need for ongoing intersubjective assessment that could be thought of as a collaborative auto-ethnographic inquiry, where both the therapist and the client keep close account of their independent and joint experience of the therapy. In sociology and anthropology, methods in which the observer immerses themselves in the context of their subjective observations, and become a participant, have a long tradition called *participant observation*. In the endogenous research of therapy, such methods have clear relevance and encourage the therapist to draw *reflexively* on their experience as 'native' within the process of therapy with the client – who then draws on and represents their own insider view of their own 'native' cultural experience. Therapists and clients can become co-witnesses and ethnographic co-researchers of these relational territories, both inside and outside simultaneously. Art therapists are 'inside' enough to empathise and yet partially abstracted in their role, so as to still provide an 'outside' to the client's dilemmas whilst inviting the client into 'our' world of artists/makers. These participatory elements all help to build a bond of trust and a working relationship dedicated to resolving the client's dilemmas. It must not be forgotten that a majority of art therapists in private practice are working in their own homes (as is evidenced by the survey that follows in the next chapter). This could be seen to encourage the client's role as a participant observer of the therapist's native existence also. Julia Ryde, in exploring the limits of privacy in Chapter 1, also pays attention to this issue. The complexity and layered nature of the therapeutic relationship is also thoroughly explored by Clarkson (1995).

3.1.2 Heuristic Research – Discovery
Post assessment, the client may now have tentatively begun to make further representations of their world, both verbally and through the artwork. This creative aspect of research is identified by Moustakis (1990) as being a central part of heuristic research methodology: a cycling process of *pushing*

forward, deepening, questioning, rephrasing that reveals the dialectical, dialogical and interactive nature of *discovery* in artistic production. This process of research is largely ignored by scientistic research discourses in the pursuit of 'objectivity' and 'value free' information. Yet, as Polanyi and Schön would claim, this process is necessarily at the heart of all exploration and research. Polanyi (1962), himself a chemist, investigated the importance of 'personal' and 'tacit' knowledge in scientific research, contradicting both popular assumptions and positivist mythology. He shows how the practical scientists find that

> it is customary today to represent the process of scientific inquiry as the setting up of a hypothesis followed by its subsequent testing. I cannot accept these terms. All true scientific research starts with hitting on a deep and promising problem, and this is half the discovery. (Polanyi 1969, p.118)

Moustakis (1990), on heuristic research, pointed to the importance of the 'illumination of a puzzlement' (p.55) and indicates that research usually begins with the discomforting crisis of knowledge and an encounter with a limitation. This contrasts strongly with positivist scientific discourse which seeks certainty and security of knowledge and also contrasts with the notion that research evolves from proving or disproving a hypothesis. He also counters the idea that research necessarily requires the formation of clear questions for testing in advance of the research and places the researcher's self and his/her subjectivity back at the heart of all scientific research projects. Moustakis, following Polanyi, shows that if we preclude the 'tacit dimension' we also preclude the possibility of both knowledge and of learning, suggesting that what would be left is an empty rehearsal of ideological positions predetermined and prescribed by the state, representing everything Polanyi, as a refugee from Stalinist Russia, would have wished to avoid.

Following a moving personal disclosure, Moustakis relates how he began his heuristic research into loneliness. He exemplifies an emergent heuristic methodology and presents it as an example of heuristic research. He also reveals how a critical incident in the life of the researcher can provide a starting point and motivation for research, and that the author and/or client can follow this path of research through the stages he outlines as follows:

- the initial engagement
- immersion
- incubation
- illumination
- explication

- creative synthesis

- validation.

He also proposes 'heuristic therapy' as a collaborative research project and describes this endogenous therapy research with its method of intersubjective dialogical validation as follows:

> Through methods of immersion, indwelling, intuition and the tacit dimension, the therapist arrives at subjective knowledge of the person in therapy and of the relationship. The therapist offers this knowledge; it is either accepted, altered, or rejected. When it is verified, the therapist continues to explore the problem, facilitates the other person's understanding, and eventually grasps its basic constituents. The process of dialogue continues until a mutual position is reached. (p.116)

Most practising therapists will recognise how this 'heuristic attitude' is present as a research method in their practice. The American art therapist Rappaport clearly draws on this tradition in *Focusing-Oriented Art Therapy* (2009) and shows directly how art therapy in practice can be informed by the heuristic process of discovery.

3.2 Action Research, Social Action Research and Systemic Inquiry – Situated Experiments in Therapy

It is also possible to envisage therapy as a more rigorous laboratory for experimentation, in line with more behavioural approaches. For some clients and for some therapists this research approach may be more attractive. It is worthwhile to reflect on how and why we shift 'modes' as practitioners, since 'taking action' can sometimes be a defence against the exploration of feeling.

Action research has its roots in the field research of Lewin (1951) and the social action research of Freire (1996) and is here outlined by the health care practitioner and trainer Tina Tilmouth. In health care settings it can be used as a practice-based research method focusing on an ongoing inquiry into the effects of practical actions. This research method can clearly be useful within the collaborative work of therapy and also in the investigation of the 'problems' of practice that arise in its provision. It is similar in its action-orientated approach to the neuro-linguistic programming TOTE strategy – test-operate-test-exit – which was borrowed from cybernetics (Dilts *et al.* 1980) and also echoes the practical stepped processes of material art making.

Tilmouth, Davies-Ward and Williams (2011) outline the steps in the action research process as follows:

1. identifying a focus of interest or a problem

2. collecting data

3. analysing data and generating hypotheses

4. planning action steps

5. implementing action steps

6. collecting data to monitor change, analysing and evaluating.

This brings the action research cycle to its conclusion and also back to the beginning. At this stage, the action researcher describes the situation as it stands at the end of the first action steps and is then in a position to explain the new situation. By doing this, the next stage is put into place and the change is set off again on a seemingly never ending cycle. New data will be generated providing a different perspective on the situation. (Tilmouth *et al.* 2011, pp.164–165)

This experimental approach is present in most attempts to solve problems in and outside therapy. CBT actively promotes the notion of client and therapist actively involved in joint empirical research and testing. Solution-focused therapy, as described by de Shazer and Dolan (2007), also seeks to use the sessions for active problem-solving research and 'learning by doing'. Nardone and Portelli (2005) offer a history of brief strategic therapy which focuses on 'knowing through changing' and also sees therapy as active research. In an edited volume of art therapists' writing on 'brief time-limited art therapy', Hughes (2016) comments on how financial pressures in the statutory provision of art therapy is leading art therapists to develop similar, brief and focused approaches with identifiable goals and identifiable achievements. The variety of clients with a wide range of difficulties in private practice offer numerous opportunities for brief approaches, dependent on the client's wishes and needs. Some clients may seek a brief focused therapy for a specific problem – and though it is a possibility in private practice to offer long-term depth work, it is sometimes neither desirable nor appropriate. These circumstances encourage therapists in private practice to work integratively based on the client's wishes. These brief and experimental approaches can also be usefully employed to resolve the personal and practical management problems identified by the practitioner in their service provision. This again highlights the complex systemic parallels that can exist between the solutions of practical issues of the provision and the layered symbolic 'meanings' discovered in a holistic perspective of the work.

3.2.1 Social Action Research, Emancipatory Theory and Practice

The sociologist Habermas, following the American pragmatist G.H. Mead and the phenomenologist Husserl, points to the social origin of the human subject and our 'communicative action'. Habermas (1972) counters positivism with a well-argued case for the recognition of other significant domains of knowledge beyond that of technical rationality. In further consideration of Dilthey's notion of 'human science' (1976), he adds the 'social' and the 'emancipatory' domains of knowledge to that of 'technical rationality'. This reengages science with wider social concerns and reconnects research with the emancipatory aims of human knowing which are often pushed aside in positivism. Likewise in *social action research*, following Freire (1996), action and research are brought together within the therapeutic and social context but with a more emphatically political and emancipatory aim. This community-based social action research methodology is apparent in Chapter 3 in the context of a non-statutory community engagement. Social action art therapy and research are also explored as a method of provision and research by Hogan (2016), Kaplan (2007) and Levine and Levine (2011). In the spirit of this approach, Hogan points out that 'in art therapy we cannot undo discriminatory practices that exist outside the art therapy arena, but we can actively interrogate them, and explore our multiple and often contradictory selves – and the tension between these' (Hogan and Pink 2010, p.166).

Political and personal freedom and congruence are important concepts in art therapy and have often been sidelined within the medically orientated health service discourses. It is my experience that clients in private practice are often seeking freedom through art, hoping that art may help them free themselves from personal and social restraints, as well as the physical symptoms that have often followed as a consequence. The notion of 'incongruence' in Rogers and 'conflict' in Freud imply a sense of conflicting agencies at work in the lives of the clients that therapy, broadly speaking, aims to address. The private practitioner must have their eyes, ears, minds and hearts open to these internalised social struggles within their clients and be attuned to the sense of bondage clients often feel with regard to these social constraints, physical symptoms, psychological limitations and contradictions they find themselves confronting. This is a rich territory for a critical practice, and many art therapists have explored, written and published with regard to gender, race, religion, class, age and disability. In 1994 I published an article (West 1994) citing the evidence of a visual culture that pointed to such historical and cultural tensions of race, class and identity in Mexico City.

Therapists in private practice will encounter many tests of their own cultural positioning, and it is important to appreciate the value of extending ourselves towards the Other because the power dynamics at play in therapy, both real and fantasied, exist in the data represented by word, image and action in therapy between us. These dynamics must be met with compassion, congruence and integrity and an understanding of the potential for both formation and de-formation within therapy. The therapist in this sense has a complex obligation to protect both the client's best interests and themselves as the vehicle of change. Hephzibah Kaplan also explores some of the complex cultural interactions of private art therapy in Chapter 4. The BAAT Art Therapy, Race and Culture Special Interest Group (ARCSIG) and the texts it has produced (Campbell *et al.* 1999) also provide a useful forum for reflection and research.

3.2.2 Systemic Inquiry

The writings of Simon and Chard (2014), Shotter (2016) and Vetere and Stratton (2016) reveal the developing field of systemic research and how it has good fit with the action research agendas described above. They represent various means to reengage practice with research through collaborative local enquiry, research and personal and professional development. Simon lists the many forms this research is currently taking, reuniting both theory/practice and practice/research.

The systemic resonances and parallels that are evident in private practice supervision mentioned above encourage art therapists into systemic inquiry and collaborative sense-making. I recall my excitement in training when I first read Agazarian and Peters' *The Visible and Invisible Group* (2010) and was introduced to systems and field theory. Systems theory asks therapists to hold a multi-levelled view of the therapy process, gauging the process in numerous ways depending on our focus of attention and its relevance to the forming clinical picture. Adding the image to this inter-systemic pattern, we develop a multi-levelled systemic view of art therapy practice that recognises all the potential cross-referencing and intertextuality that occurs between these live resonating fields – where the image, the individual, the group role, the group as a whole, family roles, and organisational dynamics all reflect each other isomorphically. In private practice we consider the image in relation to the individual, the therapeutic relationship, transferential relationships and the larger social groupings (family, workplace, etc.) and develop an understanding of the complex ongoing patterns of systemic relationship, which can make abstractions and generalisations from therapy so difficult, but nonetheless present us with a need to study these very specific qualitative processes over time. Nili Sigal draws on systemic family work to understand the complex interactions around the work and the negotiations of the fee in Chapter 5. Systems theory also draws on the work of Virginia Satir, a founder of family therapy.

New developments in this field present a rich seam for art therapists to mine. A systemic view is in tune with our practice and draws together the potential for the collaborative experiments of action and social action research that can impact on broader issues of social justice and emancipatory practices within and beyond the therapy.

3.3 Case Study Research – Making a Case or Painting a Portrait?

The notion of the scientist practitioner in psychotherapy (McLeod 1999) clearly has its roots in Freud's case studies and is often a first and useful research step for therapists. All art therapists will have been asked to represent their work in a case study format as part of basic training, so it is a research format with which we are accustomed. Though there is a risk of the case study format representing a form of naïve realism, where the truth of the narrative is laid out as a 'self-evident' truth telling, it nonetheless remains an important varied form of research, painting a detailed portrait of a single case or series of cases. As a method, it spans various research methodologies, from the relativistic narrative and constructivist traditions to the more positivistic scientific experimental approach. The art therapist Hackett (2016) gives an example of N=1 case study research (a case study with one individual) in art therapy, seeking to exemplify cause and effect that might contrast with the more typical storytelling approach that also has its place and a long tradition in art therapy. The case study is interesting as a research method, since it can evidently take many forms and so asks us to be reflexive in considering the epistemology and the justifying methodology for its use. Stake (1995) and Yin (1994) are key texts in understanding this form of research. The art therapist Edwards (1999) also writes eloquently about the case study as an essential research tool in art therapy practice research. All authors in this book have drawn on this research method and some have added interviews to further validate the portrait and represent client feedback.

Here is Freud, in many ways the founder of this practice research method, considering the value of the case study:

> I was trained to employ local diagnoses...and it still strikes me myself as strange that the case histories I write should read like short stories and that, as one might say, they lack the serious imprint of science... Case histories of this kind...have, however, one advantage...namely an intimate connection between the story of the patient's sufferings and the symptoms of his illness. (Freud and Breuer 1974 [1895], p.231)

3.4 In-Therapy and Post-Therapy Interviews and Reviews

The interview – both structured and unstructured – is an essential research method. Importantly, it potentially yields both quantitative and qualitative research data which can be analysed independently through discourse, narrative and grounded research methods. Used within therapy as a retrospective review, it can also offer an opportunity to stand back and offer a reflective pause regarding the course of therapy, receiving feedback and then potentially to re-commissioning the project. In Appendix 2 there is a copy of the United Kingdom Council for Psychotherapy semi-structured post-therapy interview which exemplifies a semi-structured interview format, with a flexible approach to probing for additional spontaneous comments, which aims to gain a perspective on the client's and therapist's experience of 'moments of meeting' in therapy (Stern 2004) as well as other significant events in sessions (Hardy *et al.* 1999).

Interviews can be used within therapy as part of a review, but can also provide an opportunity to gather more 'objective' scaled measures of therapeutic efficacy and explore the interior of the therapeutic dynamic through testing theoretical ideas by active 'in-house' investigations. In this way they can bridge the practice/research gap, uniting exogenous and endogenous research approaches. This sort of research project could be developed relatively easily to explore specific art therapy themes within a practice research network of private practitioners. We will return to the interview as potentially part of the retrospective review of the artwork.

3.5 Literature Review and the Critical Review of Theory in Prioritising Practice

3.5.1 Literature Review

We are asked as evidence-based practitioners to found our practice on the latest relevant research represented in research journals that our professional bodies take pains to present in digestible form through practice guidance. This does not exclude critical reflections on research, but practitioners are also faced with a number of difficulties in first finding the research, then assessing its relevance, and finally in applying it congruently in practice. The best way to understand the language of research is to be involved in it. My own involvement as a peer reviewer for the *International Journal of Art Therapy* has certainly helped me to understand both the aims and languages of many different research projects. The HCPC requires, as a standard of practice, that art therapists 'be aware of the principle and applications of research enquiry, including the evaluation of treatment efficacy and the research process' (HCPC 2013, 13.2); 'recognise the value of research to the critical evaluation of practice' (HCPC 2013, 14.14); and 'evaluate research and other evidence to inform their own practice' (HCPC 2013, 14.16).

It is therefore clear that involvement in research is a professional requirement, as well as something that should be welcomed as part of our personal and professional development. Literature review in relation to practice is maybe a first step that begins as an integral part of the master's training.

3.5.2 Critical Review of Theory: Potential Data Loss Again

Theory structures how we see what we offer and guides our actions and interactions as therapists. Our ideas will have potential implications for our clients. Theory should not be displayed as a badge of professional club membership, but should be critically considered in how it guides our praxis and should be held provisionally until the data of practice conflicts with it and then leads us to revise or change our theories; we may then seek out a new structure of understanding which has better fit to the data of practice. The metaphorical adaptability and playfulness of artists should be an identifiable feature and primary resource for art therapists in this process. However, the therapists' theoretical constructions can lead to premature filtering of the data, which can preclude an appreciation and evaluation of its wealth within the therapy engagement. It was on this basis that Husserl encouraged the bracketing of prior knowledge in order to retain an openness to new data of experience; this open stance is fundamental both to the scientific and artistic orientation. Private practitioners have an obligation and an incentive to value the data of practice, as the success of the project is determined by the quality of this attention. It is also true that no business should ignore its customers. It would be seen as careless by the client/funder if information that is sometimes so reluctantly and painfully brought to therapy is not fully appreciated because the therapist is distracted by 'higher' theoretical or research aims. It would also show a professional disregard for the unique local research agenda that is endogenous to therapy.

Hogan (2016) outlines some of the main theoretical bases of current art therapy practice. She identifies cognitive behavioural, solution-focused brief, psychoanalytical (Freudian), analytical (Jungian), gestalt, person-centred, mindfulness, integrative and feminist approaches to art therapy in addition to art therapy as social action and art therapy as a research tool.

In this book, some of the theoretical constructs identifiable in guiding practice are Freudian and post-Freudian psychoanalytical theory, object relations theory, group analytic theory, Jungian analytic psychological theory, attachment theory, behaviourism and cognitive behavioural theories, neurological theory, art and aesthetic theory, pragmatism, ecology, horticultural theory, holism, specific art therapy theory, integrative theory, gestalt theory, systems and field theory, social action theory, symbolic interactionism, phenomenology and empiricism. The survey in Chapter 14 uses the approaches suggested by the PPSIG (often representing art therapists' post-qualification continuing professional development (CPD) trainings): attachment-based, cognitive analytical, cognitive behavioural, dialectic behavioural, existential, gestalt, integrative, Jungian, mentalisation-based, pastoral, person-centred, psychoanalytical, psychodynamic, psycho-educational, psycho-synthesis.

It is worth remembering that Freud's work – and the roots of all psychotherapy practice and theory – drew deeply on private practice as endogenous research. In researching his own dreams and developing theory in relation to the manifestation of his clinical practice and exploration of his own material, Freud built a theoretical structure from practice research. Despite the criticisms that can be made of psychoanalytic constructs and the 'objectivity' of this model of practice research, it remains valid as a form of endogenous research evolving from the actual intersubjective engagement of practice.

3.5.3 Taking Pleasure in Reality (Testing)

In 1906 Freud (2006 [1906]) proposed two contesting principles of mental functioning: the pleasure principle and the reality principle. In art therapy private practice these are evident in both the client's and therapist's process as we both 'wish' and 'test realities'. We both construct possible worlds and find their limitations in reality as co-researchers. The client constructs and reconstructs their own reality within the boundaries set by their imagination and their reality, and the therapist likewise creates and tests theoretical constructs and seeks to satisfy epistemological wishes and discovers the reality of these constructions over time. In Freud's writings his humour often appears to mask an omnipotent arrogance but also, more importantly, a deeper and complex awareness of the problems of verification in therapeutic practice that remains a reality for practitioners today. Though he lived in a time of simplistic positivism which has largely fallen away, it is often only time and the slow movement of cultural paradigms that test our theories and reveal whether they are the illusory products of collective wishing or of real assistance to our ongoing endeavours of living and knowing. If I ask the question 'Where does art lie between these two principles?', I find that it coyly but stubbornly sits between 'pleasure' and 'reality', as a vehicle for building illusions and a primitive tool of scientific reasoning and investigation. Art – and therefore art therapy – is now, as it always has been, a bridge between knowing and wishing. We cannot help but wish, but neither can we help but be continually confronted by, the realities that test the limitations we find in our constructed and re-presented worlds. This tension and dialectic was Freud's greatest 'discovery' as he relentlessly, and sometimes at great personal cost, pointed to the way we seek to build illusions and then inevitably find them causing tensions, and even physical and mental ill health, through our resistance to engage in 'reality testing'. He pointed to this in the lives of individual paying clients, but also in the larger landscape of psychology, politics and religion. We might have to add to this analysis the discourse of science itself, as it is clear that the scientific community is not immune to these tensions of wishing and testing. Social constructivists point to the historical, social and political realities that influence the construction of scientific 'realities' and paradigms. A consistent part of the picture is that 'power' frequently denies itself in its own discourse as 'knowledge'. Michel Foucault's writing (1972) and the discipline of discourse analysis (Wetherell 2001) provide a thorough critique of this academic vanishing act and some useful tools of the analysis of discourse, both verbal and visual (Gee 2011).

Freud's request was that we live without opposing the two principles of pleasure and reality and attempt to find our pleasure more congruently within our tested reality. This understanding suggests a pluralistic approach that is respectful of, and promotes, all our diverse and inherent capacities for research. A practice research that diminishes the fuller perspective of our research capacities as researching subjects runs contrary to itself and, through consequent data loss, necessarily invalidates its own outcomes.

3.6 Grounded Theory

As a counterbalance to constructivist concerns it seems important now to consider an approach that aims to keep us close to the data of practice and 'listens' to what the data itself has to say. The open and flexible handling of data was the primary drive in the development of grounded theory (Glaser and Strauss 2008) as a form of research. Its virtue as a method is its respect for 'the data' and the promotion of novel theoretical construction and hypotheses in relation to it. It also promotes the notion of 'emergence', where the process of research and the data are seen to yield theory, rather than research being seen conservatively as the testing of 'ready-made' theory and hypotheses. This seems in tune with the spirit of the art process, where the activity is often seen to yield meaning and the 'unknown' is invited in as a welcome guest on the journey into novel productions. In therapy, as clients and therapists, when the data fits the theory it supports its ongoing value; however, sometimes the most valuable moments in therapy are moments of unique discovery from the data. These explorations of theoretical blind spots warrant ongoing enquiry to enrich and revitalise both theory and practice as evolving social phenomena.

3.7 Reflectively Practising towards Research: Reflective Journals

The HCPC Standards of Proficiency for art therapists states that we should 'understand the value of reflection on practice and the need to record such reflection' (HCPC 2013, p.11). Donald Schön in *The Reflective*

Practitioner (1983) and *Theory in Practice* (Argyris and Schön 1974) examined the current crisis of professions and the gap that often exists between theory of action and theory in use. He implores us to 'search, instead, for an epistemology of practice implicit in the artistic, intuitive processes which some practitioners do bring to situations of uncertainty, instability, uniqueness, and value conflict' (Schön 1983, p.49). He goes on to outline the notion of 'reflection in action' and counterposes it with a critique of 'technical rationality', and then offers it as a way of looking at, and resolving, various real-world problematic situations that are encountered by various professions in the course of their daily practice.

The research process of reflection in action he identifies includes:

1. framing and reframing the problem

2. drawing on experience

3. 'on the spot' experiments

4. the use of 'virtual worlds' (identified as drawing in architecture and transference in therapy).

Art therapists will notice interesting parallels in both these working scenarios that bring together design and psychotherapy. Art therapy draws on both the exploration of transference and the creative art processes within our practice. What is vital to our considerations here is that 'problems' in these two scenarios are faced and resolved within the practice context, through a process of reflection in action. Schön promotes this as a valid form of practice research and his work provided a foundation of the development of reflective practice, now seen as essential in professional and organisational development.

Ghaye and Lillyman's (2006) *Learning Journals and Critical Incidents* uses Schön's ideas as a resource for health care practitioners. They encourage an active research stance initiated by the problematic situations and the critical incidents of practice, suggesting that these incidents, far from being something to hide, are seen as the best source of questions and research. Similarly both Dave Rogers (Chapter 8) and David Edwards (Chapter 11) point to the apparent value of 'error' in practice. The writings of Patrick Casement (1985, 1990, 2002) suggest we make emphatic and more conscious use of 'mistakes' in therapy and supervision.

Tracing the origin of 'reflective practice' to the American pragmatist John Dewey (1981), Ghaye and Lillyman (2006) thoroughly explore and identify a route from reflective practice towards research. Promoting the use of learning journals and critical incident analysis, they make reference to Carper who, like Habermas mentioned above, identifies the following domains of knowledge: the *scientific*, the *personal*, the *aesthetic* and the *ethical*, all evident in good practice. They represent them also as a way of redressing some of the imbalance found in health service discourses that inflates the scientific paradigm as the sole and guiding epistemology of practice. In the absence of the external accounting in post-qualification private practice, the process of reflective practice provides a clear and practical route to collaborative research which would encourage the private practitioner to think through critical incidents, therapeutic ruptures and moments of doubt to transform them into individual and collective explorations for personal and professional development, forming the kernels of new questions for further individual, collaborative and collective research projects. Most importantly for the lone practitioner, it reengages the private practitioner with research, reflective practice and the broader research agenda of the profession. The collective work of private practice-based research could be envisaged as a subgroup of larger professional research groups that already exist for art therapists considering research. (The BAAT Private Practice Special Interest Group and the Art Therapy Practice Research Network already provide forums for reflective practice and research development. This book is a result of such reflection in these fora of research.)

3.7.1 Research Journals

Creative writing can be its own form of research, as is acknowledged by both Clarkson (1995) and McLeod (1999, 2011). Having chosen a topic and begun to write, authors notice a particular process occurring that in many ways follows a course akin to the 'work of therapy' itself. Moustakis outlines this process in his study of heuristic research (1990) which draws together the general process of scientific invention, creative writing and the therapeutic process. This form of research fits well with art therapy private practice research, as it points to a form of research that is endogenous to the therapy process and involves skills which are already occurring in the scenario by deepening and honing them. Ghaye and Lillyman (2006) show that writing journals is an essential part of personal and professional development; they outline the importance of this re-presentation of practice through writing and other forms of representation. Though written for the nursing profession, it is the best account I have encountered of the use of journals in the process of professional reflective practice through 'reflection in action' and 'reflection on action'. The keeping of a research journal, in meeting the obligations set by the HCPC for us to make artwork and also make a 'record of reflective practice', should therefore become part of every practitioner's routine. Writing and art making in a journal develops a narrative of research which can then support further cycles of research which, when 'analysed', 'coded' and 'memoed', can take practice and research themes to deeper levels of refinement and understanding – but most importantly it maintains the link between clinical practice and research. The use of 'visual response' is currently taught as a technique of reflection in art therapy trainings, but post-qualification this should be taken into the process of journal writing, making active research part of ongoing practice and PPD. Most researchers would identify that writing, and in our case art making also, are themselves a method of research, which unites tacit and intuitive knowing into explicit exploration, enhancing the self-esteem and confidence of the practitioner and helping us to *show* our practice to ourselves, our clients and then others by revalidating practice research methods for art therapy. Ghaye and Lillyman (2006) point out how journal writing has cognitive, affective and clinical/competency benefits as an essential act of re-presentation. Schön showed how it is only by attending to the reality of practice that a crisis of the professions can be resolved and the link between theory and practice re-established.

3.8 Pictured and Storied Lives: Art and Narrative Therapy and Research

I am enough of the artist to draw freely upon my imagination. Imagination is more important than knowledge. Knowledge is limited. Imagination encircles the world.

Albert Einstein 1929, p.117

In the exploration of the interior of art therapy private practice we can now move to the arts-based research methodologies that are central to art therapy practice. Cresswell (1998) notes that three of the five identified qualitative research traditions, biography, ethnography and the case study, have the portrait as their central focus. Studies that provide a picture of something tend to use the suffix '-graphy' from the original Greek meaning 'to scratch, to scrape or to graze' (Liddell and Scott 1889). For the Greeks it is clear that these scratchings do not only involve writing but open up a broader range of signifying possibilities. Photography, topography, geography, ethnography, infographic, biography, monograph, autograph and graph, and of course graphics, all imply visual graphic means of research through picturing. Without labouring the point, the notion that research means representation in words or numbers alone is clearly false. Our scratchings and re-scratchings should involve all the modalities native to our understanding.

An impromptu investigation of contemporary train station newsagents reveals a quiet revolution occurring in image-based research that now includes sketch notes, info doodles, infographics, mind maps and of course the endless calls for business people to think like 'artists'. This revolution of graphic means to productive thinking seems to have been largely ignored by the academic research community and art therapists, yet as art therapists we support clients to employ similar graphic means through which they attempt to re-vision their worlds in a determined effort to re-establish fresh, art-based forms of research and thinking through mapping, sketching and emotional colour maps. Art therapists should be leading the way in this process and linking up with the parallel endeavours of visual sociology and visual ethnography, as the image regains momentum as a research methodology and begins to be seen as a very productive means for research. Pink, Hogan and Bird (2011) have drawn attention to this rich potential for cross-pollination. A good example of photographic ethnography would be Zuccotti (2015), who requested her subjects to take images of the things they touched in the course of a day and then produced the images in a book as an ethnographic archive. Rose (2016) offers a useful way of appreciating the various sites through which an image can be considered: the site of *production*, the site of *the image itself*, the site of *circulation* and the site of *audiencing*. The interdependent interplay of these 'sites' can usefully be employed in the research of any image in its context.

3.8.1 Visual Re-Search in Art Therapy Private Practice

The recurrence of the prefix 're-' suggests that all research involves re-flective re-presentation of the data of experience with the aim of discovering new knowledge. The art process and its objects demand reflective re-presentation. The action of re-search suggests a reflective doing again or re-making and re-presenting as part of the research process, which brings our attention to some thing or some detail, as yet taken for granted or unnoticed. It re-introduces agency into passive viewing and encourages reality testing. This phenomenon is a common ground for both research and art making. The effective research paper or artwork bring our attention to neglected experience or usefully reframe reality. Though it is rare to find art practice represented as research, this suggests there is a common aim in both processes. Recognising this, Barrett and Bolt (2010) and Nelson (2013) attempt to unite practice and research within the art school context. Both research and art practice interrogate reality, though they do it in different ways. Art does it concretely, whilst traditional research does it logically and conceptually. The 're-' in research suggests that we turn back mindfully to experience and question what happens generally or what has happened in our world. Art gives us an experience in the world, whereas research attempts to give us sound knowledge of it. But is this distinction really so clear? Art informs in some way, and research surely only has value through its live and situated application.

Saldaña (2013) considers the use of visual data in his book on coding in qualitative research:

A slippery issue for some is the analysis of visual data... Despite some pre-existing coding frameworks for visual representation, I feel the best approach to analysing visual data is a holistic, interpretive lens guided by intuitive inquiry and strategic questions. Rather than one-word or short phrase codes (which are still possible if desired for such approaches as content analysis), the researcher's careful scrutiny of and reflection on images, documented through field notes and analytic memos, generate language-based data that accompany the visual data. Ironically, we must use words to articulate our 'take' on pictures and imagery. So any descriptors and interpretations we use for documenting the images of social life should employ rich, dynamic words.

Gee (2011) suggests that the same tools used in discourse analysis can be applied to analysing visual materials, and Clark (2011, p.142), quoted in Saldaña (2013, p.52), considers that visual artefacts should not be thought of 'as "nouns" (i.e., things analyzed by a researcher *after* their production) but as "verbs" – processes co-examined with participants *during* the artistic product's creation, followed by participants' reflections on the interpretations and meanings of their own work'.

These research perspectives fit with our understanding of the need to consider this rich form of data in practice research, whilst also considering its particular generative qualities in research generally. The sociologist Stuart Hall, whose thoughts on the 'circuit of culture' we considered earlier, likewise beautifully describes the way to interpret images within research:

It is worth emphasising that there is no single or 'correct' answer to the question, 'What does this image mean?' ...since there is no law which can guarantee that things will have 'one true meaning', or that meanings won't change over time, work in this area is bound to be interpretive – a debate between, not who is 'right' and who is 'wrong', but between equally plausible, though sometimes competing and contesting, meanings and interpretations. The best way to 'settle' such contested readings is to look again at the concrete example and try to justify one's 'reading' in detail in relation to the actual practices and form of signification used, and what meanings they seem to you to be producing. (Hall 2013, p.xxv)

Gilroy (2011) made an assessment of four visual research methods used by art therapists, involving looking, writing, curating and making. I will elaborate loosely on these, and curatorial research will have its own section later in the chapter.

a. Retrospective Review and Art Historical Research
As Schaverien (1996) points out, many of the ways art therapists view pictures are borrowed from art history. Hatt and Klonk (2006) explore the

theoretical constructs and methods of art history. Gilroy (2013) identifies the importance of the art historian Panofsky, who suggested three ways to look at pictures:

- ekphrasis: artful description

- iconographic analysis: looking at motifs

- iconological interpretation.

It is useful for an art therapist to consider these phases of art historical research and honour clients with this close attention to their artwork. This art historical research approach has good fit with the idea of endogenous private practice research. Schaverien's notion of 'retrospective review' asks us to attend periodically to the artwork and draw on these art historical skills, and to provide a moment to stand back and reflect on the *oeuvre* as a whole; to notice gestural, colour and iconographic trends and developments, and to reconsider also the changing landscape of feeling that accompanied its production. In private practice it also provides a moment for readjustment of the therapeutic contract, when appropriate, as well as a moment of accountability of the therapist to the client with regard to the process, progress and change – evidenced by the work and the client's recollections of the process. This reflective pause in therapy can also provide an opportunity for *interview*, within the session or independent of it, to encourage reflection and interpretive (hermeneutic) depth for both parties involved in the research. The UKCP Semi-Structured Post-Therapy Interview mentioned in Section 3.4 exemplifies the sort of research that may be possible and beneficial for both the client and the profession. Springham and Brooker (2013) explore the value of bringing together the research potential of audio-image recording (AIR) and the reflect interview (RI), uniting image and speech in research.

B. ART WRITING AND ART SPEAKING AS RESEARCH

In ancient times art was used as a means for rhetorical training called *ekphrasis* (and also corresponds with Panofsky's first level of understanding pictures). Those learning the art of rhetoric would use images to improve the quality of their speech. Finding eloquence around images clearly remains an important part of art therapy both in therapy and in training. We have also pointed to the widely recognised generative capacity of images in research to produce novel perspectives and insight. Research writing around images is also gaining momentum as a form of qualitative and visual research. We have already considered the importance of creative writing and art making, in parallel to practice, as a way to generate and reflect upon theory, and also as a means to develop reflective practice through keeping research journals.

c. Art Making as Research – Visual Response

The notion of aesthetic countertransference and the importance of our visual response to the work are built into our training and are discussed by Schaverien (1995, 2000). Some art therapists make work alongside clients, and others make work after. The notion of making work 'after' another artist has a long tradition in the arts and has been a way of honouring and reflecting on technique. When I redrew Dr Rey's drawing, above, I learned through the process of re-production that it is not a drawing of Van Gogh's ear but a doctor's generalised representation of a male ear drawn to illustrate the incision made by the artist. His drawing was not meant to be an expressive artwork but an anatomical illustration. The copying process nonetheless reveals his care for his patient and his wish to represent a history accurately. Drawing 'like' another and exploring countertransference through parallel art making is highly informative to the practitioner. Even when we are not aware of it initially, we will find clients' motifs and styles invading our own production in ways that are informative to practice and worthy of further research. This process of parallel production is explored by Havsteen-Franklin and Camarena Altamirano (2015). In private practice, the joint monitoring of productivities is another area for further inter-systemic, intertextual and holistic exploration, providing us with a means to attune our aesthetic antenna.

3.8.2 Knowing the Signs – Semiotics

Charles Peirce, a scientist, and a founder of pragmatism and the science of signs (known as semiotics), realised, like Kant, that our scientific endeavours are always mediated through symbolic representation. He believed that this required a specific attention to the process of signification in order to fully understand the world, the meanings we draw from it and the means by which we share our ideas. Understanding the nature of signification became his quest. Scientists, art historians and sociologists have all adopted what has shown to be a particularly useful theorisation of the field of visual signification. He divided sign types into three main groupings:

- symbolic signs: governed by convention

- indexical signs: governed by observation

- iconic signs: governed by perception.

These sign types relate to the three main forms of logic mentioned earlier: the symbolic sign with deduction, the indexical sign with induction, and the iconic sign with abduction. These signs and logics are evident in the products of art therapy and in its analysis. Rosalind Krauss's (1981) art historical study of the modern sculpture's movement from *symbolic* and *iconic* signification towards *indexicality* is a good example of a Peircian semiotic analysis of art. Further research in this area could be invaluable to art therapist practitioners. Robin Tipple (2012) alone in art therapy has referenced Peirce as part of a discourse analysis with a child client.

3.8.3 Narrative Research and Discourse Analysis

White and Epston (1990) outlined a clear agenda for narrative therapy as a process of constructive questioning, reframing and externalisation of our 'storied lives' which has relevance for art therapists, who hear so many stories around the campfire of the image. Offering clients the possibility to deconstruct oppressive and restricting narratives and supporting them to try out alternative tellings of new or repressed narratives adds to the potential honing of the therapist's skills, and a research attention to *discourse* (Wetherell 2001; Willig 2008) and *narrative* (Lieblich, Tuval-Mashiach and Zilber 1998) *research*. It also may attune us to a more critical listening of the variety of discourses we may hear in clinical meetings and draw attention to the discourses of research itself and the scientific narratives presented to us as 'fact'. We need to see the sequences and listen more closely, using these skills to attend to our clients and recognise the potential retellings we are witnessing, encouraging and/or possibly avoiding. Kate Rothwell (in Chapter 9) recognises and draws upon the anthropological notion of 'emplotment' in considering narrative developments in therapy.

4. Researching the Ending

Therapeutic endings in therapy are always important, and endings in private art therapy have not yet been researched. They may represent a symbolic loss that may provoke strings of associations to the losses encountered in a lifetime. They are generally difficult to predict and require sensitive and open facilitation by the therapist. The ending of private art therapy could be researched through surveys or through structured, semi-structured or unstructured interviews which may provide a more nuanced understanding of this important area.

In the course of the last authors' meeting, prior to concluding our work, this area was highlighted as an area for potential research, for both clients and therapists. It was also acknowledged that tensions can exist between the business interests of the therapist and the realities and needs of the client around ending in a private art therapy practice intervention. Non-payment of fees was also raised as an area of particular concern, both with regard to understanding it within the transference and through the practical reality of running a business. An impromptu list was formed around some of the reasons for endings in private practice which could be followed up with further client and therapist research.

Some possible reasons for ending in art therapy private practice:

- achievement of therapeutic goals

- stuckness – e.g. no progress

- change of circumstance (for either the therapist or the client)

- funding issues and non-payment: real financial hardship, transferential issues or both, possibly calling on the therapist to make a sliding scale adjustment of the fee or a delayed payment schedule

- significant deterioration in mental or physical health and/or the therapist referring on to another professional.

In our discussion endings fell into these three main headings in relation to who initiates them:

- led by therapist

- led by clients

- led by carer/parent.

The survey in Chapter 14 found that 95 per cent of art therapists in private practice 'negotiate endings with clients'.

Supervision is recommended as the appropriate forum for any art therapist 'in puzzlement' over any ending issues, but further research would also be very helpful.

5. Researching After: What Is There to Show?

The ending provides an opportunity to assess the outcomes set at the start of therapy, and this also tends to occur naturally and informally as part of ending conversations. Research has shown that clients who reflect on what has happened in therapy may be able to make better use of it going forward, therefore suggesting that these final reflections on ending can determine the future beneficial therapeutic effect (Gendlin and Zimring 1955).

The ending also represents an opportunity for a final reflective review of the therapeutic work as a whole, including the artwork. It is a time to ask clients to make concrete powerfully symbolic decisions about what artwork to take, what to leave, or even destroy. These rituals around the disposal of the therapeutic artefacts in ending could be researched further ethnographically. Therapists' practices, policies and contracts around ending and ongoing storage of work and justifications could be also usefully explored.

5.1 The Show: Curatorial Research

Endings for artists are often associated with a show, and increasingly it is now considered an important potential for art therapy clients, especially in community group contexts. In art therapy, Schaverien (1996) writes of the 'retrospective exhibition', suggesting the importance of a 'show' within therapy and as part of the therapy as a collaborative reflective and research event. Showing work can be the final opportunity to explore the evidence of the collaborative research endeavour in art therapy; whether it is the more traditional final review within the confidential boundary of therapy, or a collaboratively curated exhibition (as described in Chapter 3), the show or the final showing of the reflective review, or in combination, is central to research in art therapy.

The curator Hans Ulrich Obrist (2015) writes eloquently on curating as a form of research. He states, 'Collection-making, you could say, is a method of producing knowledge' (p.39). Co-curating also represents an opportunity for the collaborative re-authoring of personal narratives as social action research. As art therapists broaden their horizons, we are asked to question the prohibition that exists on the display of the client's artwork, which has traditionally been seen as contained within the boundary of confidentiality. This is being challenged with respect to the benefits it may have in building the client's self-esteem, the technological developments of digitalisation and communicability of the image and its copies, and also in its use as data for the research of art therapy. We also note the dovetailing of curatorial research methods that appear in Roam's notion of visual research that culminates in *showing*. Rose's phased notion of the sites in visual research also culminates with the sites of 'circulation' and of 'audiencing'. These visual fields are all rich research territories, especially as we move in art therapy towards an increasingly digitised and visual culture (Garner 2017).

5.2 The Gallery

When Marcel Duchamp placed a urinal in a gallery space he was 'objectively' re-presenting an aspect of reality by de-contextualising and then re-contextualising it. This act raises questions about the meaning of the object within the context in which it was first found and removed from, and in the context in which it was subsequently rediscovered as Art. The artist here used the object to force reflexivity onto the viewer. This object, taken from a set of objects related to our basic needs, is then used to question the high values of art and simultaneously invite aesthetic attention to a disregarded and devalued porcelain object of public use. This process therefore appears to be an exploratory research action. Similarly, in Warhol's screen prints, through the re-production of the subjects of mass reproduction he places value on the common place and reframes it for our attention. What implications are there in considering such re-presentation as actions of re-search within the art therapy session, in supervision and into the forum of formal academic research? This artful and aesthetic re-search, play and toying has always provided the soft underbelly of research within the natural sciences, as is evidenced by numerous historical accounts of scientists who have used imaginative play, dreams and occult fascination as part of the process of generating innovative ideas and new envisionings of reality.

The BAAT Museums and Galleries Special Interest Group (MAGSIG) currently explores some of these curatorial and archival edges to art therapy fruitfully.

Ethics of Inquiry
What Are Practice Research Ethics?

Following the Second World War, there was a need to reconsider the relationship of science and ethics due to great technological innovation during the war. In Germany and America, active scientific experiments took place on human subjects without their consent, leading to physical and psychological damage and death. This was coupled with discourses of scientific efficiency and efficacy used in a drive to develop technologies for mass killing in warfare initially, and then of civilians through eugenic policy-making and its subsequent execution. The 'final solution' of Nazism was couched in scientific terms of technical 'efficacy and efficiency'. These events of relatively recent history contribute to our ongoing sensitivity and caution with regard to research and experimentation 'on' human subjects.

Within a fully collaborative and consensual practice research, many of these ethical concerns are diminished. There nonetheless are still risks for all participants in research – but when it is reflexively, reflectively and collaboratively approached with the overview of supervision and in relation to free and open debates within professional and patient forums, the ethical risks of practice research can be significantly lessened. Practice research is research 'with', not 'on', clients. Clients seeing art therapists also have the protection of the HCPC, which exists to protect the public and ensures art therapists abide by its standards of proficiency and ethical codes in practice and in research. BAAT also has its own code of ethics and expectations of its members that are specific to our profession, where matters of research are considered in terms of ethics and best practice.

Although the idea of practice research is not new, it clearly requires a reorientation in a profession that has largely lost sight of this phenomenon. It provides another field for ethical exploration and a consideration of whether our contracts need to be rewritten and other consents gained in the light of this reorientation towards practice seen as research. Private practice research also requires us to consider what it means to actively reintroduce our human intersubjectivity into the discourses of research. I have shown that the 'interestedness' of art therapists in private practice raises important questions around 'interest' and 'investment' in the process of research more generally – and this then leads to an appropriate questioning of the assumption of 'scientific' disinterested and 'objective' research borrowed from the natural sciences and medicine without sufficient consideration. In this way art therapy in private practice can provide a critical forum within the context of the other art therapy practice groupings. The suggestion from private practice research is that we embrace 'interestedness' and explore it thoroughly as part of a reflexive ethical stance. Craig (1999), Van Manen (1990, 2014) and Moustakis (1990) likewise all suggest that an ethical and reflexive stance is an integral expectation of a phenomenological and heuristic collaborative research.

Conclusion for Part 1 and Part 2

I have shown how art therapy private practice research can embrace both the newly emerging and the more traditional qualitative and quantitative research methods within the different phases of understanding and deepening in the course of therapy. Whether this research is written up as formal research or not, the research traditions represented above are a considerable resource for ongoing private art therapy practice research with clients. Although qualitative methodologies don't tend to produce generalisable knowledge, what they provide are research aims, interest, engagement and material for further collaborative research that are likely to help practitioners in their therapeutic engagement, supporting the notion of practice as a form of research and encouraging them to reflexively and reflectively examine their interventions.

The size and highly contextualised nature of an art therapy private practice can reveal the beauty of a small-scale intervention because it enables a focus on quality and a clear view of all the resonating and systemically related elements of practice, encouraging a holistic and integrated way of working. It is my hope that art therapists can lead the way in helping to bridge the gap that has opened up between research and practice which has been identified by numerous commentators (Ferguson 2005; Finlay 2011; McLeod 1999; Schön 1983). The contextual particularities of art therapy in private practice undoubtedly provide a challenge to a profession accustomed to statutory provision but also provide opportunities to test ideas in a different context of practice and to challenge and independently test research findings, and provide an alternative independent forum for debate.

Though the circumstances remain very challenging for all art therapists in the statutory provision, and in independent and private practice, I remain hopeful that as a small profession we can work together (trainings, professional association and practitioners and clients) to use the current challenges to reshape the profession in creative ways that are helpful to clients and ourselves.

Some Recommendations

A Private Practice Specific Research Network

Due to the relative isolation of private practice, it is vital that practitioners pool their data and resources to stimulate further research and provide critical feedback to the profession from this field of practice and also develop methods and methodologies for practice research. It may be that a subsection of the current PPSIG and Art Therapy Practice Research Network could accommodate a forum specifically for private and independent practice research.

Ongoing Development of Practice Guidelines for Private Practitioners

Art therapists in private practice should continue to develop and research the themes, phenomena and issues of their working context as they relate to clients' needs and their own professional development.

Research Journals

Practitioners should continue to explore the value of keeping research journals in order to identify the pressing questions arising from practice that often follow from critical incidents, recognising that writing and art making are their own form of research. Research journals, using the rich data of art therapy practice and lived experience, can help to develop the skills of endogenous research, enhancing personal and professional autonomy, and can become an essential part of personal and professional development.

References

Agazarian, Y. and Peters, R. (2010) *The Visible and Invisible Group.* London: Karnac Books.

Argyris, C. and Schön, D.A. (1974) *Theory in Practice.* San Francisco, CA: Jossey-Bass Publishers.

BAAT (2014) *Code of Ethics and Principles of Professional Practice for Art Therapists.* London: BAAT.

BAAT (2017) *Core Skills and Practice Standards in Private Work.* London: BAAT. (Appendix 1)

Barrett, E. and Bolt, B. (2010) *Practice as Research: Approaches to Creative Arts Enquiry.* London: L.B. Tauris & Co Ltd.

Bateson, G. (2000) 'The Cybernetics of "Self": A Theory of Alcoholism.' In *Steps to an Ecology of Mind.* London: University of Chicago Press.

Betensky, M.G. (1987) 'Phenomenology of Therapeutic Art Expression and Art Therapy.' In J.A. Rubin (ed.) *Approaches to Art Therapy.* New York: Brunner/Mazel.

Blumer, H. (1989) *Symbolic Interactionism.* Los Angeles, CA: University of California Press.

British Psychological Society (2011) *Good Practice Guidelines on the Use of Formulation.* Leicester: BPS.

Campbell, J., Liebmann, M., Brooks, F., Jones, J. and Ward, C. (1999) *Art Therapy, Race and Culture.* London: Jessica Kingsley Publishers.

Cartwright, N. (2007) *Are RCTs the Gold Standard?* Centre for Philosophy of Natural and Social Science Contingency and Dissent in Science Technical Report 01/07. London: LSE.

Casement, P.J. (1985) *On Learning from the Patient.* London: Tavistock Publications.

Casement, P.J. (1990) *Further Learning from the Patient.* London: Routledge.

Casement, P.J. (2002) *Learning from Our Mistakes.* London: Routledge.

Clark, C.D. (2011) *In a Younger Voice: Doing Child-Centered Qualitative Research.* New York: Oxford.

Clarkson, P. (1995) *The Therapeutic Relationship.* London: Whurr Publishers.

Craig, R.T. (1995) 'Grounded practical theory: The case of intellectual discussion.' *Communication Theory 5,* 3, 248–272.

Craig, R.T. (1999) 'Communication theory as a field.' *Communication Theory 9,* 2, 119–161.

Cresswell, J.W. (1998) *Qualitative Inquiry and Research Design.* London: Sage.

de Shazer, S. and Dolan, Y. (2007) *More Than Miracles.* London: Routledge.

Dewey, J. (1981) *The Philosophy of John Dewey.* London: University of Chicago Press.

Dilthey, W. (1976) 'An Introduction to the Human Sciences.' In W. Dilthey and H.P. Rickman (eds) *Dilthey: Selected Writings.* London: Cambridge University Press.

Dilts, R., Grinder, J., Bandler, R. and DeLozier, J. (1980) *Neuro-Linguistic Programming, Volume 1.* Cupertino, CA: Meta Publications.

Dufrenne, M. (1979) *The Phenomenology of Aesthetic Experience.* Evanston, IL: Northwestern University Press.

Edwards, D. (1999) 'The role of the case study in art therapy research.' *Inscape 4,* 1, 2–9.

Einstein, A. (1929) 'What life means to Einstein: An interview by George Sylvester Viereck.' *Saturday Evening Post,* 26 October.

Ferguson, J. (2005) 'Bridging the gap between research and practice.' *Knowledge Management for Development Journal 1,* 3, 46–54.

Finlay, L. (2011) *Phenomenology for Therapists: Researching the Lived World.* Oxford: John Wiley and Sons.

Foucault, M. (1972) *The Archaeology of Knowledge and the Discourse on Language.* New York: Pantheon Books.

Frankl, V.E. (2008) *Man's Search for Meaning.* London: Rider.

Freire, P. (1996) *The Pedagogy of the Oppressed.* London: Penguin.

Freud, S. (1980) *The Interpretation of Dreams.* London: Pelican.

Freud, S. (2006 [1906]) 'Beyond the Pleasure Principle.' In *The Penguin Freud Reader.* London: Penguin.

Freud, S. and Breuer, J. (1974 [1895]) *Studies on Hysteria.* Reading: Pelican Books.

Gadamer, H.-G. (1975) *Truth and Method.* New York: Seabury.

Garner, R.L. (2017) *Digital Art Therapy.* London: Jessica Kingsley Publishers.

Gee, J.P. (2011) *How to Do Discourse Analysis.* London: Routledge.

Gendlin, E.T. and Zimring, F. (1955) 'The qualities or dimensions of experiencing and their change.' *Counselling Center Discussion Paper 1*, 3. Chicago, IL: University of Chicago Library.

Ghaye, T. and Lilyman, S. (2006) *Learning Journals and Critical Incidents.* London: Quay Books.

Gilroy, A. (2011) *Art Therapy Research in Practice.* Oxford: Lang.

Gilroy, A. (2013) *Art Therapy, Research and Evidence-Based Practice.* London: Sage.

Gilroy, A., Tipple, R. and Brown, C. (eds) (2012) *Assessment in Art Therapy.* London: Routledge.

Glaser, B.G. and Strauss, A.L. (2008) *The Discovery of Grounded Theory.* London: Aldine Transaction.

Goldacre, B. (2013) *Bad Pharma.* London: Fourth Estate.

Habermas, J. (1972) *Knowledge and Human Interest.* Boston, MA: Beakon.

Habermas, J. (1984) *The Theory of Communicative Action, Volume 1.* Boston, MA: Beacon Press.

Hackett, S.S. (2016) 'Art Psychotherapy with an Adult with Autistic Spectrum Disorder and Sexually Deviant Dreams: A Single-Case Study Including the Client's Responses to Treatment.' In K. Rothwell (ed.) *Forensic Arts Therapies.* London: Free Association Books.

Hall, S. (2013) *Representation.* London: Open University Press.

Hardy, G., Aldridge, J., Davidson, C., Rowe, C., Reilly, S. and Shapiro, D. (1999) 'Therapist responsiveness to client attachment styles and issues observed in client-identified significant events in psychodynamic-interpersonal therapy.' *Psychotherapy Research 9*, 36–53.

Hatt, M. and Klonk, C. (2006) *Art History: A Critical Introduction to Its Methods.* Manchester: Manchester University Press.

Havsteen-Franklin, D. and Camarena Altamirano, J. (2015) 'Containing the uncontainable: Responsive art making in art therapy as a method to facilitate mentalization.' *International Journal of Art Therapy 20*, 2, 54–65.

HCPC (2013) *Standards of Proficiency: Arts Therapists.* London: HCPC.

HCPC (2016) *Standards of Conduct, Performance and Ethics.* London: HCPC.

Heidegger, M. (2010) *Being and Time.* Albany, NY: State University of New York Press.

Heidegger, M. (2011) 'The Question Concerning Technology.' In D. Krell (ed.) *Basic Writings.* London: Routledge Classics.

Hogan, S. (2016) *Art Therapy Theories.* London: Routledge.

Hogan, S. and Pink, S. (2010) 'Routes to interiorties: Art therapy and knowing in anthropology.' *Visual Anthropology 23*, 158–174.

Huet, V. and Springham, N. (2013) *Audit Pack.* London: British Association of Art Therapists and Art Therapy Practice Research Network.

Hughes, R. (2016) *Time-Limited Art Psychotherapy.* London: Routledge.

Husserl, E. (1962) *Ideas.* New York: Collier Books.

Husserl, E. (1970) *The Crisis of European Sciences and Transcendental Phenomenology.* Evanston, IL: Northwestern University Press.

Kant, I. (2012 [1781]) *The Critique of Pure Reason* (trans. (1896) F.M. Muller). London: Forgotten Books.

Kaplan, F.F. (2007) *Art Therapy and Social Action.* London: Jessica Kingsley Publishers.

Korzybski, A. (2010) 'On Structure.' In *Selections from Science and Sanity.* Fort Worth, TX: The Institute of General Semantics.

Krauss, R. (1981) *Passages in Modern Sculpture.* Cambridge, MA: MIT Press.

Levine, E.G. and Levine, S.K. (eds) (2011) *Art in Action.* London: Jessica Kingsley Publishers.

Lewin, K. (1951) *Field Theory in Social Science.* New York: Harper & Row.

Lewis, C.S. (2013) *A Grief Observed.* London: Faber & Faber.

Liddell, H.G. and Scott, R. (1889) *An Intermediate Greek–English Lexicon.* Oxford: Clarendon Press.

Lieblich, A., Tuval-Mashiach, R. and Zilber, T. (1998) *Narrative Research.* London: Sage.

McLeod, J. (1999) *Practitioner Research in Counselling.* London: Sage.

McLeod, J. (2011) *Qualitative Research in Counselling and Psychotherapy.* London: Sage.

Mead, G.H. (2015) *Mind, Self and Society.* London: University of Chicago Press.

Merleau-Ponty, M. (1962) *Phenomenology of Perception*. London: Routledge and Kegan Paul.

Moustakis, C. (1990) *Heuristic Research*. London: Sage.

Murphy, B. (2016) *Van Gogh's Ear*. London: Chatto & Windus.

Nardone, G. and Portelli, C. (2005) *Knowing Through Changing*. Carmarthen: Crown House.

Nelson, R. (2013) *Practice as Research in the Arts*. New York: Palgrave Macmillan.

NICE (2011) *Alcohol-Use Disorders: Diagnosis, Assessment and Management of Harmful Drinking and Alcohol Dependence* (CG115). London: NICE.

Obrist, H.U. (2015) *Ways of Curating*. London: Penguin.

OECD (2015) *Frascati Manual 2015: Guidelines for Collecting and Reporting Data on Research and Experimental Development. The Measurement of Scientific, Technological and Innovation Activities*. Paris: OECD Publishing.

Panofsky, E. (1983) *Meaning in the Visual Arts*. Chicago, IL: University of Chicago Press.

Payne, H. (ed.) (1996) *Handbook of Inquiry in the Arts Therapies*. London: Jessica Kingsley Publishers.

Pink, S., Hogan, S. and Bird, J. (2011) 'Intersections and inroads: Art therapy's contribution to visual methods.' *International Journal of Art Therapy 16*, 1, 14–19.

Polanyi, M. (1962) *The Tacit Dimension*. Chicago, IL: University of Chicago Press.

Polanyi, M. (1964) *Science, Faith and Society*. Chicago, IL: University of Chicago Press.

Polanyi, M. (1969) *Knowing and Being*. Chicago, IL: University of Chicago Press.

Rappaport, L. (2009) *Focusing-Oriented Art Therapy*. London: Jessica Kingsley Publishers.

Roam, D. (2009) *Unfolding the Napkin*. London: Penguin.

Rose, G. (2016) *Visual Methodologies*. London: Sage.

Saldaña, J. (2013) *The Coding Manual for Qualitative Researchers*. ebook. London: Sage.

Sartre, J.P. (2003) *Being and Nothingness*. London: Routledge.

Sartre, J.P. (2004) *The Imaginary*. London: Routledge.

Schaverien, J. (1995) 'Researching the Esoteric: Art Therapy Research.' In A. Gilroy and C. Lee (eds) *Art and Music: Therapy and Research*. London: Routledge.

Schaverien, J. (1996) 'The Retrospective Review of Pictures: Data for Research in Art Therapy.' In H. Payne (ed.) *Handbook of Inquiry in the Arts Therapies*. London: Jessica Kingsley Publishers.

Schaverien, J. (2000) 'The Triangular Relationship and the Aesthetic Countertransference in Analytical Art Psychotherapy.' In A. Gilroy and G. McNeilly (eds) *The Changing Shape of Art Therapy*. London: Jessica Kingsley Publishers.

Schön, D.A. (1983) *The Reflective Practitioner*. New York: Basic Books.

Schopenhauer, A. (2012 [1819]) *The World as Will and Representation* (R.B. Haldane and J. Kemp trans.). Plano, TX: Lexicos Publishing.

Schumacher, E.F. (2014) *Small Is Beautiful*. New York: Harper Perennial.

Searle, J.R. (1977) *Speech Acts*. London: Cambridge University Press.

Shotter, J. (2016) *Speaking, Actually*. Farnhill: Everything is Connected Press.

Simon, G. and Chard, A. (2014) *Systemic Inquiry*. Farnhill: Everything is Connected Press.

Skaife, S. (2001) 'Making visible: Art therapy and intersubjectivity.' *Inscape 6*, 2, 40–50.

Springham, N. and Brooker, J. (2013) 'Reflect interview using audio-image recording: Development and feasibility study.' *International Journal of Art Therapy 18*, 2, 54–66.

Stake, R.E. (1995) *The Art of Case Study Research*. London: Sage.

Stern, D.N. (2004) *The Present Moment in Psychotherapy and Everyday Life*. New York: W.W. Norton & Company.

Tilmouth, T., Davies-Ward, E. and Williams, B. (2011) *Foundation Degree in Health and Social Care*. London: Hodder Education.

Tipple, R. (2012) 'The Subjects of Assessment.' In A. Gilroy, R. Tipple and C. Brown (eds) *Assessment in Art Therapy*. London: Routledge.

Unger, R.M. (2004) *False Necessity: Anti-Necessitarian Social Theory in the Service of Radical Democracy. Politics, Volume 1*. London: Verso.

Uttley, L., Scope, A., Stevenson, M., Rawdin, A. *et al.* (2015) 'Systematic review and economic modelling of the clinical effectiveness and cost-effectiveness of art therapy among people with non-psychotic mental health disorders.' *Health Technology Assessment 19*, 18, 1–120.

Van Manen, M. (1990) *Researching Lived Experience*. New York: The State University of New York.

Van Manen, M. (2014) *Phenomenology of Practice*. Walnut Creek, CA: Left Coast Press.

Vetere, A. and Stratton, P. (2016) *Interacting Selves*. London: Routledge.

Waller, D. (2013) *Becoming a Profession*. Psychology Revivals. New York: Routledge.

Wertz, F.J., Charmaz, K., McMullen, L.M., Josselson, R., Anderson, R. and McSpadden, E. (2011) *Five Ways of Doing Qualitative Analysis*. New York: The Guilford Press.

West, J.D. (1994) 'Aquellos ojos verdes.' *Third Text 8*, 26, 33–42.

Wetherell, M. (2001) 'Debates in Discourse Research.' In M. Wetherell, S. Taylor and S. Yates (eds) *Discourse Theory and Practice*. London: Sage.

White, M. and Epston, D. (1990) *Narrative Means to Therapeutic Ends*. New York: W.W. Norton & Company.

Willig, C. (2008) *Introducing Qualitative Research in Psychology*. Maidenhead: Open University Press.

Yin, R.K. (1994) *Case Study Research*. London: Sage.

Zuccotti, P. (2015) *Every Thing We Touch*. London: Penguin.

14

PAINTING A PICTURE OF ART THERAPY PRIVATE PRACTICE

Data from a UK Survey

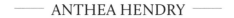

—— ANTHEA HENDRY ——

Introduction

This chapter presents some key findings from a UK survey of art therapists in private practice. The survey was conducted by the British Association of Art Therapists (BAAT) Private Practice Special Interest Group (PPSIG) in 2015–2016 to collect current demographic data about private and independent art therapy practitioners.

The chapter is divided into the following sections:

- background

- inclusion criteria for the data analysis in this chapter

- clarification of the similarities and differences between private practice and independent practice

- findings

- discussion.

Background
Reasons for the Survey

It was agreed at a PPSIG meeting in 2012 that a demographic survey would provide useful data as there was very little information about the extent and nature of private art therapy practice in the UK. A preliminary questionnaire was designed and discussed at several meetings but the PPSIG had other priorities over the next few years, particularly developing guidelines for practice. The survey was finally prioritised in 2015. It was decided to broaden the survey to include those who work independently as well as private practitioners. The reason for this was an awareness that as jobs in the NHS dwindle increasing numbers of art therapists are working independently and needing support in doing so. We made a pragmatic decision to use the term 'independent practice', which includes both those who may call themselves 'sessional workers' and those who describe themselves as 'freelance'. This is also in line with the UK Council for Psychotherapy's (UKCP) terminology.

Method

The questionnaire was finalised by a research group of four members of the PPSIG and converted into an electronic online format using web-based survey software. Permission for the survey was granted by BAAT, who provided support and administrative assistance. It was piloted in October/November 2015. Minor modifications to some of the questions were made before an invitation to participate by completing the survey was sent out by BAAT to all their members on 1 December 2015, accompanied by a letter from the private practice research group outlining the purpose of the survey. The inclusion criteria were: being a qualified art therapist, a BAAT member, and currently working as a private or independent art therapy practitioner.

The questionnaire consisted of 36 fixed-choice questions. After capturing information about age, gender, sexual orientation and ethnicity, questions included information about location of work, payment, client groups, models of intervention, theoretical orientation, and evaluation. Questionnaires were completed between 1 December 2015 and 7 March 2016.

Inclusion Criteria for the Data Analysis in This Chapter

The total number of respondents completing the survey was 404. This represents approximately a quarter of the total BAAT membership of 1609 qualified art therapists in March 2016. Not all BAAT members work either privately or independently, so the response rate of over 25 per cent of the total BAAT membership is very high.

This chapter is an analysis of some of the data only. It is specifically looking at the data relating to art therapists working as private practitioners. Within the questionnaire itself we did not define the difference between private practice and independent practice, but the inclusion criteria for the analysis in this chapter is based on cross-referencing two questions: first, 'How would you describe your practice?', and second, 'Who pays you?' This follows BAAT's definition of private practice as 'a contract for art therapy agreed strictly between the client and art therapist, who is paid directly by the client'[1].

Table 14.1 shows how respondents answered the first of these questions.

Table 14.1 Question: How would you describe your art therapy practice? Tick all that apply

Answer choices	Percentage of respondents	Number of respondents
Private	51	180
Independent	24	87
Freelance	19	67
Self-employed	58	202
Sessional	28	97
Other	23	80
		351 Respondents 53 Non-respondents

It is difficult to know exactly why there was a non-response rate of 13 per cent to this question. Possibly it was because we did not provide definitions of each answer choice. There was a request to 'Tick all that apply' as clearly there are overlaps between the answer choices. For example, both private and independent practitioners are self-employed. Providing definitions may have been helpful. Of the 351 respondents, 180 described themselves as working in private practice. Their answers to the question of 'Who pays you?' were then analysed to see if these matched the understanding of the client paying the therapist directly in private practice. Table 14.2 shows the results.

---

1   This definition can be found at www.baat.org/membershipPrivatePractice. This link is password-protected, and is only available to BAAT members.

Table 14.2 Question: Who pays you? Tick all that apply

Who pays you?	Number of respondents
Client	155
Carer	12
Parent	37
Claim through benefits	4
GP	1
Insurance	9
Other third party	50

The table tells us that 155 of the 180 respondents describing themselves as private practitioners said they were paid directly by the client. However, there are other answers to this question that would fit with the BAAT description of private practice. For example, there are parents that pay for their children to come to therapy, and clients with disabilities who need their carers to pay. There are also clients getting the money to pay for therapy through insurance who may also fit the criteria for being 'private clients'.

Another complication arising from this question is that respondents were not asked to distinguish between different elements of their work. Of the 180 private practitioners, 78 (43%) described themselves as also working independently, sessionally, as a freelance worker or a combination of these. Examination of the data, however, indicates a good correspondence between the numbers of respondents describing their work as private practice and those involving payment by the client using the broader criteria of including parents and carers and payment through private insurance. The data analysis in this chapter therefore includes these 180 respondents. Before moving on to that analysis, the section that follows is an attempt to represent diagrammatically (Figure 14.1) the significant differences between private practice and independent practice.

Clarification of the Similarities and Differences between Private Practice and Independent Practice

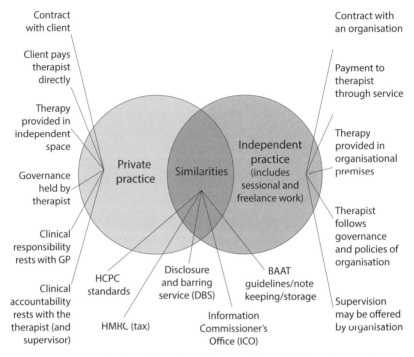

Figure 14.1 Similarities and differences between private and independent practice

At a meeting in November 2016 the PPSIG discussed the similarities and differences between independent and private practice in order to address the question of where independent practitioners might look for support from within BAAT. The above Venn diagram indicates the significance of the client paying the therapist directly. Most importantly, this is because all aspects of governance then fall on to the private therapist's shoulders. In other words the private practitioner has to represent all areas that in a larger organisation would be represented by different individuals or departments, such as safeguarding, health and safety, occupational health, and complaints. For independent practitioners the organisation that contracts them to carry out a particular piece of work will hold these aspects of governance. This is the important difference between private and independent practice but, as Figure 14.1 clearly indicates, there are significant similarities between the two in terms of following Health and Care Professions Council (HCPC) and BAAT guidelines, tax self-assessment, and taking responsibility for data protection.

Survey Findings
Age, Ethnicity, Gender and Sexual Orientation
Age
The average age of an art therapist in private practice is mid-fifties. The survey found that 93 per cent of private practitioners are over 40 and 70 per cent over 50.

Ethnicity
Table 14.3 shows that 140 (77.7%) of the respondents were 'White British' and 26 (14.4%) identified themselves as 'White Other'. There are very small numbers of private practitioners in other ethnic groups and some identify themselves by country of origin rather than ethnicity.

Table 14.3 Question: What is your ethnicity?

Answer choices	Number of respondents
White British	140
White Other	26
Irish	4
Black African	1
Black Caribbean	1
White Asian	1
Chinese	2
Other	1 Swede, 2 American, 3 Welsh

Gender
The gender split was 88 per cent female and 12 per cent male, with no respondent identifying as transgender.

Sexual Orientation
Table 14.4 indicates that approximately 12 per cent of private practitioners are not heterosexual. Of these, the largest group are bisexual (5%).

Table 14.4 Question: What is your sexual orientation?

Answer choices	Percentage of respondents	Number of respondents
Bisexual	5	9
Gay	4	7
Heterosexual	88	155
Lesbian	2	3
Pansexual	2	3
Other	2	3
		Number of respondents 177

This question was cross-referenced with a question asking respondents what client groups they offer services to. This found that a smaller percentage of therapists identifying as LGBT specified an LGBT provision to clients compared with the heterosexual therapists. Overall 15 per cent of heterosexual private practitioners stated they positively did provide for LGBT clients, whereas only 10 per cent of LGBT therapists stated they positively provided for LGBT clients.

Work Experience

Number of Years since Qualifying and Number of Years in Private Practice

The majority of private practitioners (59%) have been qualified for over 13 years and only 20 per cent under six years. However, many art therapists gain experience working in other settings before they start working privately, as the majority (58%) have only worked as private practitioners for six years or less, with 21 per cent who have worked for 7 to 12 years and 21 per cent over 13 years.

Working Hours in Private Practice

The majority (75%) of art therapists work less than eight hours a week with private clients, and only 2 per cent work 21 hours or over a week with private clients. Figure 14.2 gives the percentage for each answer choice.

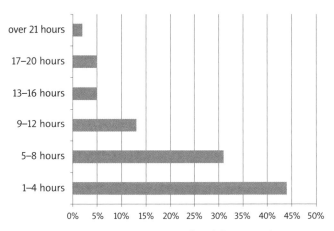

*Figure 14.2 Question: In a typical week how many hours
do you spend working in private practice?*

Location

Figure 14.3 indicates the responses to the question 'Where do you locate your practice?' This has 11 options and asked respondents to tick all that apply. Over 60 per cent of art therapists locate some of their practice in their own homes. Approximately 35 per cent of those use other premises at times as well. Respondents frequently ticked more than one location. For some this will be more than one location specifically for their private practice, but for others it may include the location of their work as an independent practitioner, which could include supervising, sessional work and/or freelance work. The question did not ask people to clearly distinguish the locations of their different types of work or highlight where the majority of their work was located, so it is not possible to be absolutely precise about what categories of work take place where.

Some of the 106 'other' answers could perhaps have fitted into other categories such as various holistic, beauty and complementary clinic rooms, and charity and voluntary sector premises were quite frequently an option; but there was an interesting range of other possibilities including woodland, village and church halls, at the client's home, residential and hospital settings for the elderly, sick and disabled and art gallery and museum spaces.

The majority of private practice takes place in towns, cities and their suburbs, but 28 per cent of art therapists in private practice spend some of their time working in villages or rural settings. In terms of regional distribution, 24.5 per cent of private practice takes place in the London region and the rest is relatively evenly spread across the BAAT regional groups.

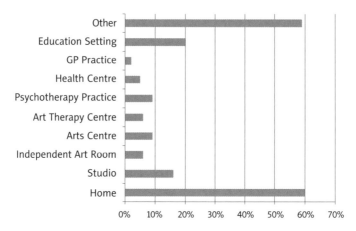

Figure 14.3 Question: Where do you locate your practice?

Charges

Approximately half of the sample operate their charges within one band of payment. The majority of this group charge between £41 and £50 per session. The other half of the sample have a range of charges, mostly between £31 and £60. Of those charging more than £61, 5.5 per cent charged between £61 and £70, 5.5 per cent between £71 and £80, and just under 4 per cent over £81. Only 4 per cent of art therapists provide sessions in the £0–£20 range and 8 per cent in the £21–£30 range.

The majority of private practitioners (68%) operate a sliding scale, lower rates for trainees (81%) and concessionary rates for those on low incomes (80%).

Client Groups

Art therapy trainees are seen by 65 per cent of private practitioners, but we cannot estimate from the survey what proportion of private practice work is made up from this group. Group work is done by 46 per cent of private practitioners, and smaller numbers see couples (14%) and do family work (22%).

Most private practitioners work with a range of age groups. The vast majority work with adults between the ages of 24 and 64 years some of the time. Figure 14.4 summarises the percentages working with each age group.

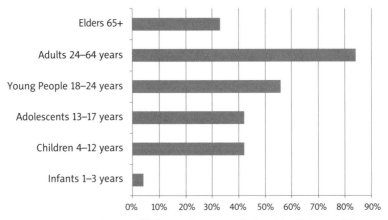

Figure 14.4 Client profile (respondents were asked to tick all that apply)

The Service Offered

The majority of art therapists offer weekly sessions to clients. Thirty-eight per cent provide weekly sessions only, while 18 per cent offer twice weekly, 35 per cent offer fortnightly and 18 per cent offer monthly. We cannot tell from the data collected how these variations in frequency of the sessions correlate with the different age groups and client groups.

The number of sessions offered spreads relatively evenly between 21 and 80 sessions per client, with 45 per cent of practitioners offering over 80 sessions to some clients.

Fifty per cent of private practitioners carry out assessments beyond a client's suitability for therapy. Twenty-four per cent do mental state assessments and 40 per cent do risk assessments. Some therapists confirmed that they did an informal assessment of safety for themselves as a lone worker and others assessed suicide/self-harm risk, ability of a parent to support a child in therapy, domestic violence, and addiction.

Respondents were asked to state their clinical and theoretical orientation. The question made an assumption that all art therapists are informed in their work by an art therapy literature relating to art processes, materials and products, but there was no direct question about these. Respondents were asked about broader theoretical influences. Table 14.5 shows how respondents answered this question.

Table 14.5 Question: Please state your clinical and theoretical orientation (tick all that apply)

Answer choices	Number of respondents	Percentage
Attachment-based	109	63.7
Cognitive analytical	10	5.8
Cognitive behavioural	16	9.3
Dialectic behavioural	5	2.9
Existential	15	8.7
Gestalt	20	11.6
Integrative	69	40.3
Jungian	50	29.2
Mentalisation-based	38	22.2
Pastoral	10	5.8
Person-centred	52	30.4
Psychoanalytical	41	24.0
Psychodynamic	138	80.7
Psycho-educational	54	31.5
Psycho-synthesis	5	2.9
Other	34	19.9
	Number of respondents 171	

The vast majority of respondents described their orientation as psychodynamic (80.7%), and a very high percentage use attachment theory (63.7%) as a basis for their work. Most respondents ticked at least three of the choices, and some as many as six. Of those that ticked 'other', several described their approach as eclectic, and others as systemic, humanistic, transpersonal or using mindfulness.

When possible, therapists negotiate the ending of therapy with the agreement of the client (95.1%). An indicator of how many clinicians see trainee therapists as part of their private work is that 54.8 per cent of respondents ticked 'trainee completion of course' as a reason for ending therapy. The other main reason for therapy ending is client drop out.

Evaluation in Private Practice

Respondents were asked if they used outcome measures in their practice. Approximately 56 per cent said they did some of the time. The most commonly used measures are the Strengths and Difficulties Questionnaire (SDQ) (used by 20%) and Clinical Outcome in Routine Evaluation (CORE) (used by 21%). Approximately 44 per cent of respondents replied to the open-ended question 'If you use other methods of evaluating your practice, please give details below'. Approximately half of these emphasised the importance of client feedback/reviews/discussion or use of client satisfaction questionnaires. A quarter emphasised the importance of supervision in evaluating their private practice.

Supervision Arrangements

Most (88.8%) private practitioners have individual supervision and over half have this on a monthly basis. A few (7%) have weekly supervision, and 25 per cent have fortnightly supervision, while 13 per cent have six-weekly supervision dependent on how much private practice work they have.

Discussion

Clarity about who we are, what we do and why we do it is necessary in the discreet world of private practice where the client chooses the therapist and pays directly for the service. This survey provides a glimpse into this world. The survey was largely fixed-choice questions to facilitate analysis, with very little opportunity for any free text from respondents. However, in response to one of the opportunities for free text, the question 'If you use other methods of evaluating your practice, please give details below', it was evident from the 44 per cent of respondents who replied that they evaluated their work through a combination of reflection with the client and supervision. This echoes much of James

D. West's exploration of how to research art therapy private practice in Chapter 13 of this book. The differences between private practice and other forms of art therapy practice provide opportunities to ask different questions about evaluation and research.

Comparisons with Other Surveys
The 1983 BAAT Survey

The one previous survey that gathered data on self-employed art therapists was conducted following a debate at the BAAT AGM in 1983 that acknowledged 'the need to support and provide a special service for those members who were self-employed' (McNab and Edwards 1988, p.15). This was a national survey of BAAT members. It did not distinguish between different types of self-employment, so there are no comparative figures about art therapists in private practice. It was known that there were very few working in this way at this time. The number completing the survey and describing themselves as self-employed either wholly, partially or considering self-employment was only in the twenties at this time. Most art therapists where employed in the health service, and one of the concerns expressed by McNab and Edwards was the effect that more self-employment amongst art therapists would have on the provision of art therapy to 'underprivileged or very damaged clients'. It was felt that any move to expand the numbers working in a self-employed capacity would potentially be a retrograde step as it would provide therapy for relatively more advantaged clients who could afford to pay. The question in our survey about the provision of lower-cost therapy is pertinent to this issue. Only 4 per cent of respondents offer sessions between £0 and £20, although 80 per cent offer some concessionary rates to people on low incomes. The reasons for offering low rates and concessionary rates were not explored in detail in this survey.

A Recent UKCP Survey

A recent UKCP survey examined the provision of lower-cost therapies amongst its members (UKCP 2014). This data was gathered in the context of ethically working as 'socially responsible therapists' and embracing the Equality Act of 2010. The survey included both those in private and independent practice. Nearly 80 per cent of respondents in this UKCP survey offered flexibility in their pricing, and the difference between minimum and maximum charge could be as much as £30. The percentage of clients in the lower range was approximately 16 per cent. The survey found that 67.8 per cent of respondents indicated that they sometimes reduced fees below their usual fee or range of fees, and within this group 15 per cent charged £10 or under in these circumstances and 10 per cent charged between £11 and £20. This survey's focus was lower-cost therapy, so their questions were more specific than the PPSIG survey reported in this chapter. The percentages in the PPSIG survey reported here are not directly comparative; however, the issue of lower-cost therapy provision amongst private practitioners is clearly a very live one in this period of NHS cuts. How to improve access to therapy for all members of the public may be worthy of further discussion within the PPSIG. The UKCP survey report has comments on the reasons for therapists reducing costs, including consideration of the gains for the therapist and its impact on the therapeutic process.

Two Recent BAAT Surveys

The analysis presented in this chapter comes from the respondents to a BAAT survey who described themselves as working in private practice. It is difficult to make comparisons with findings from other recent BAAT surveys of other groups of art therapists. However, a survey asking qualified art therapists working with children, young people and their families what theoretical influences informed their work found that nearly three quarters of them said that attachment theory did so to a great degree (Taylor Buck, Dent-Brown and Parry 2013). In the current survey the question was not worded in the same way, but 62 per cent of those working with children and young people said their clinical and theoretical orientation came from attachment theory. We can only surmise an explanation of this difference. One possibility is that the focus of the earlier survey was exploring dyadic parent–child approaches to art therapy, and the main rationale for this way of working comes from attachment research.

Another recent national survey of art therapists in the UK undertaken to create data about ethnicity, gender and sexual orientation (Hogan and Cornish 2014) provides some interesting comparative data. Their sample size was smaller than the survey material being analysed here, and in the minority ethnic groups and the non-heterosexual groups for both surveys the numbers are very small. However, in relation to sexual orientation, only 0.6 per cent of the earlier survey described themselves as gay, whereas 3.88 per cent described themselves in this way in the private practitioner survey. In the earlier survey, 4.4 per cent described themselves as lesbian, whereas in the private practice survey only 1.66 per cent described themselves in this way. It is only possible to note these differences here rather than attempt an explanation for them.

Limitations

This survey was designed by the PPSIG. Attempts were made through consultation and a pilot survey to construct a questionnaire which would provide useful demographic information. As this chapter shows, it has done this, but the process of analysis has highlighted some weaknesses in the questionnaire design. The limitations of the findings lie particularly in the following areas:

- There was no statement at the beginning of the survey clarifying whether we wanted respondents to answer questions in relation to their current caseload or their practice generally.

- For some of the questions, asking respondents to 'tick all that apply' was not helpful. It may have been more useful to ask 'tick the most appropriate to you'.

- The decision was made to include both independent and private practice in the survey. We found that many respondents work in both capacities. What we did not do sufficiently was to ask respondents to distinguish their answers, when necessary, between their private and independent practice.

Conclusion

The aim of the survey was to produce some useful demographic data about art therapy private and independent practice. The response rate was good. This chapter has clarified the similarities and differences between independent and private practice and painted a picture from the findings of the survey of who works in art therapy private practice in 2016, and where and how they work. This has produced some useful data for the PPSIG to reflect on and decide what areas need further exploration.

References

Hogan, S. and Cornish, S. (2014) 'Unpacking gender in art therapy: The elephant at the art therapy easel.' *International Journal of Art Therapy 19*, 3, 122–134.

McNab, D. and Edwards, D. (1988) 'Private art therapy.' *Inscape*, Summer, 14–19.

Taylor Buck, E., Dent-Brown, K. and Parry, G. (2013) 'Exploring a dyadic approach to art psychotherapy with children and young people: A survey of British art psychotherapists.' *International Journal of Art Therapy 18*, 1, 20–28.

UKCP (2014) 'Provision of lower-cost therapy by UKCP members in private practice.' *Survey Report*, June. London: UKCP.

AN INCONCLUSION

As this book represents a first attempt to explore the relatively new field of art therapy in private practice, it is necessary to hold back from conclusiveness and appreciate the forming landscape that is appearing in outline before us. In reading the book you will now have a clearer sense of our topic, through the many lenses and contexts by which it has been revealed. You will now also have a better sense of the way art therapists engage in private practice, what motivates us, who we are as a profession and the role we continue to play in our many and varied manifestations as state-regulated mental health professionals in the UK's public and private health care provisions.

Etymologies

The combination of the words 'art', 'therapy', 'private' and 'practice' in the title of the book means that any picture of this particular dimension of practice can only be a partial representation of a very complex and changing set of circumstances because a private practice must remain particularly responsive to the particular needs of its clients within the larger wheels of social and economic fortune. Creativity also demands movement, social adaptation and playfulness; it can never be predetermined or merely prescribed if it is to be true to its essence; yet paradoxically we must all nonetheless work with the given norms and discourses, laws and material circumstances of our times if we are to engage meaningfully as practitioners, artists and members of the public. Etymological reflections can help us to tease out some of these discursive meanings which may initially seem self-evident.

Art in Art Therapy

There are already many texts that make useful attempts to define art therapy (e.g. Edwards 2014; Hogan 2001; Wood 2010) but, as can be seen from the chapters here, it is a psychotherapeutic intervention which includes the full range of communicative possibilities that exist around the art-making process, both the verbal means and, more importantly, a particular attention to sensual and aesthetic experience. The art object within art therapy, or what we may call the *art therapy object*, is not primarily defined as other art objects are by the art market or its having supplementary or decorative use, as are the objects of craft or design. Art therapy produces objects that appear to be defined by what 'meaning' they have within the context of therapy, and so they can be seen as art objects 'made for meaning' rather than 'made for use' or 'made for purchase'. This differentiates the art therapy object from other art objects. Discourses of 'Art' are referenced in these objects but they do not limit or determine them. The art therapy object is sometimes taken from therapy and 'shown', with the client's consent, and we have explored the importance of this within art therapy research, but it should never be forgotten that the primary function was the 'meaning made' within the context of therapy.

Any artist who has drawn in public will know that art is seen as open to the public gaze. If you write a diary in a public place no one comes and looks over your shoulder and says 'What's that?' or 'Isn't that nice?' The art seems emphatically public, and in this sense it has little privacy. It invites aesthetic judgement. Artists themselves often struggle with this dance of public and private showing, its meaning and its resonances. The public showing of art therapy objects has been discouraged by therapists because the power of the wider discursive meanings of 'art' and 'research' can diminish and overwhelm the client's specific meaning, which is so central to the therapy, and so vital to the client. The art therapy object is therefore fragile in its signification, and so if it is shown as 'art' or in 'research' it is done with great caution and with a thorough consideration of ethics and timeliness in relation to the course of therapy. The need for privacy and confidentiality in all therapy remains primary despite changing contexts and the potential for display through 'a show' or in research. The psychological need for a certain privacy is no less important than the physiological need for skin. The art therapy private practitioner can consider this as a virtue that evolves naturally from the title of their practice where privacy is necessarily in the foreground.

Practice

The freedom and creativity of the arts require artists to make meaningful statements (not necessarily in words or pictures) that enhance our experience of the phenomenal and sensual world and, where we can, re-encounter ourselves and a richer and more deeply textured reality. As both artists and therapists we should be better able to appreciate unexpected atypicality through a close attention to difference and a talent for pattern recognition that supports creative change and growth in ourselves and our clients. One of the things that clients seek in a private practice is the freedom to consider who they 'are' uniquely, beyond bureaucratic structures and the tendency of human thought to typify, limit and reduce experience through the process of making sense of it.

Schön (1983) in his study of reflective practice makes a powerful critique of the technical rationality:

> In the varied topography of professional practice, there is a high, hard ground where practitioners can make effective use of research-based theory and technique, and there is a swampy lowland where situations are confusing 'messes' incapable of technical solution. The difficulty is that the problems of the high ground, however great their technical interest, are often relatively unimportant to clients or to the larger society, while in the swamp are the problems of greatest human concern. Shall the practitioner stay on the high, hard ground where he can practice rigorously, and he understands rigor, but where he is constrained to deal with problems of relatively little social importance? Or shall he descend to the swamp where he can engage the most important and challenging problems if he is willing to forsake technical rigor? (p.42)

Private practice by definition places an emphasis on practice. Schön asks us to re-evaluate the burgeoning and messy world of practical engagement and suggests it has greater practical and professional value than the pure and airy heights of abstracted knowledge. Artists and experimental scientists clearly both enjoy playing in the swamp, gleefully seeing 'what happens', whilst technical rationalists may even deny its value and inadvertently and sometimes unknowingly divorce theory from its application in practice. It has been an aim of this book to encourage practitioners to re-evaluate this practice/research dilemma and seek a better balance between the muddle of practice and the necessary abstractions of theory and research, reestablishing a productive interplay that has sometimes appeared to be at risk. This has necessarily involved questioning some false dichotomies of necessarily related terms: theory and practice, practice and research, subjective and objective, and mind and body, increasingly uncoupled from their productive association or placed in unhelpful hierarchies that have undoubtedly contributed to a devaluation of the notion of practice as research.

Husserl (1970) in his last works, like Schön, pointed to the exponential growth of both bureaucracies and professions in the last century and the consequent crisis of practice that has ensued. Many art therapists now find themselves setting up in private practice partly as a consequence of losing work within the statutory sector but also, more positively, through a drive to find an alternative way to practise that respects their artistic skills and instincts which allows them to re-enchant the heart of their practice.

This historical shift in practice requires professional adjustment and a reassessment of the discourses which may have served us well in the past. Art therapy as it appears in these chapters shows itself to be a social, symbolic and relational approach to therapy and, though it clearly has identifiable health benefits, it does not appear to be a technical medical intervention. The concerns of clients seen from the perspective of private practice more frequently evolve from discursive and normative conflicts that require joint relational reflections rather than the performance of a technical procedure.

Within the state sector therapists are frequently caught between necessary management and finance agendas and a burgeoning 'service users' voice, but this sadly has often left therapists themselves voiceless and devalued as valid witnesses to the therapy they are in fact offering. In the context of private practice this is a ludicrous and dangerous prospect, especially when we consider that the roles of organisational management and accountancy are abruptly reallocated here to the therapist and the client. In this context the therapist is highly motivated to be attentive to the client as customer, but it is also vital that they re-evaluate the voice of their own witness as a vital source of information. Research that values both these voices seems now very necessary to provide the best outcomes.

The self-governance and autonomy of a private practice have some clear advantages to both clients and therapists, as has been outlined in the book, but this comes with additional responsibilities, particularly with respect to the self-care of the therapist who is frequently the sole service provider and who now holds multiple management and administration roles in surprising and new combinations alongside and within the transference relationship. It is vital to be aware of the different hats you may be wearing, sometimes separately, and sometimes all at once, because when properly managed this contributes to the quality and benefit of a private provision.

This raises the question of the meaning of 'practice' as a complex performance of roles, which is acknowledged by Schön (1983) and Craig (2006), who engage with the eternal tussle between the notions of *theoria* and *praxis* which go back, at least, to the ancient Greeks. Is theory a representation of practice? Is practice a theory in action? What constitutes an art therapy private practice? A revision of the previous chapters will undoubtedly provide some answers.

Schön defines practice as follows: 'In the first sense, "practice" refers to performance in a range of professional situations. In the second, it refers to preparation for performance' (p.60). Craig, a communications theorist, defines practice as follows, emphasising its relationship to theory:

> Practices involve not only engaging in certain activities but also thinking and talking about those activities in particular ways. Practices have a *normative* – sometimes, even, *artistic* – aspect. They can be done well or badly, and people tend to evaluate the conduct of practices in which they participate or take an interest… By the same token, practices also have a *conceptual* – sometimes, even, a *theoretical* – aspect. (2006, p.39)

It is one of the aims of this book to reveal the discourses that have formed and continue to form around art therapy private practice so that we can deepen this discussion, critically evaluate it, and reflect upon it in ways that support the therapist's practice and the clients facing their dilemmas. The place of ongoing research, practice research, supervision and training have been shown within these pages to be key to bringing us to a greater awareness of our practice and our understanding of the perceived and actual benefits for clients in therapy.

Private

Having looked at 'art therapy' and 'practice' it is now necessary to return to the word 'private' and its positive and negative connotations, exploring some of the myths and realities of private practice. The etymological root of 'private' in Latin (*privatus*) means 'withdrawn from public life' (Waite 2013), but we may also have other quite bizarre associations to the word. Privy, private club, private parts, private soldier, privateer and privatisation all provide contending meanings. The private practitioner may not want these associations in their practice, but it seems necessary to evoke them in order to understand the visceral reaction to the term 'private' that is sometimes encountered. It is useful to explore these unconscious fantasies suggestive of shame, secrecy and exclusive privilege. We can note also through the association of sounds how easily the word 'private' becomes 'pirate' and 'privacy' becomes 'piracy'!

By way of contrast, if we contemplate what a life lived permanently in the 'public' gaze may be like, this can help us to re-evaluate the need for 'privacy' as if our very sanity depends upon it, and then we discover that the word 'privacy' also holds contrasting associations to ideas of pleasant retreat and of home. 'Private' therefore appears to be an extremely paradoxical and contradictory term that can lead us, through association, to the very extremes of our experience, from blissful reverie to total alienation. It also seems necessary to recognise their interdependent relationship, as it appears that in their meanings, 'public' needs 'private' and 'private' needs 'public'. They are necessarily related terms that make sense of each other through their association and divergence. They are not opposites but rather complementary terms in constant dialogue. We will always need privacy and a public life!

A Word on Profit

Our reflections on 'privacy' do not deny the potential for abuse suggested by the 'privateer', who through self-interest profits at the cost of the other. 'Privacy' does not evoke notions of profit in the way that 'privatisation' undoubtedly does, and these words have echoes and resonances that have consequences for practitioners who present themselves to their profession and to the public as private practitioners. Misunderstandings easily occur when words have multiple meanings, and so it is necessary to contrast 'making a profit' in order to 'make a living' through 'a fair exchange of goods' (a process that goes back to the origins of human community) with capitalist 'profiteering', where Marx showed how 'value' can be extracted from an exchange of goods to the detriment of one party and to the sole advantage of the other. It is my impression as coordinator of the BAAT Private Practice Special

Interest Group (PPSIG) since 2010 that art therapists in private practice are involved in 'a fair exchange of goods' and in fact often struggle to value their 'service' adequately in order to 'make a living'. This identifies a significant challenge for the prospective practitioner who is required to 'work through' these issues of self-value and professional identity in order to be clear about the 'value' of what they offer in the exchange of goods that requires them to 'take a fee'.

Weitz (2006) frames this challenge in a book that offers a useful guide to therapists entering private practice and asks, 'Do I see my clients' hours as a unit for sale?' She acknowledges that private practice is not for everyone and suggests that it comes down to whether this question can be answered unambiguously.

In *David Copperfield*, Dickens' Mr Micawber's adage 'Annual income twenty pounds, annual expenditure nineteen pounds nineteen shillings and six pence, result happiness. Annual income twenty pounds, annual expenditure twenty pounds ought and six, result misery' shows in material terms why the notion of the exchange and the fee in private practice must be thought through and is suggestive of the very simple maths that are involved in keeping account and of the reality testing involved in a small art therapy private practice.

In the course of this book we have given many examples of a 'fair exchange' and then gone on to illustrate and explore the meaning, value and ethics of this exchange and provide some depth and reality to a professional debate which has sometimes been thin and uninformed. This book should therefore help practitioners now contemplating this work to consider Weitz's challenge in a more informed and considered way.

The discussion about private and public work will no doubt go on and help us to clarify our ethics, values and principles in all sectors and provisions. We will also continue to consider how the client, through the exchange of a fee, requires something for their money and how the therapist also has the right through exchange of goods to make a living through offering a professional service. This exchange can provide a binding of needs that can enhance the motivation of both parties and promote a depth of therapy and a willingness to explore rich themes that may lead the client and therapist to consider other comparable exchanges and interactions, offered and received, which can include gifts and gift giving, charity offered and received, prostitution, sadism and control, and the symbolic equivalence of love and money, to name a few. In the state provision these economic and interactive realities can be sidestepped by the discourses of the objectivity and neutrality promoted by medical and technical knowledge. Private practice allows and necessitates a more thorough exploration of the intense intersubjectivities that are native to it and requires an epistemological shift to occur in the therapist as they move towards private practice. Art therapists in private practice can offer insights to the broader profession from this unique field that raise questions and can inform, enrich and revitalise the therapeutic engagement and the professional debate in the same way that all the work of art therapists in all its other contexts can inform and enlighten the private practitioner.

Limits

A private practice is usually a relatively isolated community resource (with the therapist more often working from home, according to the survey represented in Chapter 14). The private practitioner is therefore unlikely to encounter or agree to provide therapy to highly vulnerable clients. However, I hear many therapists new to private practice express surprise at what clients who work and are able to pay for therapy can 'contain' within their lives before, after and during the therapeutic 'holding'. This book illustrates the broad range of interventions and contexts possible within a private community provision. The broad training of art therapists with clients who have often experienced or are experiencing extreme states is a strength in private practice as it means that they may be better prepared and not fearful of the edges that clients may find in more serious mental health issues and they may be better equipped therefore to 'contain' and recognise their 'normality' in a community context.

Accountability of Art Therapy in Private Practice

In a recent (2016) email I outlined what an HCPC-regulated and BAAT-registered private practitioner has 'signed up to' over the course of a number of years. I have précised it below:

> An art therapist in private practice is necessarily HCPC regulated and has signed up to the HCPC Standards of Proficiency and the Code of Ethics. An awareness of these two documents is vital as they are the documents to which we are held to account if asked to appear before

the HCPC. Then, as a member of BAAT (though not all art therapists are BAAT members), we have signed up to the BAAT Code of Ethics which also has a section with requirements for private practitioners, and where it is also outlined that BAAT members should join the BAAT register for private practice (a process that requires them also to register with the Information Commissioner's Office (ICO) which makes a tick box list of requirements on its registrants). We are also required by BAAT to make a 'living will'. The BAAT private practice registration process asks you to fulfil other specific requirements and now also requires that you are acquainted with the BAAT Core Skills and Practice Standards in Private Work. As a BAAT member and a private practitioner and self-employed you are also agreeing to abide by the BAAT Guidelines for Undertaking Self-Employed Practice as an HCPC Registered Art Therapist (2014). Therefore be aware of all these seven documents and processes when considering your private practice, as possibly, over the course of a number of years, you may have forgotten that we have all agreed to abide by, and be guided by, them. What has dawned on me is there is no single document regarding private practice but an array of agreements that we have entered into often over quite a long period of time, which can easily be forgotten, but are nonetheless worth revisiting from time to time.

This shows how art therapists are held to account through their BAAT registration and state regulation. Research has been discussed at length in the book and it cannot be underestimated how audit, evaluation and research help us in our accountability to our clients, to the public, to the research community and, most importantly, to ourselves in our work.

Materia

I will end with a story which in some ways illustrates the necessarily inconclusive but endlessly productive nature of materiality in an art therapy practice. When the BAAT Private Practice Special Interest Group was completing its work on the first Core Skills and Standards for Private Practice, we realised that we had inadvertently omitted any reference to the provision of art materials and the storage of the art work. We had somehow managed to disavow the material means of our profession (a little like Schön's swamp). We quickly added the following section:

The materials in art therapy (including both the objects made and the art materials offered) are a concrete reality and are also a dimension of symbolic, projective and transferential significance for both client and therapist. They must therefore be given particular attention through the provision and storage of the art materials and the storage and disposal of the work. Appropriate and clear boundaries must be actively negotiated and worked through with the client bearing in mind this significance. (Appendix 1)

This statement remains an arrow pointing enigmatically to the dynamic and ultimately inexpressible heart of the profession, which is the material process of art, its particularity and uniqueness, and its polysemic and intertextual multiplicity which resists interpretation and reduction. Art opens things up! I believe this incident represents what is sometimes taken for granted in the profession and yet is its most precious gift. It is in the material and symbolic transformation of materials that clients hone a capacity for play and adaptability which provides the symbolic and transformative power of the therapy. It is a paradox for us that it also presents to us the greatest challenge in representing art therapy to others, and so we often resort to 'showing' rather than describing as it seems to do a disservice to the art therapy intervention to reduce it verbally in this way. When the poet T.S. Eliot was asked to state the meaning of a poem he had read, he resorted to simply rereading it, suggesting to the enquirer that it was not open to the conceptual retranslation that was being sought. 'Do it, don't talk about' is often the rule of practice; stop describing and preparing and allow yourself to experience this active mode of communication which evolves from a place close to your body and feelings and yet sometimes so far from your mind. If you trust this process, some time later, the right words will usually come.

References

BAAT (2014) *Code of Ethics and Principles of Professional Practice for Art Therapists.* London: BAAT.

Craig, R.T. (2006) 'Communication as a Practice.' In G.J. Shepherd, J. St. John and T.G. Striphas (eds) *Communication as...Perspectives on Theory.* London: Sage.

Edwards, D. (2014) *Art Therapy.* London: Sage.

Hogan, S. (2001) *Healing Arts.* London: Jessica Kingsley Publishers.

Husserl, E. (1970) *The Crisis of European Sciences and Transcendental Phenomenology.* Evanston, IL: Northwestern University Press.

Schön, D.A. (1983) *The Reflective Practitioner.* New York: Basic Books.

Waite, E. (2013) *Pocket Oxford English Dictionary.* Oxford: Oxford University Press.

Weitz, P. (2006) *Setting Up and Maintaining an Effective Private Practice: A Practical Workbook for Mental Health Practitioners.* ebook. London: Karnac.

Wood, C. (2010) *Navigating Art Therapy.* London: Routledge.

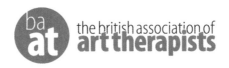

Appendix 1

Core Skills and Practice Standards in Private Work[1]

BAAT Private Practice Special Interest Group

Contents

---

1   These standards were cross-referenced with the BAAT Code of Ethics and the HCPC Standards of Proficiency. In addition to this document, members in private practice *must* also refer to the BAAT Code of Ethics, including Sections 21, 22 and 23 on private practice. **Members working with children must refer to the BAAT ATCAF (Art Therapists Working with Children and Families) Principles of Best Practice available on the BAAT website.**

1.0 Clinical governance

1.1 Duty of care

There is a tacit agreement within all caring professions regarding 'duty of care'. In art therapy the moral and ethical responsibilities we hold in relation to providing treatment, professional conduct and the review and termination of therapy are defined by the BAAT Code of Ethics (COE), the HCPC Standards of Proficiency (SOP) (2016) and the HCPC Standards of Conduct, Performance and Ethics (SCPE) (2016). These documents provide the profession with the construct of an art therapist's duty of care. The duty of care that therapists owe to themselves in private practice should also be borne in mind and developing strategies of self-care can be included as part of your CPD and 'you must make changes to how you practise, or stop practising, if your physical or mental health may affect your performance or judgement, or put others at risk for any other reason' (HCPC SCPE 6.3).

1.2 Clinical responsibility

The concept of clinical responsibility is finite and is described in law. In institutions and in secondary mental health care clinical responsibility is held by a consultant. Outside institutions and in primary care it is held by the patient's general practitioner (GP). In private practice it is our clients' GP who will hold this role and in effect hold clinical responsibility for the clients we see in private practice.

Members in private practice must try to ensure that they obtain the client's GP contact details wherever possible (as they are responsible for the client's medical welfare) and those of a partner, carer or next of kin should it be necessary to do so (BAAT COE 21.3). Clients who are students or trainees may well be registered with the university medical centre and there will be other variations, but these are the basic parameters. In terms of clinical accountability, it is doubtful whether a client's GP would exercise influence over the assessment and the treatment plan of a client in private practice though this may change as GP commissioning develops.

1.3 Clinical governance and professional responsibility

Clinical governance and questions regarding professional responsibility and clinical accountability are the responsibility of the practitioner (HCPC SOP 4, 10, 11, 12, 13).

1.4 Supervision

It is essential that art therapists who work privately employ an approved clinical supervisor who is registered and complies with the HCPC Standards of Proficiency. The supervisory contract should be explicit about the role and limitations of the supervisor–practitioner line of accountability. It may be helpful to clarify the extent to which a supervisor would be prepared to endorse any proposed treatment decision and clinical intervention carried out by an art therapist in private practice. This is in addition to the central purpose of supervision which is to provide a supportive and reflective space for the critical scrutiny of one's practice.

1.5 Professional indemnity insurance

In terms of claims of malpractice and public liability in private practice it is a legal requirement that any HCPC-registered practitioner carry full legal indemnity cover from an insurance company recognised within the therapy industry. Recommended providers will provide legal representation and advice at all stages of an HCPC investigation and may well call on third-party representation that could include the clinical supervisor (BAAT COE 4).

2.0 Advertising & marketing

Marketing and advertising in the therapies field is necessary and should seek to strike a balance of providing information about services to the general public as well as making services accessible, affordable and accountable. A marketing strategy may make use of the web-based media. All advertising must follow the BAAT Code of Ethics guidance, which is as follows:

> Members must ensure that all advertisements and publications, whether in directories, business cards, newspapers or conveyed on radio or television or by electronic media, are formulated accurately to convey their services to the public so that clients can make an informed decision about therapy. (BAAT COE 20.3; see also HCPC SOP 2.1 on acting in the client's best interests and 2.6 on gaining informed consent)

> Members must not use any description that is likely to mislead the public about their identity or status and must not hold themselves out as being partners or associates of an organisation if they are not. (BAAT COE 20.4)

> Members who practise privately may advertise their services. However, advertising should be limited to a statement of name, address, qualifications and type of therapy offered and such statements should be descriptive and not evaluative. (BAAT COE 20.9)

Members must adhere to professional rather than commercial standards in advertising their services. They must notify related professions and referring agencies of their practice and should promote and facilitate public awareness and understanding of the profession with dignity and discretion. (BAAT COE 20.10)

3.0 Fees, financing and personalised budgets

It is important to set fair and accessible fees and be clear about all charges and costs in one's advertising, referral and assessment processes. The cost of the therapy must be formally written into the initial contract with the client and the possibility of fees rising must also be included. It is essential that one is explicit from the start about payment for missed sessions and arrangements for breaks and holidays and be consistent (BAAT COE 19).

Therapists can provide bank details for standing orders or invoice weekly/monthly. Clients can pay either directly or through another party (parent or sponsored funding or other stake holder) and this factor involves broader dynamics that should be considered.

A clear, consistent and ethical approach must be underpinned by the following BAAT Code of Ethics guidance:

Members in private practice must make financial arrangements with clients, their agents, and supervisees that are clear, easily understood and conform to accepted professional practices. (BAAT COE 19.03)

Members in private practice must disclose their fees at the commencement of service and give reasonable notice of any changes in fees. (BAAT COE 19.5)

4.0 Referral, assessment and risk assessment processes

The importance of establishing a considered approach to referral, assessment and risk assessment strategies is essential (HCPC SCPE 6). Developing clear and professional protocols with your clinical supervisor ensures that elements of risk have been considered and managed as well as informing your proposed art therapy interventions and clinical decision making.

4.1 Referral process

Referral and acceptance of clients in private practice should be arranged in consultation with your clinical supervisor, although ultimate responsibility lies with the clinician. Many referrals with adults in private practice are self-referrals and so any formal acceptance will be between the practitioner and the client.

When working with children and adolescents or when receiving referrals for adults from secondary care services you will be able to request formal referral information which will aid in your assessment and art therapy provision:

- Always get written referral information via email or letter
- Clarify who is paying
- If the client is paying – their ability to pay
- Professional support – clinical responsibility for the client
- Key professional for liaison.

The level of liaison required to write up evaluation reports, or attend review meetings, must be clarified and costed into the agreement with client or funder.

4.2 Assessment skills

Initial contact

A self-referral assessment checklist is essential for assessment purposes but also for managing risk, particularly if you are working alone, in isolation at home. It may include:

- personal details
- practical implications – fees, location, times
- reason for seeking therapy now
- previous experience of therapy
- drugs/medication history
- who they live with/family/relationships
- why they chose the therapist and what they are looking for
- sleep patterns/physical health.

Some therapists ask for a lot of information at this initial stage; others simply make an appointment to make an assessment at an initial session.

With regard to equal opportunities it is good practice to ask the same set of basic questions to all clients regardless of ethnicity, age, gender, sexuality, disability, etc.

The initial face-to-face meeting

It is helpful to clarify that this initial assessment is a mutual process of deciding whether the referral is appropriate. The basic questions from the self-referral assessment checklist can be asked and enlarged upon.

Members must develop and use assessment methods that help them understand and serve the needs of their clients. Such assessment methods should only be used within the context of a defined professional relationship (BAAT COE 6.1; HCPC SOP 8.3, 9.3, 13.7, 13.15, 14.6, 14.7, 14.10).

Ensure that you obtain the client's permission to contact the client's GP, who is responsible for the client's medical welfare, and also their partner, carer or next of kin should it be necessary to do so (BAAT COE 21.4).

Additional questions may be important:

- support networks – formal and informal

- significant relationships

- significant life changes, bereavements or losses

- current employment situation

- type of therapy required

- why are they choosing art therapy?

4.3 Informed consent

The assessment process is an important part of ensuring that clients are able to give informed consent to undertake therapy (HCPC SOP 2.6, 7.1; BAAT COE 7). Ensuring informed consent means giving, *both verbally and in writing*, details of the art therapist's qualifications and professional memberships, HCPC registration and its remit to respond to complaints, and the agreed frequency of sessions, fees and payment (see Section 4.6 below).

4.4 Risk assessment

During an initial assessment it is important to establish the parameters of the service required and the limitations of one's practice within the private setting. One should only work within the limits of one's knowledge, skills and experience and, if necessary, refer on to another professional (HCPC SCPE 3.1, 3.2). It is therefore important to identify levels of risk as well as clinical complexity during the initial assessment meeting. This will inform treatment planning. The following criteria may be considered in the assessment:

- history of self-harm/suicidal ideation

- any formal diagnosis

- details of any current or past treatment plan

- details of any current or past treatment team or named medical practitioner

- potential number of sessions/length of therapy

- make potential client aware of the confidentiality policy (BAAT COE 10).

4.5 Some considerations for children and adolescent referrals

With children and adolescents there needs to be consideration around what information from the parents might be helpful or not, and whether or not it is appropriate to meet with the parent(s) and/or the child, and potentially the school. The practitioner needs to be clear about why they are undertaking any particular approach in contacting parents/schools (or not) as well as the implications for keeping boundaries (BAAT COE 11.1, 11.2).

It is also important to be clear with the parent(s) about their role (e.g. bringing child to therapy), confidentiality and also invoicing/payment, so that the child does not get caught up in these negotiations.

Practitioners should also familiarise themselves with relevant child protection and safeguarding legislation (HCPC SOP 2.5; BAAT COE 11.3; The Children Act 2004).

On the telephone:

- Option to hear *less* information from the parents before the first session

- Over 12s – check that they are happy to make a first appointment

- Face-to-face assessment

- Child's understanding of therapy

- Length of sessions (e.g. 50 minutes)

- Confidentiality – what information is shared with parents, schools, etc.

- Any issues or requirements regarding safeguarding or child protection monitoring.

4.6 Client contracts

Members in private practice must, on accepting a client, explain to the client their terms and conditions that may be written into a formal agreement or contract for personal therapy. This may include the following:

- fee

- method of payment

- session times

- notification of holidays

- notice of cancellation

- boundaries

- information relating to confidentiality and its limits (BAAT COE 10; HCPC SOP 7)

- duty as a therapist to report infringements against minors or violent risk to others (BAAT COE 22.1; HCPC SOP 7.3).

The management of the physical artwork/object in art therapy includes its storage, confidential recording and its return and/or disposal. All agreements in relation to these provisions within art therapy need to be made in relation to the practice context and specified clearly in the clinical agreement at the beginning of therapy. The materials in art therapy (including both the objects made and the art materials offered) are a concrete reality and are also a dimension of symbolic, projective and transferential significance for both client and therapist. They must therefore be given particular attention through the provision and storage of the art materials and the storage and disposal of the work. Appropriate and clear boundaries must be actively negotiated and worked through with the client bearing in mind this significance (BAAT COE 14.1, 15).

4.7 Data protection and record keeping

In line with the Data Protection Act 1998 and 2003 if you are intending to hold any information about clients on your home computer, you will need to register with the Information Commissioner's Office (ICO) (https://ico.org.uk) (formerly the Data Protection Agency). It is therefore an expectation that private practitioners will need to register with them.

There is a general guideline originating in the laws of tort that therapists may need to keep their records for up to seven years, but this must be balanced with the fact that the HCPC has no time limit for complaints, and the ICO requests therapists to continually purge their records of data (see also HCPC SOP 10). Members must also bear in mind that clients have a right to access their records; the Department of Health states:

> The Data Protection Act 1998 is not confined to health records held for the purposes of the National Health Service ('the NHS'). It applies equally to the private health sector and to health professionals' private practice records. It also applies to the records of employers who hold information relating to the physical or mental health of their employees, if the record has been made by or on behalf of a health professional in connection with the care of the employee.[2]

If art therapists keep process notes they should therefore be aware that they may be requested by clients, and they should dispose of them when they are no longer needed. It is also advisable that if they do choose to keep them they should be anonymised in case they are mislaid (BAAT COE 21.5).

4.8 Treatment planning in private practice

The plans must also adhere to the following principles in the BAAT Code of Ethics (BAAT COE 23.1; see also HCPC SOP 14.2, 14.3, 14.4).

- Seek to attain and maintain the client's optimum level of functioning and quality of life.
- Delineate the type, frequency and duration of art therapy.
- Set goals that, wherever possible, are formulated with the client's understanding and permission and reflect the client's current needs and strengths.
- Allow for review, modification and revision.

Treatment plans should also include an understanding of how any risks will be managed.

4.9 Termination of therapy

> Wherever possible, members should terminate art therapy services in agreement with the client and in a planned manner and must do so when therapy is no longer helpful or appropriate. When it is not possible to discuss termination of therapy with the client, others close to the client, such

---

2 This quotation can be found in the National Archives at http://webarchive. nationalarchives.gov.uk/+/http://www.dh.gov.uk/en/Managingyourorganisation/ Informationpolicy/Patientconfidentialityandcaldicottguardians/FAQ/DH_065886.

as a parent, carer, guardian or case manager, should ideally be involved. (BAAT COE 24.2)

An underpinning ethical position with regard to ownership of the artwork or object made during the course of therapy in private practice is that they belong to the client and will be handed to the client on termination of therapy. (BAAT COE 14.1)

It is important to note that ending the therapeutic relationship is a sensitive time and so the considered and sensitive handling of the return or continued storage or disposal of artworks needs to be negotiated on a case-by-case basis.

5.0 Evaluation, audit and review

To be able to assure the quality of their practice. (HCPC SOP 12)

In private practice it is good practice to represent the process of evaluation at the contract agreement stage. You may choose to specify an initial assessment period, followed by a time-limited intervention or ongoing therapy with evaluation reviews set at agreed intervals.

The evaluation of outcomes in private practice is based on client feedback and it is considered good practice to hold a regular retrospective review of the art and therapeutic work. This review can occur at the agreed review date, before or after an agreed break, at six-monthly intervals or on the anniversary of an ongoing intervention.

With regard to the audit of one's practice (HCPC SOP 12.3) this will require the use of clinical supervision and should occur at agreed intervals. The value of engaging in this process in art therapy private practice is to ensure that one's practice adheres to the principles of quality assurance used within the field.

6.0 Research and evidence-based practice

understand both the need to keep professional skills and knowledge up to date and the importance of career-long learning (HCPC SOP 3.30)

understand the value of reflection on practice and the need to record the outcome of such reflection (HCPC SOP 11.1)

be aware of the principle and applications of research enquiry, including the evaluation of treatment efficacy and the research process (HCPC SOP 13.2)

recognise the value of research to the critical evaluation of practice (HCPC SOP 14.14), and to evaluate research and other evidence to inform their own practice (HCPC SOP 14.16)

There are currently few articles or case studies of art therapy in private practice here in Britain. As a specialism in art therapy we should be looking at ways to record, structure, share and reflect on best practice.

The client-led and arts-based methodologies that are currently being developed include:

- user-led and client-centred methodologies
- use of audio image recording (AIRs) focusing on the art process
- retrospective review of the art and therapy process during therapy and at the end
- post-therapy feedback and interviews
- measurement of outcomes.

7.0 Equality of access and non-discriminatory practice

Art therapists in private practice are required to provide equality of access and non-discriminatory practice to the public and should also understand the concept of 'reasonable adjustments' as it applies to their working context. They should be acquainted with the following relevant laws (see also HCPC SCPE 1.5, 1.6, SOP 5, 6):

- **The Equality Act 2010**
- **The Mental Health Act 2014**
- **The Care Act 2014**
- **The Human Rights Act 1993.**

Art therapists working with any clients whose capacity to consent may be compromised by their situation, condition or diagnosis, for example dementia, learning disability, acute mental health problems, post-traumatic stress disorder, etc., should be aware of the **Mental Capacity Act 2007**.

All documents can be found at www.legislation.gov.uk

First published by the British Association of Art Therapists in 2015 and revised in 2017.

Appendix 2

Semi-Structured Post-Therapy Interview for Clients at 40 Weeks or at End of Therapy[1]

Moments of Meeting Project – UKCP Practice/ Practitioner Research Network (UKCP PRN)

Correct utilisation of this measure requires a short training to fill in the rating schedule with the help of the Manual of Rating Examples.

Can you tell me the story of how you decided to start therapy with your therapist? What was happening in your life?

Initial feelings

Was the person you saw first the same as your therapist? If not, how were you feeling when you saw that first assessor person? Depressed? (Probe how severe) *Anxious?* (Probe severity) *Stuck or trapped or blocked? Low self-worth?* (Probe severity) *Concerned about feelings of anger? What about drinking, drugs?* (Probe severity; probe re mood, sleep, appetite, energy, rumination, social withdrawal)

When you started therapy proper, can you describe how you were feeling? Depressed? (Probe how severe) *Anxious?* (Probe severity) *Stuck or trapped or blocked? Low self-worth?* (Probe severity) *Concerned about feelings of anger? What about drinking, or drugs?* (Probe severity; use probe to contrast with how client felt earlier with assessor)

---

1   There is a second version of this interview, with similar wording, for therapists.

Hopes

What did you want to achieve in your therapy? Did you discuss this with your therapist?

Did you have any sense that going to a therapist was something you would want to keep secret? Why was that? (stigma)

How would you describe what has happened during your therapy with your therapist so far?

Current feelings

How are you feeling now in your life after a period of therapy? Depressed? (Probe severity) *Anxious? Tense?* (Probe severity) *Stuck or blocked or trapped? Low self-worth? Concerned about feelings of anger?* (Probe severity; probe re mood, sleep, appetite, energy, rumination, social withdrawal)

What, if anything, do you think your therapy has changed in your life?

Significant events,[2] including MOMs or Moments of Meeting[3]

Focusing on specific therapy sessions now or on moments/turning points/key interactions[4] in these sessions:

- *Were there any that stand out for you as being particularly important (either in a positive way or negative way)?*

- *If yes, can you describe what happened at those points, e.g. tone of voice, facial expression, the rhythm of the dialogue?*

What made these sessions or moments/turning points/key interactions important to you?

Do you think these important sessions or moments/turning points/key interactions led to changes in your life, e.g. in relation to your feelings about yourself, other people, etc.?

---

2   Llewelyn, S.P., Elliott, R., Shapiro, D.A., Firth, J. and Hardy, G. (1988) 'Client perceptions of significant events in prescriptive and exploratory periods of individual therapy.' *British Journal of Clinical Psychology 27*, 105–114.

3   Stern, D. (2004) *The Present Moment in Psychotherapy and Everyday Life.* New York: W.W. Norton.

4   Timulak, L. (2010) 'Significant events in psychotherapy: An update of research findings.' *Psychology and Psychotherapy: Theory, Research and Practice 83*, 421–447.

- *If yes, how do think these sessions or moments/turning points/key interactions led to these changes?*

How did these sessions or moments/turning points/key interactions affect how you felt about your therapist?

Can you tell me about any other things that happened in your therapy sessions that you think made a difference either positively or negatively?

Disruptions[5]

Were there any occasions when you felt your therapist had somehow left your wavelength; that his/her understanding of you had been disrupted?

- *Can you tell me a little about those occasions?*

Repair to disruptions

Did you feel that you and your therapist got back on the same wavelength again?

- *Can you tell me how that came about?*
- *How long did that take?*

Therapist's manner as perceived by client

How did/do you perceive your therapist? What do/did you think about her/his manner? (or age, gender, nationality/ethnic features)

If mentalisation[6]/capacity to view things from the point of view of others not covered already

Do you feel you now look at things from a different point of view?

In what way? Has your capacity to listen to others changed?

---

5   Safran, J.D., Muran, J.C. and Eubanks-Carter, C. (2011) 'Repairing alliance ruptures.' *Psychotherapy 48*, 1, 80–87.

6   Bateman, A. and Fonagy, P. (2009) 'Randomized controlled trial of outpatient mentalization-based treatment versus structured clinical management.' *American Journal of Psychiatry 166*, 1355–1364; Llewelyn, S.P., Elliott, R., Shapiro, D.A., Firth, J. and Hardy, G. (1988) 'Client perceptions of significant events in prescriptive and exploratory periods of individual therapy.' *British Journal of Clinical Psychology 27*, 105–114.

Can you now see things from other people's perspectives in a way you didn't before? For example from your partner's perspective?

Is that things about how they see you, or just how they see the world?

Fresh start experiences

Can you tell me about any things happening outside the sessions that you also think have made a difference in how you are feeling now compared to when you started therapy? (For example changes at work, or changes in your relationships with people you know?)

Achievement of hopes in therapy

So, all in all, how much do you feel you achieved what you had hoped for in the therapy?

Thank you so much for participating in this research project. I wonder, if I find there is anything I haven't covered fully today, whether I might contact you by phone for a few minutes to clarify?

The Moments of Meeting Project Semi-Structured Post-Therapy Interview is published here with the kind permission of the UKCP Practice/Practitioner Research Network – Moments of Meeting Project group. All inquiries relating to this document should be directed to the UKCP PRN.

Contributor Biographies

David Edwards is an art therapist and a UKCP-registered psychoanalytically informed psychotherapist. He currently works as a therapist and clinical supervisor in private practice in Sheffield.

Andrea Heath is a psychotherapist and supervisor based in North London. She trained with the Philadelphia Association and as an art therapist at Goldsmiths College. She has a particular interest in self-organised community groups and currently works as a house therapist with the Philadelphia Association and Arbours communities.

Anthea Hendry is an art psychotherapist in private and independent practice, a clinical supervisor and trainer working in the UK. She has previously worked in education as a further education lecturer and teacher abroad, in social services as a social worker, in the voluntary sector as a manager and the NHS as Principal Art Psychotherapist in a Child and Adolescent Mental Health Service.

Hephzibah Kaplan is an art psychotherapist in private practice, a clinical supervisor and also lectures and runs art therapy workshops internationally. She has worked in education, adult mental health, bereavement, with arts therapy trainees and as a supervisor for many organisations. She is founder and director of the London Art Therapy Centre, which has been at the heart of establishing protocols and models for art therapy in private practice.

Themis Kyriakidou currently works as a private practitioner and supervisor, as a senior clinician for a CAMHS service as well as an associate lecturer for the Art Therapy Northern Programme in Sheffield. She has worked as an art therapist with a variety of contexts with clients with brain injuries, learning disabilities, visual impairments, addiction and in forensic mental health.

Stephen Radley is an art psychotherapist in full-time private practice in London. He qualified in 1996 at the University of Western Ontario. He is training in psychoanalytic psychotherapy at the British Psychotherapy Foundation at the time of publication.

Dave Rogers is an experienced art psychotherapist, supervisor and trainer. He has worked with clients in community settings, the Prison Service, an HIV/AIDS Hospice and Neuro Rehabilitation Services, and now works entirely in private practice. A significant part of this work is with art therapy trainees, as supervisor, mentor and trainer. A particular area of interest to Dave has been the continuing development of best practice in art psychotherapy.

Kate Rothwell is Head of Arts Therapies for the Forensic Directorate in the East London Foundation Trust. She has worked for over 30 years in forensic settings, and has a private practice working with children, adolescents and adults. Supervising arts therapists across a range of services, Kate is also a published author and editor of the *Forensic Arts Therapies Anthology of Practice and Research*.

Julia Ryde has been a trained art therapist for many years with experience of teaching, supervising and working in different settings including the NHS. She also trained as a Jungian analyst and currently works in private practice in London.

Nili Sigal has a background in fine art and psychology. She has experience of working with children and adults in private practice, in the voluntary and education sectors and in mental health services. She coordinated the monthly clinical meetings and wrote a blog for the London Art Therapy Centre for several years. Nili currently works for the NHS, where she specialises in trauma-focused art therapy.

Colleen Steiner Westling is an art psychotherapist and supervisor who works in private practice in London. Born in America, her first degree was in Toy Design, where she studied Developmental Psychology in addition to the design, safety and production of internationally sold toys. Colleen is also a minded yoga therapist working within the NHS teaching inpatients diagnosed with depression, anxiety disorders and psychosis.

Catherine Stevens has worked as an art therapist since 1994. She has worked in the voluntary sector with children and families, in mainstream schools, and in residential settings for looked after children. Her work with adults has been in community-based charities and in the NHS. Most recently she has been developing her private practice and supervisory work.

Frances Walton has been employed as an art therapist since 2001, developing an individual and group work practice within the charitable sector and NHS specialising in mental health rehabilitation and community art therapy groups. Her interest in the transitions between the institution and the community led her to develop a private art therapy practice and to explore unconscious psychological and systemic group processes. She subsequently completed a masters in working with groups at the Tavistock and Portman NHS Trust.

James D. West completed his first degree in Fine Art and Art History. He then trained as an art psychotherapist and has been in self-employment and private practice since 1994 working with elders, adolescents, people with learning disabilities and also in addiction services and staff support. He is a clinical supervisor to therapists working in a wide variety of practice contexts and modalities. He offers talks and workshops on related topics and is a peer reviewer for the *International Journal of Art Therapy*. He is the current coordinator of the BAAT Private Practice Special Interest Group and was co-founder and coordinator of the BAAT Addictions Special Interest Group. He is also a registered clinical hypnotherapist and a master practitioner of NLP.

Joan Woddis trained as an art therapist in the late 1970s after a substantial career as an art teacher in London's special education service. She has had an active role in the development of the profession of art therapy and has worked in private practice for many years, both as an art therapist and a group analyst. Joan is also Honorary Vice-President of the British Association of Art Therapists.

Chris Wood (PhD) is an educator with the Art Therapy Northern Programme, an art therapist in different settings and research fellow with the University of Sheffield. She is interested in art, urban living, the politics of mental health and in the ways in which people manage to live well.

Subject Index

Author Index